Cardiology

3/97

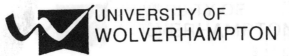

UNIVERSITY OF
WOLVERHAMPTON

LR/LEND/001

Cardiology

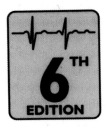

6TH EDITION

Desmond G. Julian MA MD FRCP FACC

Consultant Medical Director
The British Heart Foundation
London, UK

J. Campbell Cowan MA DPhil MRCP

Consultant Cardiologist
The General Infirmary at Leeds
Leeds, UK

Baillière Tindall
London   Philadelphia   Toronto   Sydney   Tokyo

Baillière Tindall   24–28 Oval Road,
W. B. Saunders   London NW1 7DX

The Curtis Center,
Independence Square West,
Philadelphia, PA 19106—3399, USA

55 Horner Avenue,
Toronto, Ontario M8Z 4X6, Canada

Harcourt Brace & Company (Australia) Pty Ltd,
32–52 Smidmore Street,
Marrickville, NSW 2204, Australia

Harcourt Brace (Japan) Inc.
Ichibancho Central Building, 22–1 Ichibancho
Chiyoda-ku, Tokyo 102, Japan

First published 1970
Fourth edition 1983
Fifth edition 1988
Sixth edition 1992
Second printing 1993

Typeset by Columns Design & Production Services Ltd, Reading

Printed and bound in Great by
Mackays of Chatham PLC, Chatham, Kent

This book is printed on acid-free paper

A catalogue record for the book is available from the British Library

ISBN 0–7020–1644–6

Contents

Preface

The first edition of this little book was written in 1970 with the purpose of explaining the heart and its diseases in a way that was readily understood by the student embarking on clinical medicine. Over the succeeding years, it has increasingly attracted a much wider audience, especially general practitioners and junior hospital staff, and has been extensively used as the cardiological text for those studying for higher examinations, such as the Membership of the Royal College of Physicians. It has also been popular with specialist cardiac nurses. In order to reflect this broader readership, the book has been enlarged so that it now contains more practical information, including sections on managing cardiac emergencies and on cardiac drugs. It is recognized that, in a book as short as this, oversimplification and dogmatism are inevitable. Those who wish to go more deeply into a specific subject are advised to consult the references provided at the end of each chapter or one of the several large textbooks available.

We are also aware that the book has reached an international readership. This success poses a problem, as the manifestations of cardiovascular disease differ in different countries. Rheumatic heart disease, once a major cardiac problem, has become rare in the United Kingdom, whilst it is an increasing cause of morbidity and mortality in the rapidly growing cities of Asia, South America and Africa. By contrast, in most Western countries, coronary heart disease is the major cause of mortality. Although deaths due to coronary disease have been falling in the last decade, this has not led to a reduction in the number of patients requiring medical care — on the contrary the number of interventions, such as angioplasty and coronary bypass surgery, have been increasing. To cater for the diverse interests of an international audience, we have sought both to maintain coverage of the more traditional aspects of cardiology (such as rheumatic heart disease), whilst at the same time extending the book to include an account of more recent diagnostic and therapeutic developments.

Cardiology has progressed rapidly since the publication of the fifth edition of this book in 1988. In the intervening years, much has been learned about the function of the heart, as a result of which there is a better understanding of the mechanisms of heart failure and disorders of cardiac rhythm. This, in turn, has led to much improved management of these conditions. Knowledge of the causes, pathophysiology, prevention and treatment of coronary disease has resulted in a striking reduction in the morbidity and mortality exacted by angina pectoris and myocardial infarction. High blood pressure can usually be controlled by the many types of drug now available, although the prevention of coronary disease in hypertensive patients is a remaining problem. New investigatory techniques, such as oesophageal echocardiography and magnetic resonance imaging, are continuing to improve diagnosis, and interventional procedures, such as balloon valvotomy and angioplasty, and ductus closure are challenging the established surgical treatments. Because of these advances, we have undertaken a radical revision and restructuring of the text.

We are again indebted to Dr J. I. Hall and to Mr D. P. Hammersley for providing the illustrations, and to many colleagues for providing clinical recordings particularly Drs S. Hunter, R. J. C. Hall and A. Zezulka. We are grateful to Mrs S Rutter for assistance in typing the manuscript.

In preparing this new edition, we have been helped by the comments and criticisms of many colleagues and friends, to whom we express our gratitude.

D. G. Julian and J. C. Cowan

Normal Myocardial Function

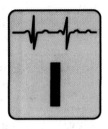

The primary function of the heart is to provide the tissues and organs of the body with a flow of oxygenated blood sufficient for their metabolic needs. In order to do this, it must pump a cardiac output of about 5 litres/min at rest (in the adult), and be able to increase this to 15 litres/min or more on exercise. It must also adjust to great variations in peripheral resistance and venous return without substantially altering arterial, venous or intracardiac pressures.

The ways in which the ventricles as a whole respond to changing demands can be, to a considerable extent, explained by the structure and function of the sarcomere, the fundamental unit of cardiac contraction.

The structure and function of the sarcomere

Each muscle cell contains, amongst other structures, a nucleus, numerous mitochondria, and a number of parallel fibrils. Each fibril is made up of functional sub-units or sarcomeres. The sarcomere is composed of parallel actin and myosin filaments, arranged with the thin actin filaments attached to its limiting membrane (or Z line) and interdigitating with the thicker myosin filaments which are placed centrally (Fig. 1.1).

The myosin filaments are lined with a series of 'heads', which can flex, thus bringing them into contact with the actin filaments. The filaments are propelled past each other by the repeated making and breaking of cross-bridges between the actin and myosin filaments. In addition to actin the thin filaments contain two regulatory proteins, troponin and tropomyosin (Fig. 1.1). The thread-like tropomyosin molecules lie in the trough between the two twisting strands of actin molecules. Troponin molecules are attached to the tropomyosin molecules at regular intervals. In the resting state, when the calcium level is low, the myosin-binding sites on the actin filament are blocked by tropomyosin, preventing cross-bridge formation. When

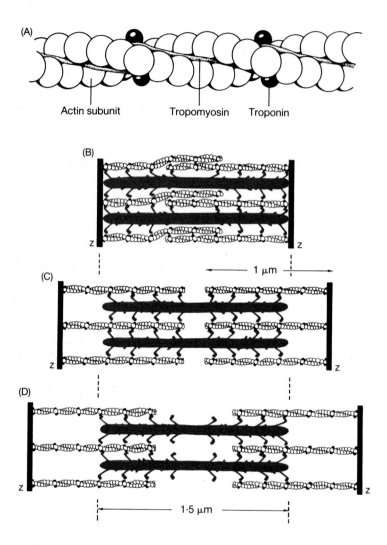

Fig. 1.1 (A) Diagram of actin filament, showing relationships of actin, tropomyosin and troponin. (B,C,D) Relationships of actin (thin horizontal lines) and myosin (thick horizontal bars) in the sarcomere. In (B) the actin filaments are overriding each other. In (C) all bridges (vertical lines) are available for binding. In (D) the sarcomere is overextended; some sites are not engaged. Contraction is maximal when the greatest number of sites are available for interaction as in (C).

activation causes a rise in calcium level, calcium ions bind with troponin, altering the position of the adjacent tropomyosin molecule and exposing the myosin-binding sites on the actin filament. Following cross-bridge formation there is a change in the angle of the cross-bridge, following which the cross-bridge disengages. The repeated making and breaking of many cross-bridges causes the thick filament to row itself into the space between the thin filaments. The energy for cross-bridge recycling is provided by adenosine triphosphate (ATP).

The number of cross-bridges that develop is dependent upon the number of calcium molecules available; the more bridges there are for interaction, the more forceful will be the resulting contraction.

Starling's law

The law of the heart, as enunciated by Starling, states that the more myocardial fibres are stretched (or the greater the diastolic volume of the heart) within physiological limits, the greater the energy of the ensuing contraction. Beyond these limits, the energy of contraction falls off. Two aspects of sarcomere function contribute to Starling's law:

- as the sarcomere is progressively stretched to its optimal length, and the diastolic fibre lengthens proportionately, the force of contraction progressively increases. This is partly due to the fact that over the normal operating range the opposing actin filaments overlap, interfering with actin–myosin cross-bridge formation (Fig. 1.1). With stretch the degree of overlap decreases and hence force generation increases;
- recent evidence suggests that calcium sensitivity of the contractile proteins increases with increase in length, providing a greater degree of activation for a given calcium concentration.

Excitation–contraction coupling

During systole there is a 50-fold increase in intracellular calcium concentration. The cardiac action potential is responsible for the increase in intracellular calcium in two ways:

- calcium ions enter the cell from the extracellular space during the plateau phase of the action potential (see Chapter 2);
- the spike of the action potential triggers the release of calcium from intracellular stores within the sarcoplasmic reticulum.

The energy supply of the myocardial cell

Energy is produced in the heart by the process of oxidative phosphorylation. This results from the conversion of the energy produced by the oxidation of substrates such as glucose, lactate and fatty acids into the energy of adenosine triphosphate (ATP) and creatine phosphate (CP). These substances provide the energy source for muscular contraction. Normally, free fatty acids are the main substrate, but in ischaemia the glycolytic pathway is stimulated. This, however, cannot substitute for oxidative-phosphorylation and inevitably ischaemia leads to a fall in ATP levels and a consequent impairment of myocardial function.

The mechanics of the myocardium

Two important characteristics of heart muscle are the force with which it contracts, and the velocity with which it shortens, for these determine the volume of blood expelled during systole. Three major factors are responsible for the force and velocity of cardiac contraction:

- 'preload' — the extent to which the muscle is stretched prior to contraction
- 'afterload' — the load that the ventricle faces during contraction;
- the contractile state of the myocardium.

Preload

If other factors are held constant, the force with which the heart contracts depends on the extent to which it has been stretched prior to contraction (Fig. 1.2). This is a restatement of Starling's law. In effect, the preload is the volume of the ventricle at the end of diastole, i.e. the *end-diastolic volume*. The end-diastolic volume is largely determined by the venous return, which is, in turn, dependent upon a number of influences including the blood volume and venous tone. Another important factor affecting venous return is the distensibility (compliance) of the ventricle. Atrial contraction contributes appreciably to ventricular end-diastolic volume as it occurs immediately before ventricular systole. This atrial component of ventricular filling assumes particular importance when the ventricle is hypertrophied because passive filling is then impeded by the indistensibility (lack of compliance) of the ventricle.

Afterload

The ventricle has to develop sufficient tension during systole to expel blood into the aorta in the face of the resistance (or, more correctly,

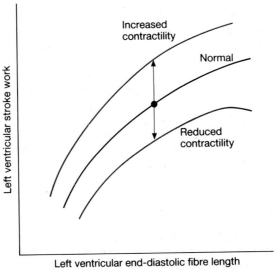

Fig. 1.2 The relationship between end-diastolic fibre length and the left ventricular stroke work. For any given end-diastolic fibre length, increased contractility, such as is produced by sympathetic action, produces more stroke work. Reduced contractility, as occurs in cardiac failure, produces less work. Similarly, if the arrows were drawn horizontally instead of vertically, it would be seen that for any given amount of work, increased contractility enables this to be performed at a smaller end-diastolic fibre length. In cardiac failure, a given amount of stroke work can only be achieved with a greater end-diastolic fibre length.

impedance) imposed by the aortic valve, aorta and peripheral arterial vessels.

The contractile state of the myocardium

If the end-diastolic volume and the aortic impedance are held constant, the force and velocity of contraction of the myocardium depend upon its contractile state. For a given end-diastolic volume, therefore, changes in contractility can alter the performance of the ventricle (see Fig. 1.2). Myocardial contractility is largely dependent upon the activity of the cardiac sympathetic nerves, but it can also be increased by circulating catecholamines, tachycardia, and inotropic drugs such as dopamine and dobutamine. Myocardial contractility is depressed by ischaemia and by a number of drugs, particularly antiarrhythmic agents.

Mechanisms which lead to an increased ventricular performance, such as an enlarged end-diastolic volume or sympathetic stimulation, also cause an increase in myocardial oxygen consumption. The greater ventricular performance does not necessarily, therefore, mean an increase in cardiac efficiency. Indeed, the increase in myocardial oxygen consumption is disproportionately great in relation to the increase in work performed.

The effect of exercise

Cardiovascular changes take place as soon as exercise is anticipated — as a result of vagal inhibition and a generalized sympathetic discharge. Both heart rate and myocardial contractility increase. The resistance vessels in the muscles dilate whilst those supplying the kidneys, abdominal viscera and skin constrict. The overall effect is to increase cardiac output and, specifically, the blood supply to the muscles.

With the onset of exercise, further dilatation of muscular arterioles and capillaries occurs and venous return is augmented by the pumping action of the muscles. The systolic blood pressure rises, the increase roughly corresponding to the severity of the exercise. Diastolic pressure changes little.

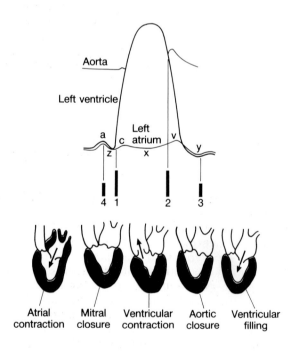

Fig. 1.3 Pressure pulses in the left atrium, left ventricle and aorta (see text).

The pressure and volume changes in the heart and great vessels during the cardiac cycle (Fig. 1.3)

The pressure and volume changes of the cardiac cycle fall into a number of phases:

Isovolumetric contraction.   With the onset of left ventricular systole, the mitral valve closes and the pressure in the ventricle rises rapidly. Until the aortic valve opens, the volume of the ventricle remains unchanged.

Ejection.   As soon as the aortic valve opens, blood is rapidly ejected from the ventricle into the aorta. This phase is followed by one of relatively slow ejection.

Isovolumetric relaxation.   Shortly after ejection ceases, the aortic valve closes. As the ventricle relaxes, the pressure within it falls rapidly, but until it has fallen to the level present in the left atrium, the volume in the ventricle remains unchanged.

Ventricular filling.   When the pressure in the ventricle falls below that in the atrium, the mitral valve opens and a period of rapid ventricular filling ensues. This is followed by a slow phase, or diastasis, during which the pressure rises slowly. This continues until atrial contraction propels more blood through the mitral valve and causes a small increase in left ventricular volume and pressure prior to the onset of the next ventricular systole.

Atrial pressure waveform

In the left atrium, there are three waves in the cardiac cycle, the crests being designated 'a', 'c' and 'v', and the troughs 'x', 'y' and 'z' (Fig. 1.3):

- the 'a' wave is due to atrial contraction, which is followed by a 'z' trough associated with atrial relaxation;
- the 'c' wave is a result of upward movement of the mitral valve cusps, with a subsequent 'x' descent as the mitral valve ring descends as the ventricle contracts;
- the 'v' wave is due to a build up of pressure in the atrium with increasing pulmonary venous return during the latter portion of ventricular systole, with the mitral valve closed. This rising pressure is terminated when the mitral valve opens. At this point, the peak of the 'v' wave is produced. The 'y' descent follows as blood flows into the ventricle during ventricular diastole.

From the opening of the mitral valve to its closure at the onset of ventricular systole, the pressures in the atrium and the ventricle are almost identical.

Right heart pressures

Events on the right side of the heart mirror those on the left but they take place slightly later so that tricuspid valve closure occurs shortly after mitral valve closure, and closure of the pulmonary valve follows that of the aortic valve. The timing of pulmonary valve closure varies with respiration. The increased negative pressure in the thorax during inspiration results in an augmented venous return to the right side of the heart. As a consequence of this transient increase in blood flow, ejection of blood in the right side of the heart is delayed and pulmonary valve closure occurs relatively later during inspiration than it does during expiration.

Further reading

Levick, J.R. (1991) *An Introduction to Cardiovascular Physiology*. London: Butterworths.

The Electrical Activity of the Heart: the Electrocardiogram

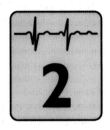

2

Electrical activity is a basic characteristic of the heart and is the stimulus for cardiac contraction. Disturbances of electrical function are common in heart disease. Their registration on an electrocardiogram (ECG) plays an essential role in the diagnosis and management of myocardial infarction, and of rhythm and conduction abnormalities. The ECG also provides important information about the presence of atrial and ventricular enlargement and can contribute to the detection of electrolyte disorders and drug intoxication.

THE CARDIAC ACTION POTENTIAL

The ECG is best understood by first considering some electrical and chemical features of the myocardial cell. Resting cells have a potassium concentration (about 140 mmol/litre) which is high in comparison with that in the extracellular tissues (about 4 mmol/litre), whereas extracellular sodium concentration is much greater than intracellular. This ionic disequilibrium between the cell and its environment is maintained by a sodium–potassium exchange pump which simultaneously transports potassium ions into the cell and sodium ions out of the cell.

During diastole there is a relative negative potential within the cell of the order of 90 mV — the *transmembrane resting potential*. This is primarily due to two factors, the high concentration of potassium ions intracellularly and the high permeability of the cell membrane to potassium ions. As a result, potassium ions tend to diffuse out of the cell down their concentration gradient, creating a negative charge in the interior of the cell, which offsets and almost balances the concentration gradient for potassium.

The cardiac action potential (Fig 2.1A) arises due to a sequence of changes in permeability to sodium, calcium and potassium ions (Fig. 2.1A and Table 2.1). At rest, the cell membrane is relatively

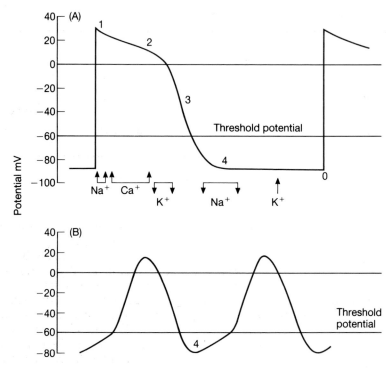

Fig. 2.1 (A) Transmembrane potential. Phase 0 corresponds with depolarization, and phases 1, 2 and 3 with repolarization. Phase 4 is the period of diastolic rest. When the cell is electrically stimulated, the transmembrane potential is reduced to the threshold potential, after which the process of depolarization is self-perpetuating. (B) Transmembrane potential in a pacemaking cell. In these cells, phase 4 is a period of slow depolarization. When the threshold potential is reached the cell rapidly becomes depolarized.

impermeable to sodium ions. The rapid upstroke of the action potential is due to a sudden increase in sodium permeability, causing a rapid influx of sodium ions. This sodium current is short-lived, because the ion channels which open to cause the increase in sodium permeability rapidly close once again. The fast inward sodium current is succeeded by a slower inward current, comprised predominantly of calcium ions and to a lesser extent sodium ions. This slow inward current is responsible for the plateau phase of the cardiac action potential, preventing the cell from repolarizing rapidly like a nerve.

During the plateau of the action potential permeability to potassium ions is reduced. Repolarization to the resting potential is achieved by a gradual increase in potassium permeability once again, accompanied by a gradual decrease in the slow inward current.

Table 2.1 Ionic currents in a myocardial cell

Current	Ion	Function
Fast inward current	Na^+	Rapid depolarization
Slow inward current	Ca^{2+} (mainly)	Plateau maintenance Excitation–contraction coupling
Outward current	K^+	Repolarization Resting membrane potential

Pacemaker activity

In a pacemaking or automatic cell (Fig. 2.1B) diastole is not stable. A gradual fall in potassium permeability causes a gradual decline in the resting potential to less negative values. When the transmembrane potential reaches its threshold, the cell automatically becomes depolarized. This characteristic forms the basis of automaticity.

The groups of automatic cells, which are present in the sinus node, the junctional tissue in the neighbourhood of the atrioventricular (AV) node, the bundle of His, the bundle branches and the Purkinje cells of the ventricles vary from each other in their rate of spontaneous depolarization. In the normal heart, the cells of the sinus node have the shortest spontaneous depolarization time (phase 4) and so have the fastest firing rate. The sinus node dominates the heart because impulses spreading from it discharge the other potential pacemakers before they are ready for spontaneous depolarization. If one of the other areas develops a faster rate, a new and 'ectopic' focus assumes the role of pacemaker. Conversely, if the rate of sinus node discharge is reduced for any reason, a pacemaker from lower in the conduction system may provide an 'escape' focus. In general terms, the more distal the location in the conduction system, the slower and less reliable is the escape pacemaker.

THE ELECTROCARDIOGRAM

The genesis of the ECG

Relation to the cardiac action potential

The ECG is the summation on the body surface of the individual action potentials from throughout the heart. To explain how the ECG arises, a single resting cell may be represented by a square with a

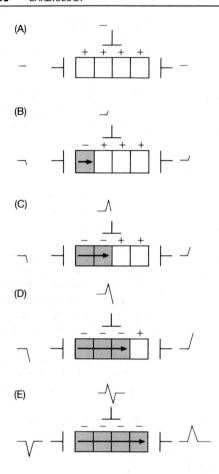

Fig. 2.2 The recording produced from electrodes during depolarization of a muscle strip. By convention, an upstroke (a positive deflection) is recorded as depolarization proceeds towards that electrode, and a negative deflection is obtained from an electrode facing the opposite direction.

positive charge on the outside and a negative one within. A muscle strip can be represented diagrammatically as a series of such squares (Fig. 2.2). If a cell at one end is stimulated, it becomes depolarized and its surface is negatively charged in relation to its fellows. As the electrical impulse spreads from one cell to the next, there is a progressively advancing negative charge. Immediately in front of it is a positive charge of equal magnitude. This combination of negative and positive charges in close proximity is termed a *dipole* with, in this case, the positive charge preceding the negative. The advancing dipole sets up an electrical field which can be detected by an exploring electrode paired with an indifferent electrode. By convention, relative positivity in the exploring electrode is represented by an upright deflection and negativity by a downward one. Therefore, as the positive front of the dipole approaches the electrode, an upright deflection is recorded; as it retreats, the deflection is negative.

The whole heart can be regarded as a large number of muscle strips arranged in a complex fashion. At any one time in the cardiac cycle there are numerous dipoles moving in different directions; as viewed from a single electrode many of these cancel each other out. The total electrical activity at any one moment in time can be summated and represented by a single electrical force of a certain magnitude and in a certain direction which is termed the *instantaneous vector*. All the instantaneous vectors occurring throughout the cardiac cycle form the *cardiac vector*.

The pathways of conduction and the ECG

The sinus node is situated in the right atrium close to the entrance of the superior vena cava. The AV node lies in the right atrial wall immediately above the tricuspid valve. The fibres of the AV bundle (of His) arise from the AV node and run along the posterior border of the septum between the ventricles (Fig. 2.3). On reaching the muscular part of the septum, they split into right and left bundle branches and then spread out in the subendocardium of the ventricles as the Purkinje system. The right bundle is a slender, compact structure. The left bundle soon splits into two or more divisions or fascicles, one of which proceeds anteriorly, sharing the same blood supply as the right bundle, and another is directed posteriorly.

In the usual sequence of events, the electrical impulse arises in the sinus node and spreads across the atria to reach the AV node. It can then only reach the ventricles by passing into the rapidly conducting AV bundle and its branches.

The first part of the ventricles to be activated is the septum,

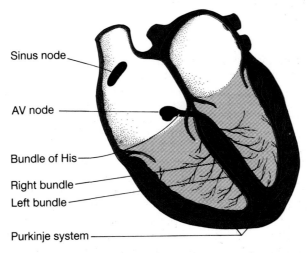

Fig. 2.3 The pathways of conduction.

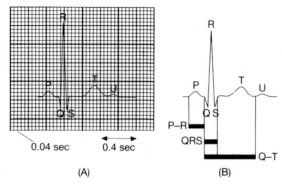

Fig. 2.4 (A) Normal ECG complexes. (B) PR, QRS and QT segments.

followed by the endocardium. Finally, the impulse spreads outwards to the epicardium.

The spread of the cardiac impulse gives rise to the main deflections of the ECG: P, QRS and T waves (Fig. 2.4):

- the *P wave* is the first deflection of the cardiac cycle and represents atrial depolarization;
- the *PR interval* represents the time taken for the cardiac impulse to spread over the atrium and through the AV node and His–Purkinje System;
- the *QRS complex* represents the spread of depolarization through the ventricles;
- the *T wave* represents ventricular repolarization.

Electrodes and leads

A conventional electrocardiogram (ECG) consists of tracings from 12 or more leads. The term 'lead' refers to the ECG obtained as a result of recording the difference in potential between a pair of electrodes.

The bipolar (standard) leads. In these leads, the electrodes are attached to the limbs. In lead I the positive electrode is attached to the left arm and the negative to the right arm. In lead II the positive electrode is attached to the left leg and the negative to the right arm. In lead III the positive is attached to the left leg and the negative to the left arm. They may thus be depicted as:

- lead I = left arm minus right arm (LA–RA);
- lead II = left leg minus right arm (LL–RA);
- lead III = left leg minus left arm (LL–LA).

It can be deduced from these equations that lead II should be

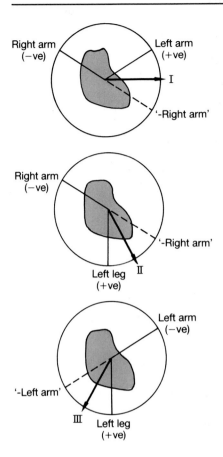

Fig. 2.5 Diagram of the effective position of the bipolar (standard) leads. In lead I, the positive electrode is attached to the left arm and the negative to the right arm. In effect, lead I is the sum of the potentials from the left arm with those that would be obtained from an electrode diametrically opposite the right arm. The resultant force is directed midway between these two points. Similar principles can be applied to derive the effective direction of the leads II and III.

equal to the sum of leads I and III.

The position from which the heart is viewed by each of these leads is shown in Fig. 2.5.

Einthoven regarded each limb used in the recording of the bipolar ECG as an apex of an equilateral triangle, equidistant electrically from the heart at the centre. Although useful, this hypothesis is only approximately true, as it assumes that the body is a homogeneous sphere, which it clearly is not.

Unipolar leads. These have an exploring electrode placed on a chosen site linked with an indifferent electrode with a very small potential. In an attempt to obtain a central terminal with 'zero potential', Wilson connected all three limb electrodes through 5000 Ω resistances to form the indifferent electrode.

Unipolar chest leads. When unipolar leads are recorded from the chest wall, the exploring electrode is connected to the positive pole of the ECG and the negative to the central terminal of Wilson (Fig. 2.6A).

By convention, the following sites are normally selected (Fig. 2.6B):

- V1, the fourth intercostal space just to the right of the sternum;
- V2, the fourth intercostal space just to the left of the sternum;
- V3, midway between V2 and V4;
- V4, the fifth intercostal space in the mid-clavicular line;
- V5, the left anterior axillary line at the same horizontal level as V4;
- V6, the left mid-axillary line at the same horizontal level as V4.

Additional leads can be taken from V3R and V4R, sites on the right side of the chest equivalent to V3 and V4. Occasionally, leads may be placed at higher levels, e.g. the second, third or fourth intercostal spaces or further laterally (V7 and V8).

Unipolar limb leads. In these leads, the exploring electrode is placed on one limb, and the negative pole is connected to Wilson's central terminal, modified by the omission of the connection from the limb under study to the central terminal (Fig. 2.7). This modification augments the voltage of the ECG, and the leads so derived are referred to as 'a' leads. They are designated as follows:

- aVR, right arm lead;
- aVL, left arm lead;
- aVF, left foot lead.

The normal electrocardiogram

Normally, ECGs are recorded at a rate of 25 mm/s and the ECG paper is printed with thin vertical lines 1 mm apart and thick vertical lines 5 mm apart (Fig. 2.8). The interval between the thin lines represents 0.04 s and that between two thick lines 0.20 s. If the heart rhythm is regular, the rate can be counted by dividing the number of small squares between two consecutive R waves into 1500 or large squares into 300. If the rhythm is irregular, one can multiply the number of complexes in 6 s (i.e. 15 cm) by 10. Special rulers simplify the calculation of rate.

There are also thin horizontal lines at 1-mm intervals and thick horizontal lines at 5-mm intervals. An ECG recording is standardized so that 1 mV gives a deflection of 10 mm on the paper. The height of a deflection therefore indicates its voltage.

The P wave

The normal P wave (Fig. 2.9A) results from the spread of electrical activity across the atria (the activity of the sinus node itself cannot be detected in the ECG). Because the impulse spreads from right to left,

(A)

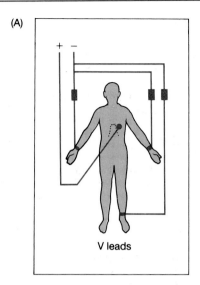

V leads

(B)

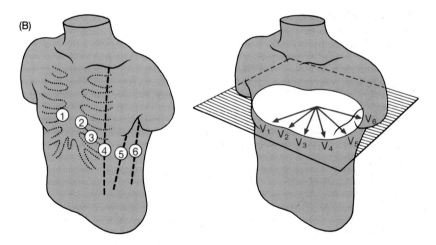

Fig. 2.6 (A) Each lead is recorded with respect to an 'indifferent' terminal, created by linking together the three limb electrodes. (B) The sites of electrode placement on the precordium.

the P wave is upright in leads I, II and aVF, is inverted in aVR and may be upright, biphasic or inverted in lead III, aVL and V1. It should not be higher than 3 mm in the bipolar leads or 2.5 mm in the unipolar leads, or greater than 0.10 s in duration.

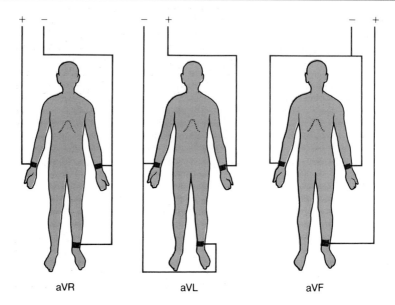

Fig. 2.7 The attachment of unipolar limb leads. Note that the limb under study is not attached to the central (negative) terminal.

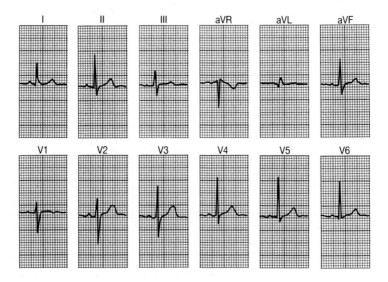

Fig. 2.8 Normal 12-lead electrocardiogram. Note the progression in the upright deflection from 'r' over the right ventricle (VI) to an 'R' over the left ventricle (V6).

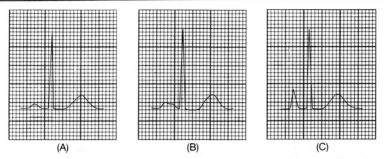

Fig. 2.9 P wave appearances in lead II. (A) Normal. (B) Broadened and notched (P mitrale). (C) Tall and peaked (P pulmonale).

When abnormal, the P wave may become:

- *inverted* (i.e. negative in the leads in which it is usually positive). This indicates depolarization of the atria in an unusual direction, and that the pacemaker is not in the sinus node, but is situated either elsewhere in the atrium, in the AV node or below this; or there is dextrocardia;
- *broadened and notched*, due to delayed depolarization of the left atrium when this chamber is enlarged (P mitrale) (Fig. 2.9B). In V1, the P wave is then usually biphasic with a small positive wave preceding a deep and broad negative one;
- *tall and peaked*, exceeding 3 mm, as a result of right atrial enlargement (P pulmonale) (Fig. 2.9C);
- *absent* or invisible due to the presence of junctional rhythm or sino-atrial block;
- replaced by flutter or fibrillation waves.

PR interval

This is measured from the beginning of the P wave to the beginning of the QRS complex (i.e. to the onset of the Q wave if there is one, and to the onset of the R wave if there is not). This interval corresponds to the time taken for the impulse to travel from the sinus node to the ventricular muscle. There is an iso-electric segment between the end of the P wave and the beginning of the QRS, whilst the impulse is passing through the AV node and the specialized conducting tissue, as an insufficient amount of tissue is being electrically stimulated to produce a deflection detectable on the body surface.

The PR interval varies with age and with heart rate. The upper limit in children is 0.16, in adolescents 0.18 and in adults 0.20 s, although it may be even longer in a few normal individuals. The faster the heart rate the shorter is the PR interval. It is regarded as abnormally short if it is less than 0.10 s. A shortened PR interval is seen when the impulse originates in the junctional tissue and in the

Wolff–Parkinson–White syndrome (see p. 189). The PR interval is prolonged in some forms of heart block (see p. 184).

The QRS complex

The QRS complex represents depolarization of the ventricular muscle. The components of the QRS complex are defined as follows (Fig. 2.10):

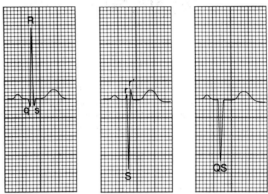

Fig. 2.10   Variations in the QRS complex (see text).

- the R wave is any positive (upward) deflection of the QRS. If there is more than one R wave, the second is denoted R'; an R wave of small voltage may be denoted r;
- a negative (downward) deflection preceding an R wave is termed Q;
- a negative deflection following an R wave is termed S;
- if the ventricular complex is entirely negative (i.e. there is no R wave), the complex is termed QS.

The whole complex is often referred to as the QRS complex irrespective of whether one or two of its components are absent.

Ventricular depolarization starts in the middle of the left side of the septum and spreads across to the right (phase 1 of ventricular depolarization) (Fig. 2.11). Subsequently, the main free walls of the ventricles are activated, the impulse spreading from within outwards and from below upwards. Because of the dominating bulk of the left ventricle, the direction of the vector of phase 2 is to the left and posteriorly. Finally, the base of both ventricular walls and the interventricular septum are depolarized. The appearances of the QRS in different leads can be largely explained by the major vectors of these phases as is seen in Fig. 2.11. In leads facing the left ventricular surface, there is a small Q wave due to septal depolarization and a

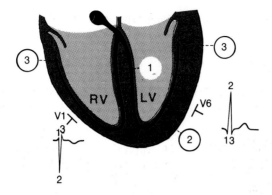

Fig. 2.11   Genesis of QRS complex. Note that the first phase, directed from left to right across the septum, produces a Q wave in V6 and an R wave in V1. The second phase, due mainly to depolarization of the left ventricle from endocardium to epicardium, results in a tall R wave in V6 and a deep S wave in V1. Finally, depolarization of the basal parts of the ventricles, may produce a terminal S wave in V6 and a terminal R wave in V1.

large R wave due to left ventricular depolarization. On the right side of the heart, as seen from V1, there is usually an r wave due to septal depolarization and a large S wave due to left ventricular forces directed away from the electrode.

Pathological Q waves.   As mentioned, small, narrow Q waves are normally to be found in leads facing the left ventricle, e.g. lead I, aVL, aVF, V5 and V6. These Q waves do not normally exceed 2 mm in depth, or 0.03 s in width. It should be noted that QS waves are normal in aVR, and are common in V1. Abnormally broad and deep Q waves are often a feature of myocardial infarction (see p. 120). Q waves in lead III are difficult to evaluate but can be ignored if there are no Q waves either in lead II or in aVF, or if they do not exceed 0.03 s. Usually, a 'normal' Q wave in lead III diminishes or disappears on deep inspiration because of an alteration in the position of the heart, whilst the 'pathological' Q wave of infarction persists.

The QRS complex should not exceed 0.10 s in duration, and usually is in the range 0.06–0.08 s. Broad QRS complexes occur in bundle branch block (p. 188), in ventricular hypertrophy and in ventricular ectopic beats.

The T wave

The wave is due to repolarization of the ventricles. If repolarization (the T wave) occurred in the same direction as depolarization (the QRS complex) the T wave would be directed in an opposite way to that of the QRS. In fact, depolarization takes place from endocardium to epicardium, whereas repolarization takes place from epicardium to endocardium. Because of this, the T wave usually points in the same direction as the major component of the QRS complex. Thus, the T wave is normally upright in leads I and II as well as in V3 to V6, is inverted in aVR, and may be upright or inverted in lead III, aVL, aVF and V1 and V2.

The T waves are usually not taller than 5 mm in standard leads and 10 mm in precordial leads. Unusually tall and peaked T waves may be seen in hyperkalaemia and in early myocardial infarction. Flattened T waves are seen when the voltage of all complexes is low, as in myxoedema, as well as in hypokalaemia and in a large number of other conditions in which it may be regarded as a non-specific abnormality. Slight T wave inversion is also often non-specific, and may be due to such influences as hyperventilation, posture and smoking. The most important causes of T wave inversion are:

- myocardial ischaemia and infarction;
- ventricular hypertrophy;
- bundle branch block.

Detailed descriptions of T wave changes will be found in the subsequent section on abnormalities of the ST segment, and also under the sub-headings dealing with ventricular hypertrophy, bundle branch block and myocardial infarction.

The QT interval

The QT interval represents the total time from the onset of ventricular depolarization to the completion of repolarization. It is measured from the beginning of the Q wave (or the R wave if there is no Q wave) to the end of the T wave. Its duration varies with heart rate, becoming shorter as the heart rate increases. In general, the QT interval at heart rates between 60 and 90 per minute does not exceed in duration half the preceding RR interval. The measurement of the QT interval is often difficult as the end of the T wave cannot always be clearly identified, and the relationship between heart rate and duration of the QT is a complex one. Tables are available in textbooks of electrocardiography giving normal QT intervals. In practice, the main importance of a prolonged QT interval is that it is associated with a risk of ventricular tachycardias (particularly torsades de pointes), and sudden death. A long QT is sometimes an inherited abnormality but may result from such drugs as quinidine, procainamide, disopyramide, amiodarone and tricyclic antidepressants.

The ST segment

The ST segment is that part of the electrocardiogram between the end of the QRS complex and the beginning of the T wave (Fig. 2.12). The point of junction between the S wave and the ST segment is known as the J point. The ST segment occurs during a period of unchanging polarity in the ventricles, corresponding with phase 2 of the action potential (see Fig. 2.1). The normal ST segment is situated on the iso-electric line but curves upwards.

Displacements of the ST segment and variations in its shape are of great importance in electrocardiographic diagnosis. The characteristic abnormalities of the ST segment are illustrated in Fig. 2.12. In some normal individuals, particularly young blacks, slight ST

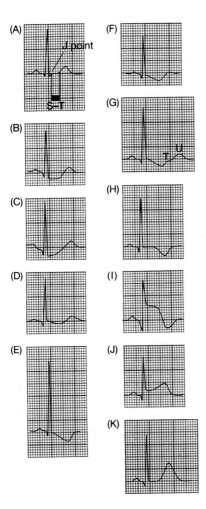

Fig. 2.12 Normal and abnormal ST segments and T waves. (A) Normal ST segment with J point. (B) Horizontal ST depression in myocardial ischaemia. (C) ST segment sloping upwards in sinus tachycardia. (D) ST sagging in digitalis therapy. (E) Asymmetrical T wave inversion associated with ventricular hypertrophy. (F) Similar pattern sometimes seen without voltage changes in hypertrophy-'strain'. (G) ST sagging and prominent U waves of hypokalaemia. (H) Symmetrically inverted T wave of myocardial ischaemia or infarction. (I) ST elevation in acute myocardial infarction. (J) ST elevation in acute pericarditis. (K) Peaked T wave in hyperkalaemia.

elevation is seen. This may be up to 1 mm in standard leads and 2 mm in the right precordial leads. Depression of more than 0.5 mm is abnormal. When ST elevation occurs in normal individuals, it is often preceded by a slight notch on the downstroke of the R wave:

- *acute myocardial infarction.* The ST segment is elevated with a curve which is convex upwards in the leads facing the infarct. At a later stage ST segment elevation becomes less pronounced as T wave inversion develops. These changes are considered in more detail on p. 122;
- *pericarditis.* This also causes ST elevation, but the ST segments are concave upwards and the changes are widespread rather than localized as in myocardial infarction;
- *digitalis therapy* depresses the ST segment, particularly in leads II and III, so that there is a gentle sagging, but the T wave remains upright or flattened;
- *ventricular hypertrophy.* ST segment depression may occur in leads facing the relevant ventricle and be accompanied by asymmetrical T wave inversion. This contrasts with the symmetrical T wave inversion seen in myocardial infarction and ischaemia;
- *acute myocardial ischaemia.* The ST segment is horizontally depressed or slightly downward sloping from the J point onwards;
- *sinus tachycardia.* There may be ST depression which slopes upwards from the J point;
- *hypothermia.* There is a prominent J wave (the junction of the S wave and the ST segment) (Fig. 2.13).

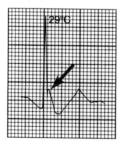

Fig. 2.13   ECG in hypothermia. The arrow indicates the characteristic prominent J wave.

The U wave

The U wave is a broad, low-voltage wave present in most normal ECGs. Its cause is unknown; it may become unusually prominent in hypokalaemia and with digitalis therapy.

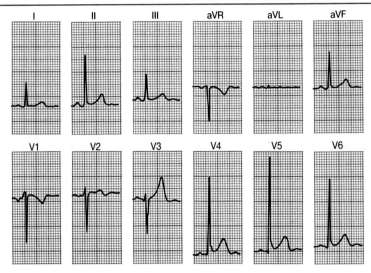

Fig. 2.14 Left ventricular hypertrophy. Note the deep S wave in lead V1 and the tall R waves in leads V5 and V6.

Abnormal ECG patterns

Left ventricular hypertrophy (Fig. 2.14)

Hypertrophy of the left ventricle increases the amplitude of R waves in left chest leads and S waves in right chest leads. Where there is septal hypertrophy, deep but narrow Q waves are seen in left chest leads. When left ventricular hypertrophy becomes advanced, the T wave may become flattened in the leads in which the R wave is tall; eventually ST depression and T wave inversion may occur.

Many efforts have been made to lay down criteria for the diagnosis of left ventricular hypertrophy. None is satisfactory as many factors contribute to the amplitude of ECG waves, including the thickness of the chest wall and the age of the patient. The following criteria have gained wide acceptance:

- R in V5 or V6 plus S in V1 greater than 35 mm. This criterion applies only in individuals over 25 years of age. In younger persons, R in V5 or V6 plus S in V1 should exceed 40 mm before the diagnosis of left ventricular hypertrophy can be made;
- R in V5 or V6 greater than 25 mm;
- R in aVL greater than 13 mm;
- R in aVF greater than 20 mm.

Right ventricular hypertrophy (Fig. 2.15)

When the right ventricle becomes hypertrophied, the leads facing the

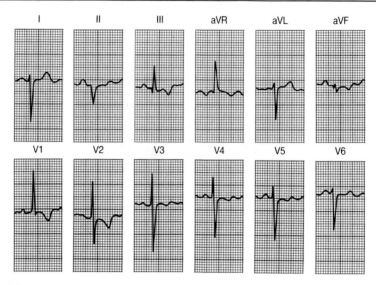

Fig. 2.15   Right ventricular hypertrophy. Note the tall R waves in leads V1 and V2, and associated T wave inversion extending across the chest leads to V5. There is right axis deviation.

right ventricle (particularly in V1, V3R and V4R) show dominant R waves instead of the usually dominant S wave. The diagnostic criterion for right ventricular hypertrophy is:

- R wave in V1 equal to or greater than the S wave and at least 5 mm tall.

As with left ventricular hypertrophy, ST depression and T wave inversion may develop in the leads with tall R waves.

Left bundle branch block (Fig. 2.16)

When the left branch of the bundle is blocked, the interventricular septum is activated from the right instead of from the left side and the initial vector (phase 1) is directed to the left. Because of this, the normal initial q wave in the left ventricular leads is lost, being replaced by a small r wave. Right ventricular depolarization, which follows, produces an r in V1 and an s in V6. The left ventricle is finally depolarized resulting in an R' in V6 and a broad S in V1. The QRS duration is increased to 0.12 s or more.

The abnormal left ventricular depolarization sequence in left bundle branch block causes secondary repolarization changes. Consequently, the ST segment and T wave are abnormal. This prevents interpretation of other factors causing ST and T wave changes, such as ischaemia and infarction.

(A)

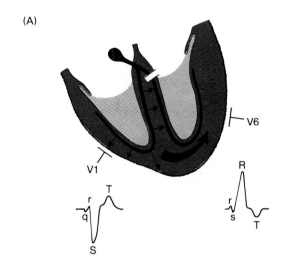

(B)

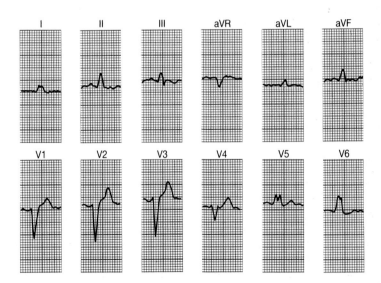

Fig. 2.16 Left bundle branch block. (A) The initial vector is abnormal in being from right to left across the septum, thus producing an initial r wave in V6 and a q wave in V1. (B) 12-lead ECG demonstrating features of left bundle branch block.

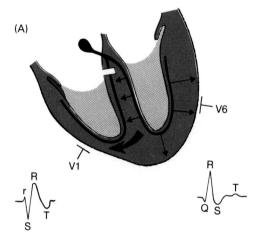

(A)

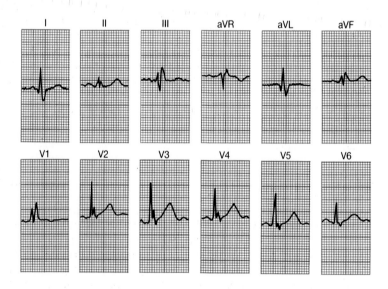

(B)

Fig. 2.17 Right bundle branch block. (A) The septum is depolarized normally from left to right and hence a small q is preserved in left ventricular leads and a small r in right ventricular leads. Left ventricular depolarization causes an s wave in V1 and an R wave in V6. Late depolarization of the right ventricle results in a prominent R' wave in V1 and broad S wave in V6. (B) 12-lead ECG showing features of right bundle branch block.

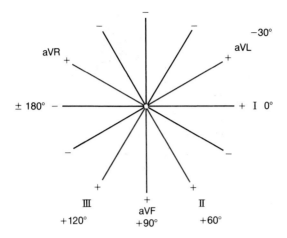

Fig. 2.18   Hexaxial reference system. The orientation of the limb leads in the frontal plane is shown.

Right bundle branch block (Fig. 2.17)

In this disorder, the right branch of the bundle is blocked, but the septum is activated from left to right, as in the normal heart. The left ventricular q wave is preserved, as is the initial r wave over right chest leads. The left ventricle is then depolarized, producing an S wave in right chest leads and an R wave in left chest leads. Finally, depolarization reaches the right ventricle, and so produces an R' in the right chest leads and a deep broad S wave in the left chest leads. An M pattern is thus seen in the right chest leads, such as V1. It is also common to see T wave abnormalities in leads V2 and V3.

The mean frontal QRS axis

As pointed out on p. 13, the total electrical activity at any one moment of time can be summated and represented by a single electrical force of a certain magnitude and in a certain direction, termed the instantaneous vector. All the instantaneous vectors occurring during the inscription of the QRS complex can be averaged, the direction of the vector so derived being called the mean QRS axis. It is customary to measure this only in the frontal plane and any two of the ECG leads which view electrical forces in this plane can be used for this purpose. This can be seen from the so-called hexaxial reference system (Fig. 2.18).

An approximate method of deriving the mean frontal QRS axis is to find in which of the leads I, II, III, aVR, aVL and aVF, the deflections of the QRS above and below the line are most nearly equal. The mean frontal QRS axis is at right angles to this lead.

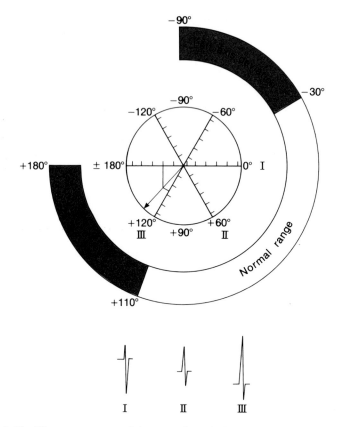

Fig. 2.19   The measurement of the mean frontal plane axis of the QRS complex. In this example, the sum of Q, R and S in lead I is −2 and in lead III is +2.5. By drawing a line through the intersection of perpendiculars drawn from these points, the axis may be derived.

To calculate the QRS axis more accurately, one should plot the difference between positive and negative QRS deflections in lead I on the lead I axis and that in lead III on the lead III axis of Fig. 2.19. By dropping perpendiculars from both points and drawing a line through this intersection from the centre point to the periphery of the curve, the axis may be determined.

Left axis deviation is present when the axis is less than −30° and right axis deviation when the axis is greater than +110°.

Calculation of the mean frontal QRS axis is of limited value except in a few conditions such as the differentiation of ostium primum from ostium secundum atrial septal defects (see p. 276).

Left axis deviation is often due to block in the anterior division (fascicle) of the left bundle branch, and when associated with right bundle branch block is a frequent precursor of complete heart block.

Right axis deviation commonly accompanies right ventricular hypertrophy, but may be due to block of the posterior fascicle of the left bundle.

ECG interpretation.

ECG interpretation is largely a matter of experience and pattern interpretation. However, while building experience, it is useful to develop a method of 'systematic' ECG analysis. This is most easily performed by asking oneself a number of questions in a logical sequence about P, QRS and T waves in turn. A simple system is presented in Table 2.2.

Table 2.2   A system of ECG interpretation

Rate and rhythm
   What is the rate (see p. 16)?
   Is it regular or irregular?

P Wave
   Are P waves present?
   Is the P wave axis normal (p. 16)?
   Is there evidence of left or right atrial enlargement (p. 19)?

PR interval (normal range 0.12–0.20 s)?
   Is the PR interval normal?
   Is each QRS complex preceded by a P wave?
   Is there evidence of a slurred QRS upstroke (delta wave) (pp. 19, 189)?

QRS complex
   Is the QRS duration within normal limits (0.08–0.11 s)
   Is there evidence of bundle branch block (pp. 20, 26, 29)?
   Is the QRS axis normal (p. 29)?
   Are pathological Q waves present (p. 21)?
   Is there a normal R wave progression across the chest leads (pp. 18, 20)?

ST segment and T wave
   Is there abnormal ST elevation or depression (p. 23)?
   Are the T waves upright (except aVR and V1)?

QT interval
   Is the QT interval normal (in general less than 0.44 s)?

Exercise electrocardiography

The main purpose of exercise electrocardiography is to determine whether a patient has exercise-induced ischaemia, as revealed by ST

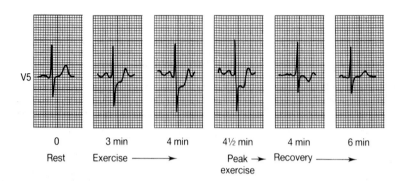

V5

0	3 min	4 min	4½ min	4 min	6 min
Rest	Exercise ⟶		Peak ⟶	Recovery ⟶	
			exercise		

Fig. 2.20 Exercise ECG. The changes occurring in lead V5 throughout an exercise test are illustrated. During exercise there is progressive depression of the ST segment, which returns to normal in the subsequent recovery period.

depression (Fig. 2.20). Exercise tests are carried out on a treadmill or stationary bicycle; if possible, the patient exercises until he develops chest pain (maximal symptom-limited test), but many patients give up because of fatigue or dyspnoea. If angina occurs, ST depression is usually present, but if the test is terminated before it does so, it may be 'false negative'. 'False positives' also occur (i.e. ST depression in the absence of ischaemia), especially in younger women.

Exercise testing is potentially hazardous as hypotension and dangerous arrhythmias (including ventricular fibrillation) may be induced. The blood pressure should, therefore, be checked regularly throughout this test and full resuscitation facilities (including a defibrillator) should always be available.

Dynamic electrocardiography (Holter monitoring)

With this technique, a continuous tape recording of one or more electrocardiographic leads is obtained, using a small portable tape recorder. Usually, the recording is made over a complete 24-h period, but some devices allow sampling only in response to activation by the patient, or when they are triggered by an arrhythmia. Special playback apparatus is required, which replays (and may analyse) the recording at many times real speed. It is an invaluable method for the study of transient episodes of arrhythmia which are unlikely to be captured by routine electrocardiography (Fig. 2.21). It is mainly used for the diagnosis of syncope and palpitation of unknown cause, but it is being increasingly employed to detect ST changes in suspected cases of myocardial ischaemia.

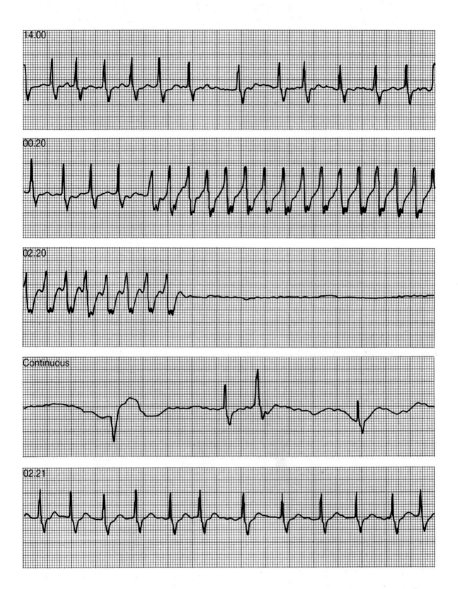

Fig. 2.21 The patient had a history of palpitations and syncope. On commencement of the tape (14.00) he was in atrial fibrillation. At 00.20 he developed sustained ventricular tachycardia. This lasted for 2 hours. On termination of the tachycardia (02.20) there was a prolonged asystolic pause followed by a ventricular escape beat. The patient subsequently continued in atrial fibrillation.

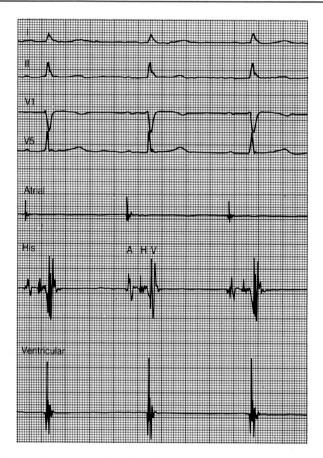

Fig. 2.22 Invasive electrophysiological testing. The traces show (from above downwards) four surface ECG channels, atrial, His bundle and ventricular intracardiac electrograms. The His bundle recording shows three wave forms, A, H and V corresponding to atrial, His and ventricular excitation respectively.

Invasive electrophysiological studies

It is possible to position electrodes in various parts of the heart, having introduced them percutaneously through a peripheral vein (or rarely an artery). Thus, electrodes may be placed in juxtaposition to several sites in the atria and ventricles, and also adjacent to the bundle of His (Fig. 2.22). The sequence of activation of the heart may then be determined, and specific sites found where conduction is accelerated (as in the Wolff–Parkinson–White syndrome) or delayed (as in heart block). Furthermore, by introducing stimuli at an appropriate time and place, an arrhythmia may be triggered in susceptible patients, and the effect on it of various pharmacological and electrical measures assessed. This technique is particularly valuable in:

- *arrhythmia diagnosis*, e.g. distinguishing the mechanisms of supraventricular tachycardias;
- identification of the origin of a ventricular arrhythmia or of the site of a bypass tract in Wolff–Parkinson–White syndrome;
- assessing the efficacy of antiarrhythmic therapy. This is of particular value in patients with malignant ventricular arrhythmias. If a drug is successful in preventing arrhythmia induction, this indicates that it is also likely to be successful in preventing spontaneous occurrences of the arrhythmia;
- *ablation* of accessory pathways or of the AV node using radiofrequency current (see p. 197).

Further reading

Campbell, R.W.F. & Murray, A. (1986) *Dynamic Electrocardiography*. Edinburgh: Churchill Livingstone.

Goldman, M.J. (1986) *Principles of Clinical Electrocardiography*, 12th edn. Los Altos, California: Lange.

Noble, D. (1979) *The Initiation of the Heartbeat*, 2nd edn. Oxford: Clarendon.

Schamroth, L. (1982) *An Introduction to Electrocardiography*, 6th edn. Oxford: Blackwell.

Task Force on Assessment of Cardiovascular Procedures (1986) Guidelines for exercise testing. *Circulation* **74**: 653A.

The Symptoms of
Heart Disease

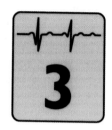

DYSPNOEA

Dyspnoea — difficulty with breathing — is the commonest symptom of heart failure. The term implies discomfort in the act of respiration, a consciousness of laboured breathing. It is, of course, also a symptom of respiratory disease and occurs in normal individuals on exercise.

No single explanation so far advanced accounts for all cases of dyspnoea. Furthermore, because it is subjective the degree of distress depends, in part, upon individual perceptions. Thus, some patients do not complain of breathlessness in spite of obviously laboured respiration, whereas others claim to be short of breath although their capacity for exercise is normal.

Mechanisms

The dyspnoea of cardiac disease may be due to the following factors:

Increased work of breathing. It is probable that in most cases of cardiac failure the discomfort arises in overworked respiratory muscles. In left-sided cardiac failure, engorgement of the pulmonary veins and capillaries occurs; if the pulmonary capillary pressure exceeds 25 mmHg, fluid may exude into the alveolar walls or even into the alveoli. These changes make the lung more rigid (less compliant) and require more respiratory work for a given volume of air inspired.

Reduced vital capacity. This is due to pulmonary venous congestion and, occasionally, to hydrothorax or ascites.

Reflex hyperventilation. The pulmonary stretch receptors may be abnormally stretched by congestion of the lungs.

Bronchial narrowing. Bronchial narrowing by spasm or fluid may occur in cardiac failure and adds to the work of breathing.

Hypoxaemia and carbon dioxide retention. These may both contribute to dyspnoea. They are seldom important factors in patients
with left-sided heart failure, in whom the carbon dioxide tension is
normal or low as a result of hyperventilation, and there is little
hypoxaemia except when there is pulmonary oedema. In cyanotic
congenital heart disease, hypoxaemia is severe.

Clinical features

The patient with cardiac dyspnoea breathes rapidly and shallowly.
This pattern contrasts with that of the anxious individual who has
deep and sighing respiration, and 'is unable to take a deep breath' or
'fill his lungs with air'. It also differs from the deep breathing of
patients with diabetic keto-acidosis or renal failure.

Dyspnoea in patients with cardiac disease is usually slowly
progressive, although it may be suddenly exacerbated by the onset of
atrial fibrillation or the occurrence of pulmonary infarction or
infection. At first it occurs only on effort, but as the disease process
advances, less and less exercise is required to provoke breathlessness
until it may eventually be present at rest.

Orthopnoea. Orthopnoea is dyspnoea when lying flat. There are
several possible explanations for its occurrence in left heart failure:

- when an individual lies flat there is increased venous return,
  which in the patient on the verge of failure may increase
  pulmonary venous congestion, and thereby decrease pulmonary
  compliance and vital capacity;
- the vital capacity is reduced in the recumbent posture by the
  relatively high position of the diaphragm, which may be further
  displaced upwards by ascites or an enlarged liver.

Orthopnoea usually occurs when there is already a considerable
limitation of exercise tolerance, but is occasionally an early symptom.
Many patients learn for themselves that they are more comfortable
propped up by three or four pillows.

Paroxysmal dyspnoea. In patients with left-sided cardiac failure,
attacks of dyspnoea may develop without an obvious precipitating
cause. They are most apt to occur during sleep (paroxysmal nocturnal
dyspnoea). The mechanism is probably the same as that of orthopnoea, but the sensory unawareness of the sleeping state prevents the
patient from correcting the situation by sitting up. The victim wakes
up intensely short of breath and frightened. He sits on the side of the
bed or struggles to the window. The attack may pass off spon-

taneously within a few minutes, or progress to acute pulmonary oedema.

Acute pulmonary oedema. In this condition, fluid accumulates in the alveoli as a result of a high pulmonary capillary pressure. Such attacks occur in patients with mitral stenosis, acute myocardial infarction and other left-sided cardiac lesions. There is often a provoking factor such as an arrhythmia or respiratory infection.

The patient is intensely dyspnoeic with noisy breathing, cough and frothy sputum which is often blood-tinged. The skin is usually moist, cold and cyanosed. The pulse is fast and may be irregular. Crepitations may be heard throughout the chest in a severe attack. In some patients, rhonchi, due to fluid in the bronchi, predominate and the clinical picture may resemble bronchial asthma. Pulmonary oedema is usually visible on a chest radiograph (see p. 73).

Cheyne–Stokes respiration. In Cheyne–Stokes respiration, there is a periodic waxing and waning in the depth of respiration, over a period of about 1 min. As William Stokes wrote in 1854:

> It consists in the occurrence of a series of inspirations, increasing to maximum, and then declining in force and length, until a state of apparent apnoea is established. In this condition the patient may remain for such a length of time as to make his attendants believe that he is dead, when a low inspiration, followed by one more decided marks the commencement of a new ascending and then descending series of inspirations.

This pattern of breathing is seen during sleep in some normal individuals, but its occurrence in the conscious patient suggests advanced left ventricular failure. It also occurs in patients with cerebral vascular disease, particularly if they have received morphine.

The cause of Cheyne–Stokes breathing is not yet established but it seems likely that the prolonged lung-to-brain circulation time disturbs the normal feedback mechanisms for respiratory control.

CARDIAC PAIN

There are two major causes of cardiac pain: myocardial ischaemia and pericarditis.

Myocardial ischaemia and infarction (see also Chapter 7)

A transient and reversible inadequacy of the coronary circulation gives rise to that type of chest pain known as angina pectoris. If the reduction in coronary blood flow is such as to cause death of an area of myocardium (myocardial infarction), the pain is usually more severe and prolonged.

The term angina pectoris was adopted by William Heberden, who described the characteristics of the syndrome in 1768. He wrote:

> There is a disorder of the breast marked with strong and peculiar symptoms, considerable for the kind of danger belonging to it, and not extremely rare which deserves to be mentioned more at length. The seat of it, and the sense of strangling, and anxiety with which it is attended, may make it not improperly called angina pectoris.
>
> They who are afflicted with it, are seized while they are walking (more especially if it be uphill, and soon after eating) with a painful and most disagreeable sensation in the breast, which seems as if it were to extinguish life, if it were to increase or continue; but the moment they stand still, all this uneasiness vanishes.
>
> In all other respects the patients are, at the beginning of this disorder, perfectly well, and in particular have no shortness of breath, from which it is totally different. The pain is sometimes situated in the upper part, sometimes in the middle, sometimes at the bottom of the os sterni, and often more inclined to the left than to the right side. It likewise very frequently extends from the breast to the middle of the left arm.

Heberden clearly described the four cardinal features of angina pectoris:

- the location — in the retrosternal region and its radiation particularly to the left arm;
- the character — often a strangling feeling;
- the relationship to exertion;
- the duration (usually 1–10 min).

For a more detailed description of angina pectoris, see p. 105.

Angina pectoris most commonly occurs in response to exercise in patients with coronary artery disease. The same symptom can be provoked by paroxysmal tachycardia, when there is insufficient time during diastole for the coronary arteries to fill and meet the increased oxygen demands of the tachycardia. Angina is a frequent symptom in aortic stenosis because of the inability of the coronary circulation to match the oxygen requirements of extreme left ventricular hypertrophy. Other conditions which may cause or exacerbate angina pectoris are coronary arterial spasm, aortic regurgitation, syphilitic aortitis, anaemia, hyperthyroidism and mitral stenosis.

There seems little doubt that the cause of angina pectoris is myocardial hypoxia secondary to inadequate coronary blood flow. The site of angina appears to be the myocardium; the stimulus to the pain has not been determined but may be due to a chemical substance related to oxygen lack or to a phenomenon analogous to cramp. The impulses arising in the myocardium pass through afferent sympathetic fibres to reach the upper thoracic sympathetic ganglia and are then directed to the upper four or five thoracic spinal nerves. In this way, the same segments of the spinal cord receive sensations from the heart as receive sensory impulses from the anterior chest wall and the inner aspect of the arm, forearm and hand. The pain is perceived as arising in the territory supplied by the corresponding spinal somatic nerves, rather than in the organ itself.

The pain of myocardial infarction is similar to that of angina pectoris in its location and character, but its duration is longer (usually more than 30 min), it is usually more severe, and it has no relationship to exertion.

Pericarditis (see also Chapter 10)

Pain is a characteristic feature of pericarditis, and appears to arise in the parietal pericardium, the visceral pericardium being insensitive. It is usually sharp, but may be of an aching nature. It is situated in the retrosternal region, and radiates to the neck, back or upper abdomen, but rarely the arms. It may be exacerbated by inspiration, swallowing and by lying down flat.

PALPITATION

Palpitation may be defined as an awareness of the heart beat. It takes several different forms includings a thumping sensation in the chest, a throbbing in the neck, a consciousness of missed or extra beats, or a racing of the heart. Anxious individuals are often distressed by the sinus tachycardia associated with emotion. Even normal individuals may be disagreeably conscious of their heart action when lying on the left side. Palpitation is, therefore, a common symptom in those without heart disease, but it is also an important complaint in patients with arrhythmias or abnormal heart action. Ectopic beats frequently give rise to the sensation of jumping of the heart, missed beats or extra beats. Patients with supraventricular tachycardia are aware of the sudden onset of rapid regular beating of the heart, whereas those with atrial fibrillation may be conscious of its irregularity.

Patients with a vigorous cardiac action due, for example, to thyrotoxicosis or aortic regurgitation, may feel the regular forceful beating of their hearts.

OEDEMA

Oedema — the accumulation of fluid in the interstitial tissues — is an important but relatively late manifestation of cardiac failure. It does not usually occur except in the presence of a raised venous pressure, and salt and water retention. Oedema is preceded by a gain in body weight of some 3–5 kg due to an increase in the extracellular fluid.

Normally, fluid exudes into the tissues at the arterial ends of capillaries because the hydrostatic pressure of approximately 30 mmHg exceeds the colloid osmotic pressure of 25 mmHg. Fluid is reabsorbed at the venous ends because the hydrostatic pressure at this point is approximately 12 mmHg. Oedema occurs when there is inadequate reabsorption of fluid from the tissues. A high venous pressure alone can, by increasing the hydrostatic force at the venous ends of the capillaries, cause oedema, as it does, for example, in vena caval obstruction. Raised venous pressure is nearly always a factor in cardiac oedema, but is seldom the sole explanation, for the retention of salt and water almost invariably antedates the appearance of the oedema.

The location of oedema in cardiac failure is determined by local factors, particularly gravity. In the ambulant patient, it occurs bilaterally in the lower legs and feet; in those kept in bed, it accumulates in the sacral area. When the oedema is very great, it may affect the whole of the lower limbs, the genitalia, the abdominal and chest walls and even the face (anasarca).

In the oedema of cardiac failure, the tissues dimple ('pit') when pressure is applied to them by the thumb.

ASCITES

The intraperitoneal accumulation of fluid is a manifestation of advanced heart disease, usually occurring later than peripheral oedema but for similar reasons. In some conditions, however, such as tricuspid valve disease and constrictive pericarditis, ascites may be even more evident than oedema and is probably then, in part, a consequence of portal hypertension secondary to cardiac cirrhosis of the liver.

CYANOSIS

Cyanosis, a blue discoloration of the skin or mucous membranes, is more a sign than a symptom of heart disease and is often first noticed by relatives when the affected individual exercises or is exposed to cold temperatures. It is usually due to a large proportion of reduced haemoglobin in the superficial capillaries and venules. It has been observed that cyanosis appears when the amount of reduced haemoglobin in the blood of these vessels exceeds 5 g/100 ml. Cyanosis results either from oxygen desaturation of the arterial blood or from an unusually large extraction of oxygen in the peripheral tissues. When the cyanosis is due to arterial oxygen desaturation, it is considered to be 'central' in origin because it is caused by a disorder in the heart or lungs. When the cause of the cyanosis is high oxygen extraction in the tissues, it is said to be 'peripheral'.

Central cyanosis is due either to blood bypassing the lungs as it is shunted from the venous side of the circulation to the arterial, as a result of congenital heart disease, or to inadequate oxygenation of the blood in the lungs, as in some varieties of lung disease. Clubbing of the digits is a common accompaniment of cyanotic congenital heart disease.

Peripheral cyanosis, a consequence of diminished blood flow through the skin and mucous membranes, occurs in normal people when they are cold, and in patients with a low cardiac output due to such conditions as mitral stenosis and acute circulatory failure.

The differentiation of central from peripheral cyanosis is usually not difficult. In peripheral cyanosis the skin is cold, and the cyanosis does not affect the warm mucous membranes such as those of the tongue. Furthermore, peripheral cyanosis can be abolished by warming the skin. The central origin of the cyanosis can be confirmed by measuring the arterial oxygen saturation which is usually less than 85%.

Rarely, central cyanosis may be due not to arterial oxygen desaturation but to methaemoglobinaemia or sulphaemoglobinaemia as a result of taking certain drugs.

HAEMOPTYSIS

The expectoration of blood is not uncommon in patients with heart disease. Several mechanisms are involved; examination of the sputum may help to determine which of them is responsible.

Frank haemoptysis — the coughing up of pure blood — occurs in mitral stenosis, due to the rupture of pulmonary or bronchial veins, or to pulmonary infarction. When there is pulmonary infection, the sputum may be purulent or rusty in appearance. In pulmonary oedema, the frothy sputum may be pink or streaked with blood.

Of course, patients with heart disease may also have haemoptysis due to other types of lung disease such as tuberculosis, bronchiectasis and bronchial neoplasm.

SYNCOPE

Syncope is a transient loss of consciousness due to inadequate cerebral blood flow or perfusion pressure. Cerebral blood flow and perfusion pressure depend upon the cardiac output, the arterial blood pressure and the resistance of the cerebral circulation. Cerebral arteries are relatively uninfluenced by the autonomic system but are dilated by carbon dioxide.

The commonest type of syncope is that of the simple faint (*vaso-motor or vasodepressor syncope*). It is often a response to emotion, but various physical factors such as blood loss, debility after infection and pain may contribute to its occurrence. It is believed to result mainly from dilatation of the arterial resistance vessels in the muscles. The fall in blood pressure causes a diminished perfusion pressure in the brain and loss of consciousness. Fainting of this kind usually develops when standing, rarely when sitting and virtually never when lying or walking. The first symptom is usually a sense of weakness, accompanied by yawning or sighing, sweating, nausea and 'a sinking feeling' in the stomach. After seconds or minutes, unconsciousness ensues; this is transient because the subject usually falls flat on the ground and this posture leads to an improvement in cerebral blood flow. In a severe attack, the face is pale, the pupils are dilated and respiration is slow. The heart rate is usually diminished and the radial pulse difficult to feel, although carotid artery pulsation can be detected without difficulty.

Micturition syncope occurs in adult men with nocturia. Consciousness is lost immediately after passing urine. It is particularly likely after considerable alcohol consumption. It may be due to reflex vasodilatation secondary to sudden relief of distension of the bladder combined with the vasodilator effects of alcohol and a warm bed.

Heart disease may be responsible for syncope. A catastrophic fall in cardiac output may result if the heart rate is either extremely slow or very fast. In supraventricular and ventricular tachycardias the ventricular rate sometimes exceeds 180/min, leaving insufficient time for adequate filling of the heart. A more important and dangerous form of syncope is the *Adams–Stokes attack*, which is a brief episode of cardiac arrest due to either asystole or ventricular fibrillation. This characteristically occurs in patients with heart block in whom either the ventricular pacemaker suddenly fails, or in whom ventricular arrhythmias are superimposed on the heart block. In most cases, effective cardiac action returns in 10–15 s, but if the attack is more prolonged convulsions may occur. The return of consciousness is accompanied by flushing as blood flows once more through vessels dilated by hypoxia.

Syncope on exertion. This is a characteristic feature of severe aortic stenosis (see p. 259), and may be due to an inability of the heart to supply an adequate blood flow in the face of the increased demands of the muscles. Patients with aortic stenosis are also susceptible to syncope due to heart block or ventricular arrhythmias.

Carotid sinus syncope. This is an uncommon condition occurring in elderly individuals in whom light pressure on the carotid sinus produces extreme cardiac slowing or reflex hypotension.

Postural syncope. When a normal individual stands up, pooling of blood in the legs is prevented by arteriolar and venous constriction, and there is an acceleration of the heart rate together with an increase in plasma catecholamine levels. Postural syncope, due to orthostatic hypotension, occurs in patients with autonomic disorders, including diabetic neuropathy and tabes dorsalis, as well as in some otherwise normal elderly individuals in whom these compensatory mechanisms do not function. Some hypotensive agents, particularly antiadrenergic drugs such as guanethidine, lead to orthostatic hypotension.

Syncope of cardiac origin also occurs in other conditions in which there may be a sudden fall in cardiac output such as massive pulmonary embolism, acute myocardial infarction and mitral valve obstruction due to left atrial myxoma or ball-valve thrombus.

FUNCTIONAL CAPACITY

On the basis of recommendations of the New York Heart Association, patients may be divided into four classes depending upon the severity of their symptoms. In class 1, the patients, although they have heart disease, can withstand normal physical activity without symptoms. If the patient develops symptoms on moderate or severe exertion but not at rest or with mild exertion, then he is classified as class 2. In class 3, symptoms are present even on mild exertion. In class 4 it is impossible to undertake any physical activity without distress, which may be present even at rest.

Such a classification is of value provided its limitations are borne in mind. Thus, many patients with severe heart disease have few or no complaints, whereas those who have an anxiety neurosis, or are anaemic or pregnant may have dyspnoea in the absence of heart disease.

Further reading

Criteria Committee of the New York Heart Association (1964) *Diseases of the Heart and Blood Vessels (Nomenclature and Criteria for Diagnosis).* Boston: Little, Brown.

The Physical Signs of Heart Disease

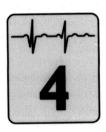

Signs are small measurable things but interpretations are illimitable.

George Eliot *Middlemarch*

THE ARTERIAL PULSE

The elastic structure of the aorta and its major branches enables them to act as both reservoirs and conduits. As a consequence, they are able to convert the highly pulsatile discontinuous blood flow from the ventricles into a more continuous flow in the peripheral vessels. The pressure pulse recorded a short distance above the aortic valve shows a sharp upstroke, produced by the rapid ejection of blood from the left ventricle, followed by a slower downstroke, as the rate of flow into peripheral arteries exceeds that from the left ventricle into the aorta (Fig. 4.1). This descending limb of the pulse wave is interrupted by the *dicrotic notch*, as the column of blood, briefly retreating towards the ventricle at the onset of diastole, is halted by aortic valve closure. As the main wave of the pulse travels peripherally, secondary waves are produced at the points of branching of the arteries. These are reflected backwards and summate with the main wave. Consequently, the peak systolic pressure in a peripheral artery may be higher than that in the central aorta.

When the arterial pulse is examined, the following characteristics should be noted:

- the rate;
- the rhythm;
- the amplitude;
- the character or wave form.

It is customary to feel the right radial artery to determine the rate and rhythm of the heart, but the amplitude and quality of the pulse is

Fig. 4.1   The normal arterial pulse
wave.

Dicrotic
notch

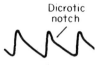

better appreciated in the carotid arteries. One should also search for pulsation in the radial, brachial, carotid, femoral, dorsalis pedis and posterior tibial arteries on both sides.

The heart and pulse rate. The rate of the pulse, if regular, can be calculated by multiplying the number of beats in 15 s by 4. If it is irregular, the number of beats in 30 s should be doubled. The pulse rate in normal resting adults ranges from 60 to 100/min. A rate of less than 60/min is most commonly due to sinus bradycardia (see p. 165), but may also be due to junctional rhythm or heart block. Rates in excess of 100/min (tachycardia) are most often due to sinus tachycardia associated with emotion or exercise; the heart rate may exceed 200 beats per minute on vigorous exercise. If the rate exceeds 120/min at rest in adults, some form of arrhythmia is likely (see Chapter 9).

Pulse rhythm. The normal pulse is regular or exhibits sinus arrhythmia. An occasional irregularity in an otherwise regular pulse suggests ectopic beats, and a coupling of beats (pulsus bigeminus or bigeminy) is due to the alternation of normal and ectopic beats. A totally irregular pulse suggests atrial fibrillation.

The amplitude and character of the pulse. The amplitude of the pulse depends on the pulse pressure, i.e. the difference between the systolic and diastolic pressures. The pulse is of small volume when the pulse pressure is small. This is the case when there is a low stroke volume and peripheral vasoconstriction as occurs in acute myocardial infarction, the shock syndrome, mitral stenosis and pericardial constriction or tamponade. In aortic stenosis, the pulse is small and prolonged and has a slow upstroke. This is called an *anacrotic* pulse if the wave has a notch on its upstroke (Fig. 4.2). *Pulsus bisferiens* is a pulse of moderate or large volume in which a double beat can be felt. This sign suggests a combination of aortic stenosis and regurgitation but is not diagnostic.

A large pulse, associated with a large stroke volume occurs in aortic regurgitation, anaemia, pregnancy and thyrotoxicosis. When a large volume pulse rises rapidly and collapses suddenly (Fig. 4.2) it is described as a *collapsing* pulse; this is also called a *waterhammer* pulse, after a Victorian toy of this name. This type of pulse is encountered when there is a rapid runoff of blood during diastole as in aortic regurgitation, persistent ductus arteriosus and arteriovenous fistulae. It is best felt by placing the palm of the hand on the patient's vertically elevated forearm, thereby increasing the retrograde flow of blood during diastole.

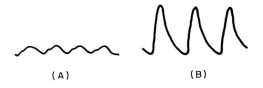

Fig. 4.2 (A) The pulse of severe aortic stenosis. (B) The rapidly rising and collapsing pulse of aortic regurgitation.

(A)   (B)

A reduction in systolic pressure of up to 10 mmHg may occur on inspiration in normal people, probably because the capacity of the pulmonary vascular bed enlarges and reduces the return of blood to the left ventricle. This is partly compensated for by a simultaneous increase in right ventricular output. A more substantial inspiratory fall, which occurs in obstructive airways disease, especially asthma, and pericardial constriction, produces *pulsus paradoxus*. In obstructive lung disease the reduction in arterial pressure is the consequence of the increased negativity of the intrathoracic pressure. In pericardial constriction and tamponade, this may be due to the right ventricle being unable to compensate for the augmented pulmonary vascular capacity by increasing its output. Another and probably more important explanation is that an inspiratory increase in the right ventricle occurs at the expense of left ventricle, as they are both confined within an indistensible pericardium.

In *pulsus alternans*, the beats are evenly spaced in time but are alternately large and small in volume. This is most readily detected when the blood pressure is being measured, for as the cuff is being deflated only alternate beats are heard at first. After a fall of a further 5 or 10 mmHg, every beat is audible. The mechanism of pulsus alternans is not well understood, but is usually associated with left ventricular failure.

The *absence* of a peripheral pulse indicates an anatomical aberration, or narrowing or occlusion of the artery proximal to it. In coarctation of the aorta, pulsation of the femoral arteries is delayed compared with that of the radial arteries.

Blood pressure recording

Precise measurement of the blood pressure can be obtained only by intra-arterial catheterization but a sphygmomanometer is sufficiently accurate for clinical purposes. This instrument consists of a manometer linked to an inflatable bag, surrounded by an inelastic cuff. The size of bag and cuff is of importance in ensuring accuracy, large cuffs being required for the obese and small for children. The cuff must fit around the arm snugly, being neither loose nor touching any article of clothing. It should be applied about 2 cm above the antecubital space with the rubber bag over the medial aspect of the arm.

Manometers are of two types: mercury and aneroid. The mercury type requires care in ensuring that there is no loss or oxidation of mercury and that the air vent at the top of the tube is open. Aneroid manometers are as accurate as mercury instruments, provided they are calibrated regularly.

It is best for the patient to be reclining comfortably, but the blood pressure can be taken satisfactorily with the patient sitting or standing provided the limb is supported and at the same level as the heart. Using a mercury manometer, one's eye should be in line with the top of the meniscus.

The patient should be warm, comfortable and in a quiet environment. He should have stayed in the same position for 5 min before the blood pressure recording; if in doubt, several recordings should be made.

The cuff should be inflated until the pulsations of the brachial artery can no longer be felt. The pressure is then raised by a further 20 mmHg and released at a rate of about 2 mmHg a second. As the pressure falls, sounds (Korotkoff sounds) are heard as blood begins to pass through the artery which has been occluded. At first these are faint and tapping; then a swishing quality is noted. The sounds become crisper and more intense and, as the pressure falls further, there is an abrupt muffling (fourth phase) and, finally, the sounds disappear altogether (fifth phase). Sometimes there is a period of silence after the first appearance of the sounds before they reappear, known as the auscultatory gap, which is particularly common in the presence of hypertension.

The systolic pressure is that at which the sounds are first heard. Intra-arterial pressure recordings suggest that the fifth phase usually represents the diastolic pressure better than the fourth but in some individuals, particularly if they are vasodilated, the sounds may never disappear; this may also be due to overextension of the elbow. To avoid inconsistency between different observers and repeated observations, the pressures both at muffling and disappearance should be noted.

When blood pressure measurements are taken in the leg, the patient should be lying on his abdomen, with a large cuff covering the mid-thigh region, and the stethoscope placed in the popliteal fossa.

Certain circumstances make blood pressure estimations difficult. In the shock syndrome, blood pressure readings from a sphygmomanometer may be grossly inaccurate. In atrial fibrillation and other arrhythmias, the blood pressure may vary from beat to beat; the average of a number of beats should be taken for both the systolic and diastolic pressures.

THE VENOUS PULSE AND PRESSURE (Fig. 4.3)

Inspection of the veins in the neck is an essential but often neglected part of cardiac diagnosis. The external jugular vein is easily seen, but

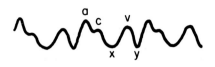

Fig. 4.3 The venous pulse. Note the 'a' wave due to atrial systole and the 'c' wave occurring at the time of tricuspid valve closure. The upstroke of the 'v' wave occurs as the atrium is filling passively during ventricular systole; the descent from the peak of 'v' to 'y' occurs as blood flows from the atrium to the ventricle after tricuspid valve opening.

is so often obstructed as it passes through the fascial plane that it cannot be relied upon as a guide to the true venous pressure. The internal jugular vein cannot be directly visualized, but it imparts a broad pulsation to the tissues of the neck overlying it. Its undulations can be seen in virtually all individuals, if the correct technique of examination is used; occasionally, especially in the obese or bull-necked, it cannot be identified.

There are normally three peaks:

- 'a' corresponding to atrial systole;
- 'c' occurring at the time of tricuspid valve closure;
- 'v' at the time of tricuspid valve opening.

There are two troughs:

- 'x' corresponding to the descent of the tricuspid valve ring as the right ventricle contracts;
- 'y' trough representing the fall in pressure as blood flows into the right ventricle.

As it is usually not possible to see the 'c' wave in the jugular pulse, the normal venous pulse in the neck is composed of two positive and two negative waves (Fig. 4.3).

It is essential to observe both the *waveform* and the *pressure level* of the jugular venous pulse. The pressure should not be determined until the characteristics of the wave form have been identified. The patient should be reclining with the chest, head and neck at 45°, and with the muscles of the neck relaxed. If venous pulsation cannot be seen with the patient at 45°, he should be placed more horizontally until it can.

The venous wave form. In differentiating venous from arterial pulsation the following points are important: the venous pulse normally shows two positive pulsations in each cardiac cycle compared with the single pulsation in the arteries; the venous pulse cannot usually be felt, although it can be readily seen, whereas the arterial pulsation is more easily felt than seen; the venous pulse wave can be obliterated by light pressure at the root of the neck. Pressure on the abdomen, by increasing venous return to the thorax, increases the venous pressure in the neck transiently and permits it to be visualized more easily.

The venous pressure. With the patient is the semi-recumbent position, the vertical height of the top of the venous column above the sternal angle is observed. In normal individuals, this does not exceed 2 cm; it is increased by factors which augment venous return including pregnancy, anxiety, exercise and anaemia. If these causes cannot be invoked, raised venous pressure is usually due to right-sided cardiac failure; it is important to exclude non-pulsating engorgement due to obstruction of the superior vena cava.

Hepato-jugular reflux. If pressure is exerted on the relaxed abdomen, venous return to the right atrium is increased, and the jugular venous pressure rises accordingly. In normals this rise is very transient; in patients with heart failure, it may remain high as long as pressure is exerted on the abdomen.

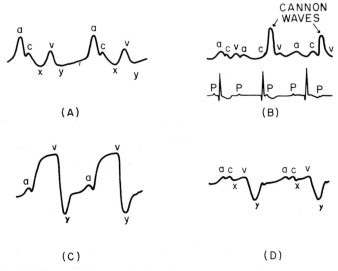

Fig. 4.4 (A) The giant 'a' wave. (B) Intermittent cannon waves in complete heart block, occurring at the time of synchronous atrial and ventricular contraction. (C) The systolic venous pulsation of tricuspid regurgitation. (D) The venous pulse in pericardial constriction, showing the rapid 'y' descent, followed by a plateau.

The timing of venous waves may be difficult; it is essential either to feel the carotid artery pulsation on the other side of the neck or to listen for the first heart sound in order to allow identification of the 'a' wave which precedes these two events.

Giant 'a' wave (Fig. 4.4). This develops when the right atrium contracts forcefully against the increased resistance provided by a stenotic tricuspid valve, or hypertrophied right ventricle.

Cannon waves. These are large venous pulsations due to atrial contraction against a closed tricuspid valve. They occur intermittently in complete heart block and in ventricular tachycardia when atrial and ventricular systoles coincide (Fig. 4.4). In junctional rhythms, atrial and ventricular contractions are synchronous and cannon waves occur with every heart beat.

Systolic venous pulsation ('cv' wave). This is due to blood regurgitating into the venous system during ventricular systole and is characteristic of tricuspid regurgitation (Fig. 4.4).

In pericardial constriction, the venous pressure is greatly raised, and there is a sharp 'y' descent as blood rushes into the right ventricle in the early part of diastole (Fig. 4.4). Another feature of this condition is elevation of venous pressure during inspiration because the increase in venous return at this time cannot be accommodated by the constricted right ventricle.

INSPECTION OF THE CHEST

Abnormalities of the thorax and lungs may cause changes in the position of the heart; they may also result from or cause heart disease. Funnel chest (pectus excavatum) and kyphoscoliosis may lead to displacement of the heart. Cardiac enlargement associated with advanced congenital heart disease in childhood may cause deformity of the sternum and ribs.

The rate and pattern of breathing should be noted. The respiratory rate is often increased in left ventricular failure. Prolonged expiration suggests obstructive airways disease.

The cardiac impulse is frequently visible, particularly when there is heart disease. It is often possible to see the exaggerated apical impulse of left ventricular hypertrophy, the displaced apex of left ventricular dilatation, the left parasternal pulsation of right ventricular hypertrophy or the abnormal pulmonary arterial pulsation in the second and third left interspaces in pulmonary hypertension.

PALPATION OF THE CHEST

The apex beat

In the normal individual, the maximal thrust of the left ventricle — the apex beat — can be felt at or just internal to the mid-clavicular line in the fifth intercostal space. If it is displaced, one should determine whether this is due to abnormalities of the thoracic cage or lungs. After the apex beat has been located and assessed, the whole precordium should be explored with the palm of the hand in the search for abnormal pulsation.

The graphic record of the movements of the apex beat shows a characteristic pattern — the *apex cardiogram* (Fig. 4.5). This commences with an 'a' wave as atrial systole causes ventricular distension. The next wave, which is the major one in the cardiac cycle, corresponds to the forward rotation of the apex due to left ventricular systole. The apex beat starts to retract as soon as the aortic valve opens and continues to do so until the 'o' point is reached, at which time the mitral valve opens and the ventricle distends rapidly. This process then slows and there is little change before the next atrial systole. Normally, only the ventricular systolic component is detectable by palpation, but in left ventricular hypertrophy, the 'a' wave can sometimes be felt immediately before ventricular systole, produc-

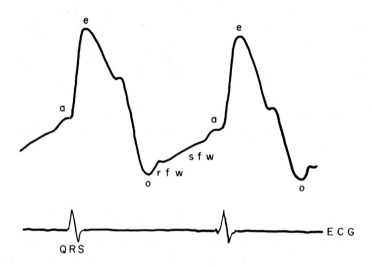

Fig. 4.5   The apex cardiogram. Note 'a' due to atrial systole, 'e' as the ventricle rotates forward with left ventricular systole, the fall from 'e' to 'o' as the ventricle empties, the early rapid filling wave (rfw) in the ventricle, followed by a slow filling wave (sfw).

ing a double impulse. More rarely, one can feel an impulse at the end of rapid filling, corresponding with the third heart sound (see below).

The ventricular impulse may be abnormal in three different ways:

- left ventricular hypertrophy produces a sustained heaving or thrusting apex beat;
- left ventricular dilatation displaces the apex downwards and outwards. If there is a large left ventricular stroke volume, as in aortic regurgitation, the impulse is vigorous, but when myocardial contractility is impaired as by ischaemic heart disease, it may be diffuse and feeble;
- in mitral stenosis, the apex beat often has a characteristic abrupt tapping quality due to the vibrations associated with the loud first sound.

Following myocardial infarction affecting the anterior wall of the heart, there is often an outward movement of the non-contracting area of the left ventricle during systole between the apex and the left sternal edge.

The right ventricular impulse in the left parasternal region is not usually palpable in health, except in children and thin adults. In right ventricular hypertrophy, as occurs in pulmonary stenosis and pulmonary hypertension (particularly secondary to mitral stenosis) there is a sustained lifting impulse along the left sternal edge. When there is right ventricular dilatation associated with a high right ventricular output (as in atrial septal defect), the impulse is vigorous but less sustained. In severe mitral regurgitation, systolic pulsation of the enlarged left atrium may also cause a left parasternal heave.

Pulmonary arterial pulsation can quite often be felt in the second left intercostal space when there is pulmonary hypertension or high pulmonary blood flow. Occasionally, the pulsation of an aneurysm can be detected in the aortic area.

Vibrations may be felt over the precordium corresponding to audible sounds and murmurs. When they are associated with heart sounds, they may be described as 'shocks'. Shocks may accompany any loud heart sound.

Thrills

Thrills are the tactile equivalent of murmurs. They do not occur in the absence of loud murmurs and have no significance beyond that possessed by the murmur. Thrills are usually best felt by the palm of the hand when the patient is sitting upright and holding his breath in full expiration. The commonest thrills are the following:

- an apical systolic thrill corresponding with the loud systolic

murmur of mitral regurgitation;
- a systolic thrill between the apex and the left sternal edge in ventricular septal defect;
- a systolic thrill in the second right intercostal space, occasionally over the sternum and the third or fourth left intercostal space, in aortic stenosis. This is often associated with a systolic thrill over the carotid arteries;
- a systolic thrill in the second or third left intercostal spaces in pulmonary stenosis;
- diastolic and presystolic thrills at the apex in mitral stenosis (best felt with the patient rotated to the left);
- a continuous systolic and diastolic thrill below the left clavicle in persistent ductus arteriosus.

It is rare for the murmurs of aortic or pulmonary regurgitation to be accompanied by a thrill.

After the chest has been palpated, the opportunity should be taken to palpate the abdomen. Particular attention should be paid to the liver. Enlargement, often tender, is a characteristic feature of right-sided heart failure. Systolic pulsation may be felt in tricuspid regurgitation, and presystolic pulsation in tricuspid stenosis.

PERCUSSION OF THE HEART

A crude estimate of the size of the heart may be made by percussion, but this is much less accurate than radiology and it has little place in diagnosis. It is sometimes of value in the diagnosis of pericardial effusion, as in this condition the area of cardiac dullness may be extended to the right of the sternum and to the second left intercostal space. In emphysema, the area of cardiac dullness may be reduced.

AUSCULTATION: HEART SOUNDS AND MURMURS

Vibrations within the heart give rise to sounds which are loud enough to be audible through a stethoscope and to be registered graphically by a phonocardiogram. If the noise is brief and transient, it is termed a heart sound; if more prolonged, it is a murmur. Careful auscultation, combined with the other methods of physical examination, provides information about the heart which even the most sophisticated modern techniques of investigation can scarcely match. A phonocardiogram is useful, however, in timing murmurs and sounds and is of value in differentiating the various types of added sound such as the opening snap and the third heart sound.

The physician should always use a stethoscope with which he is familiar. The earpieces should fit comfortably; the tubing should be short (not greater than 30 cm) and thick-walled. Both types of endpiece (diaphragm and bell) are necessary. The rigid diaphragm is best for hearing high-frequency sounds and murmurs such as the second heart sound and the diastolic murmur of aortic regurgitation. The bell pressed *lightly* on the chest is superior to the diaphragm for the low-pitched third and fourth heart sounds and the mid-diastolic and presystolic murmurs of mitral stenosis.

Traditionally, there are four areas of auscultation:-

- aortic (right second intercostal space);
- pulmonary (left second intercostal space);
- tricuspid (lower sternal);
- mitral (apex beat).

These designations are somewhat misleading, especially with regard to the aortic valve, because aortic murmurs (especially if diastolic) are often maximal at the left sternal edge at the level of the fourth intercostal space. The opening snap of mitral stenosis is also best heard in this area. Auscultation should never be restricted to the traditional areas; one should start on one side of the precordium and gradually move the stethoscope towards the other areas. One may begin in the pulmonary area in order to identify the first and second heart sounds, while palpating the carotid artery whose pulsation occurs just after the first heart sound. The aortic area may be listened to next, before moving obliquely across the sternum to the lower left sternal edge, thence to the tricuspid area, to the mitral area and into the axilla. One should then listen particularly in the aortic, pulmonary and lower left sternal edge areas with the patient sitting up and holding his breath in full expiration. The apical area should be listened to with the patient rotated into the left lateral position. If mitral stenosis is suspected, the patient should exercise by sitting forward and backwards several times, and then lie down again in the left lateral position.

Success in auscultation depends upon listening selectively for individual sounds and murmurs. Initially, the first heart sound should be identified and assessed before turning one's attention to the second heart sound and to any additional sounds. Having noted any normal or abnormal sounds, one should then listen for systolic and, later, for diastolic murmurs.

The heart sounds

The first sound

The first sound occurs at the time of closure of the atrioventricular valves. Although some have attributed the sound to the impact of closure, it seems more likely that it is due to the tensing of the cusps as they are projected into the atrium at the beginning of ventricular systole. Both tricuspid and mitral valves contribute to the sound. As these valves close slightly asynchronously, the first heart sound, in health, may be narrowly split. As the mitral component is louder, the first heart sound is usually best heard at the apex.

The intensity of the first heart sound is related to the extent of upward movement of the cusps when the ventricles contract. In the normal resting heart the valve cusps come into light contact with each other before the onset of ventricular systole which, therefore, projects them only a short distance. If the cusps are well down in the ventricular chamber, ventricular systole forces them rapidly upwards and causes a loud sound. This situation arises when the atrium contracts immediately before the ventricle (short PR interval) and when the left atrial pressure is abnormally high, as in mitral stenosis. In complete heart block, the relationship between atrial and ventricular systole changes from cycle to cycle, and the first sound varies in intensity accordingly. When the cusps are rigid, as in calcific mitral valve disease, the first sound is soft or inaudible.

The second sound

The second heart sound is related to the closure of the semilunar valves. Normally, it is single on expiration but splits into its aortic and pulmonary components during inspiration (Fig. 4.6). This phenomenon is accounted for by the prolongation of right ventricular systole associated with the increased flow into the right side of the heart occurring with inspiration. Splitting is best heard in the second left intercostal space. Abnormally wide splitting of the second sound, due to delay in pulmonary valve closure, occurs when the right ventricle is over-burdened by either a volume load (as in atrial septal defect) or a pressure load (as in pulmonary stenosis), or when there is a delay in electrical activation of the right ventricle (as in right bundle branch block). In atrial septal defect, there is usually 'fixed' splitting of the second heart sound because the increase in venous return on inspiration affects the filling of both ventricles.

When there is left bundle branch block and when the left ventricle is overburdened, as by systemic hypertension or aortic stenosis, the aortic component of the sound may be delayed. This produces 'reversed' splitting; the sound being single on inspiration and split on expiration (Fig. 4.7).

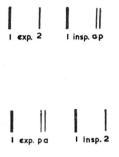

Fig. 4.6 Normal splitting of the second heart sound during inspiration, with the aortic component preceding the pulmonary.

Fig. 4.7 'Reversed' splitting of the second sound. Due to delay in left ventricular emptying, the aortic component follows the pulmonary component of the second sound on expiration. On inspiration, the pulmonary component is, as usual, delayed and is superimposed on the aortic component.

The intensity of the second heart sound may be increased by systemic or pulmonary hypertension, but this is not a reliable sign. The aortic component of the second sound may be reduced or inaudible in aortic stenosis, particularly if the aortic valve is calcified, and the pulmonary component may be soft or absent in pulmonary stension. Both first and second sounds may be soft when the heart is separated from the chest wall by fat, pericardial effusion or emphysematous lung, or when the cardiac output is low as in shock.

The third sound (Fig. 4.8A)

The third sound occurs at the end of the period of rapid filling of the ventricles. It is probably due to sudden tensing of the valve structures and ventricular walls at this time. It is usually generated in the left ventricle and is best heard at or internal to the apex. The sound is low-pitched and distant, and is often heard only with the lightly applied stethoscope bell. Although normal in the young, it is a pathological finding in the middle-aged and elderly. Its presence implies either left ventricular failure or abnormally rapid filling of the ventricle, as in mitral regurgitation, pregnancy or anaemia. Occasionally, a third heart sound can be heard over the right ventricle in

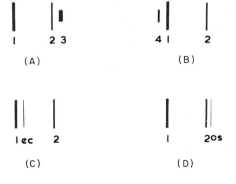

Fig. 4.8 (A) The third heart sound. (B) The fourth or atrial sound. (C) The ejection click (ec). (D) The opening snap.

right ventricular failure. In pericardial constriction, there is a very early third heart sound of higher frequency associated with the sudden limitation to ventricular filling.

The fourth or atrial sound (Fig. 4.8B)

This sound resembles the third heart sound in being low-pitched and best heard at the apex, and probably has a similar mechanism. In this instance, the ventricular distension results from atrial contraction; the fourth sound immediately precedes the first heart sound. It is rarely heard in health, and is usually a sign of either ventricular failure or hypertrophy. Thus, a fourth heart sound is heard over the left ventricle in some cases of aortic stenosis, hypertension and ischaemic heart disease. A right ventricular fourth heart sound may be heard at the left sternal edge in pulmonary stenosis and pulmonary hypertension.

Gallop rhythm

This term is applied to a cadence of three heart sounds which may be heard in the presence of tachycardia. It may be due to a third heart sound, to a fourth heart sound or to the superimposition of the two ('summation gallop').

Additional sounds in systole

Early systolic sounds (ejection sounds or clicks) occur at the time of aortic and pulmonary valve opening (Fig. 4.8C). The clicks may arise from sudden tensing of the opening cusps or from distension of the great vessels. Aortic clicks are almost invariable in valvar aortic stenosis provided the cusps are not calcified, and may be present in systemic hypertension. Pulmonary systolic clicks occur under conditions in which the pulmonary artery is dilated, as it is in valvar pulmonary stenosis and in pulmonary hypertension. They are usually heard best in held expiration.

Clicks occurring later in systole are usually due to ballooning of a mitral valve cusp (mitral valve prolapse). A systolic clicking or crunching may occur in pneumothorax.

The opening snap (Fig. 4.8D)

This is one of the most important signs in auscultation and is virtually diagnostic of mitral stenosis. It occurs at the time of mitral valve opening and is presumed to be due to sudden tension of stenosed but pliant cusps. It is soft or absent if the mitral valve is rigid from fibrosis or calcification. It is heard best at the left sternal edge in the fourth intercostal space or between this point and the apex beat and has a snapping quality. Unlike splitting of the second sound and the third heart sound with which it may be confused, it can often be heard widely over the precordium (see Table 4.1).

Heart murmurs

Murmurs appear to result from vibrations set up by turbulent blood flow. Turbulence is encouraged by high velocity of flow, by abrupt change in the calibre of a vessel or chamber and by reduced blood viscosity. Murmurs therefore develop when there is rapid flow through a valve, valvar narrowing, or anaemia.

The following features of a murmur should be noted: its timing in the cardiac cycle, its location and radiation, its intensity and its quality.

Murmurs may occur either in systole or in diastole; they may continue from one into the other.

Murmurs are usually best heard at the place on the chest wall closest to their site of origin or in the direction of blood flow. Thus, the murmur of aortic stenosis is loudest over the aortic valve (the third left intercostal space), or in the second right intercostal space, or in the neck. On the other hand, the diastolic murmur of aortic regurgitation is usually maximal at the fourth left intercostal space and is less well heard in the 'aortic area'.

The intensity of murmurs may be classified in six grades:

Grade 1   Only just audible, even under good auscultatory conditions
Grade 2   Soft
Grade 3   Moderately loud
Grade 4   Loud
Grade 5   Very loud but not audible with the stethoscope away from the chest
Grade 6   So loud as to be audible with the stethoscope lifted from the chest wall.

The quality of a murmur may be 'blowing', 'rumbling', 'harsh' or 'musical'. These are poor descriptions of what is heard; only with experience can one appreciate what is meant by such terms. Murmurs may also be described as low, medium or high-pitched.

Systolic murmurs

These are usually midsystolic or pansystolic (holosystolic) in timing.

Midsystolic murmurs start after the opening of the aortic and pulmonary valves, increase in intensity to a maximum in midsystole and decrease and disappear before the second heart sound (Fig. 4.9A).

Table 4.1 The differentiation of splitting of the second heart sound, the opening snap, and the third heart sound (of the left ventricle)

	Splitting of second sound (normal)	Splitting of second sound (fixed)	Splitting of second sound (reversed)	Opening snap	Third heart sound
Interval between first component of second sound and 'extra' sound	0–0.05 s (maximal on inspiration)	0.03–0.08 s (at all phases)	0.01–0.03 s (maximal on expiration)	0.03–0.12 s	0.10–0.16 s
Effect of inspiration	Widens	Unaffected	Narrows	None	None
Character	Abrupt — heard best with diaphragm			'Snap' heard best with diaphragm	Low-pitched heard best with bell
Site of maximal intensity	Second left intercostal space			Lower left sternal edge	At apex
Radiation	Left sternal edge			All cardiac areas	Localized (usually)

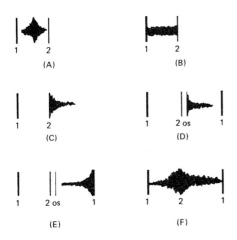

Fig. 4.9 (A) A midsystolic murmur. (B) A pansystolic murmur. (C) An early diastolic murmur. (D) A mid-diastolic murmur, following an opening snap in mitral stenosis. (E) The presystolic murmur of mitral stenosis. (F) The continuous murmur of a persistent ductus arteriosus.

Because of their configuration, they are sometimes called 'diamond-shaped', and are also termed 'ejection' because they arise during ejection of blood from the ventricles into great arteries. Murmurs arising at the aortic and pulmonary valves are characteristically midsystolic.

The murmur of aortic stenosis, which is often harsh, is usually best heard in the second right intercostal space, although sometimes it is maximal at the lower left sternal edge or even at the apex. It frequently radiates to the neck. The murmur of subaortic stenosis is loudest at the lower left sternal edge. The murmur of pulmonary valve stenosis is maximal at the second left intercostal space, that of infundibular pulmonary stenosis most intense at the third or fourth left intercostal space. The murmurs of aortic and pulmonary stenosis are often loud and accompanied by thrills.

A systolic murmur due to high flow in the pulmonary artery is characteristic of atrial septal defect but also occurs in conditions associated with a high cardiac output such as pregnancy, thyrotoxicosis and anaemia. These murmurs are usually of no more than grade 3 intensity and are not associated with thrills.

Quite frequently, particularly in children, midsystolic murmurs may be heard in the pulmonary area for which no organic cause can be found. These may be termed 'functional' or 'benign'. Such murmurs are neither intense nor accompanied by a thrill. They usually vary with position and respiration.

Pansystolic (holosystolic) murmurs persist from the first to the second heart sound and only occur as a result of mitral regurgitation, tricuspid regurgitation or ventricular septal defect, for it is only in these conditions that a pressure difference exists across the defective valve or septum throughout systole (Fig. 4.9B). In mitral regurgitation, the murmur is maximal at or just internal to the apex beat, and radiates into the axilla. It may be maximal in late systole.

The murmur of tricuspid regurgitation is usually loudest in the xiphisternal region, or at the lower left sternal edge. It frequently radiates to the apex and may therefore be readily confused with that of mitral regurgitation, but differs in becoming louder on inspiration, due to the increase in venous return at this time.

The murmur of ventricular septal defect is usually loud and is maximal at the lower left sternal edge.

Murmurs may be confined to early or late systole; those associated with a prolapsed mitral cusp characteristically follow a midsystolic click.

Assessing the significance of a systolic murmur

One can usually determine the cause of a systolic murmur by taking into account its location and radiation, its intensity, its character and its association with other abnormal findings. The duration of the murmur is also of value if one can be certain whether it is midsystolic or pansystolic, but even experts may be unsure on this point.

In aortic stenosis, there is usually a loud murmur at the lower left sternal edge and aortic area which is associated with a thrill, a small flat pulse and left ventricular hypertrophy. If the valve cusps are not calcified, there is an early systolic ('ejection') click; if the stenosis is severe, there may be reversed splitting of the second sound.

In aortic valve sclerosis, a common finding in the elderly, there is an aortic systolic murmur in the absence of any of the other features of aortic stenosis.

In pulmonary stenosis, the loud murmur in the pulmonary or lower left sternal area is accompanied by right ventricular hypertrophy, a soft and late pulmonary component of the second sound and a systolic thrill.

In severe mitral regurgitation, the apical systolic murmur, which is well heard from cardiac apex to axilla, is usually accompanied by left ventricular enlargement, a third heart sound and a mid-diastolic flow murmur. In tricuspid regurgitation, the murmur in the tricuspid area is usually increased by inspiration, and is associated with systolic pulsation in the jugular veins.

It is of particular importance to determine whether a systolic murmur is of the 'benign' variety, for the misinterpretation of such a murmur as organic may lead to unwarranted cardiac invalidism. Benign systolic murmurs are seldom of more than grade 2 intensity, are never pansystolic, are usually best heard in the pulmonary area and are not associated with cardiac enlargement or with abnormal heart sounds. Similar murmurs are encountered in pregnancy, thyrotoxicosis and anaemia, and these conditions should be excluded before a murmur is accepted as being of no significance. The pulmonary systolic murmur of atrial septal defect resembles a benign systolic murmur but is accompanied by wide splitting of the second heart sound, and often by a mid-diastolic murmur due to high flow across the tricuspid valve. One can usually be confident of the benign nature of a murmur on physical examination alone. Only if there are other features such as cardiomegaly or abnormal sounds is further investigation with ECG, radiography and echocardiography necessary.

Diastolic murmurs

Diastolic murmurs are of three main varieties: early diastolic, mid-diastolic and presystolic.

Early (immediate) diastolic murmurs

These murmurs occur shortly after closure of the aortic or pulmonary valves at the beginning of diastole (Fig. 4.9C). They are due to regurgitation through one or other of these valves when pressure in the aorta or pulmonary artery exceeds that of the related ventricle. The murmur decreases in intensity as diastole continues. The murmur is usually soft, high-pitched and blowing, and is best heard by using the diaphragm chest piece with the patient sitting forward, in full expiration. The murmur of aortic regurgitation is usually loudest at the third or fourth left intercostal space close to the sternum, but is occasionally maximal in the second right intercostal space.

The uncommon early diastolic murmur of pulmonary regurgitation (the Graham Steell murmur) is best heard in the left second, third and fourth intercostal spaces. It is similar in character to that of aortic regurgitation but is increased by inspiration and is accompanied by signs of pulmonary hypertension.

Mid-diastolic murmurs

Mid-diastolic murmurs are associated with flow through the atrioventricular valves and necessarily start an appreciable time after the second heart sound. The most important cause is mitral stenosis, in which there is a low-pitched murmur maximal in a localized area at or internal to the apex beat. The murmur is most easily heard with the bell of the stethoscope and with the patient lying in the left lateral position, preferably after exercise (Fig. 4.9D). It is frequently associated with an opening snap, a presystolic murmur and a loud first heart sound.

In tricuspid stenosis, a murmur due to a similar mechanism occurs, but in this condition it is maximal in the xiphisternal or lower left sternal region. This murmur is often of a rather scratchy character and is accentuated by inspiration. Mid-diastolic murmurs may also occur when there is a large flow through atrioventricular valves. Such flow murmurs in the mitral area occur in association with mitral regurgitation, ventricular septal defect and persistent ductus arteriosus. A high-flow tricuspid murmur occurs in atrial septal defect. Another mid-diastolic murmur is that due to rheumatic valvulitis (the Carey Coombs murmur). A mid-diastolic murmur may also be heard, in the absence of mitral valve disease, in patients with severe aortic regurgitation (the Austin Flint murmur). This may be due to the aortic regurgitant flow pushing the aortic cusp of the mitral valve across the mitral valve orifice, thereby causing turbulence as blood is also flowing simultaneously from the left atrium to the left ventricle.

Presystolic murmurs

Presystolic murmurs are produced when atrial systole propels blood through narrowed mitral or tricuspid valves. The presystolic murmur of mitral stenosis leads up to the loud first sound of that condition (Fig.4.9E); it is most easily heard with the patient lying in the left lateral position with the bell of the stethoscope placed at or internal to the apex beat. The presystolic murmur of tricuspid stenosis is maximal in the xiphisternal region or at the lower left sternal edge and is accentuated by inspiration.

Continuous murmurs

The term 'continuous' is applied to a murmur which starts during systole and continues into diastole; it is not necessarily continuous throughout the cardiac cycle. The commonest types are the venous hum and the murmur of persistent ductus arteriosus.

The venous hum is common in childhood, but may be heard in anaemic or pregnant adults. It is due to high blood flow in the jugular veins and can be diminished or abolished by lying the patient flat, or by constricting the veins by pressure. It is usually loudest in the neck, but may be audible over the upper chest.

The murmur in persistent ductus arteriosus is caused by the flow of blood from the high-pressure aorta into the low-pressure pulmonary artery. It is maximal in the left second intercostal space or under the left clavicle. It increases in intensity throughout systole, is maximal at the time of the second heart sound, and diminishes during diastole (Fig. 4.9F). It often has a 'machinery' or whirring quality. Similar murmurs are caused by systemic, pulmonary and coronary arteriovenous fistulae, and by rupture of an aneurysm of a sinus of Valsalva (see p. 316).

Pericardial friction (or rub)

As roughened visceral and parietal layers of pericardium slide over one another, they produce a harsh creaking sound which may be likened to the noise made by two pieces of sandpaper rubbing together. As the movement occurs during ventricular systole, ventricular diastole and atrial systole, the rub may be present at one or all of these times. It may be heard all over the precordium, or only at a localized site. It usually sounds superficial and can be accentuated by leaning the patient forward or by pressing the stethoscope diaphragm firmly on the chest. It can occur in acute pericarditis of any cause, as well as in uraemic pericarditis and during the course of acute myocardial infarction. In the latter condition, it is often evanescent, lasting for only a few minutes or hours.

Further reading

Perloff, J.K. (1986) *Physical Examination of the Heart and Circulation*. Philadelphia: Saunders.

Turner, R.W.D. & Gold, R.G. (1984) *Auscultation of the Heart*. Edinburgh: Churchill Livingstone.

RADIOLOGY AND OTHER TECHNIQUES OF INVESTIGATION

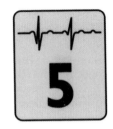

5

Radiological examination of the heart is an essential part of the full cardiological assessment as are the newer non-invasive investigations, including radionuclide studies and echocardiography.

Plain chest radiography and fluoroscopy

Plain radiographs are usually taken in postero-anterior and lateral views; oblique positions are sometimes used.

The normal cardiac contour

In the postero-anterior projection, the patient faces the X-ray cassette. In this view (Fig. 5.1) the right border of the heart consists (from above downwards):

- superior vena cava;
- ascending aorta;
- right atrium;
- inferior vena cava.

The left border of the heart is formed by:

- aortic arch;
- pulmonary artery and its left main branch;
- left ventricle.

Between the left ventricle and the diaphragm, there may be a small triangular shadow due to an epicardial fat pad. In this view, the maximum transverse diameter of the heart does not usually exceed 50% of the chest, measured from the inner aspects of the ribs, although 'cardiothoracic ratios' greater than this are sometimes seen in normal individuals.

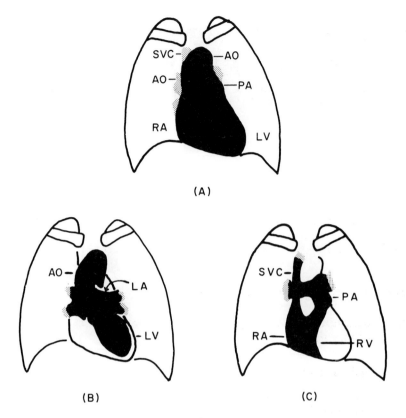

Fig. 5.1 The postero-anterior view. (A) The normal chest radiograph. (B) Appearances of the left side of the heart, after injection of radio-opaque material into the left atrium, showing the positions of the left atrium (LA), the left ventricle (LV) and the aorta (AO). (C) Appearances of the right side of the heart after injection of radio-opaque material into the superior vena cava (SVC). The positions of the right atrium (RA), the right ventricle (RV), and the pulmonary artery (PA), are shown.

In the lateral view (Fig. 5.2), the anterior border of the heart is formed by:

- pulmonary artery;
- right ventricle.

The posterior border is formed by:

- left atrium;
- left ventricle.

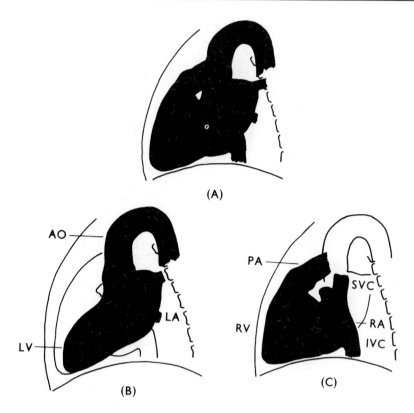

Fig. 5.2 The lateral view. (A) Normal chest radiograph. (B) Appearances of the left side of the heart, after injection of radio-opaque contrast medium into the left atrium, showing the positions of the left atrium (LA), left ventricle (LV) and aorta (AO). (C) Appearances of the right side of the heart after injection of contrast medium into the right atrium showing positions of superior and inferior venae cavae (SVC, IVC), right atrium (RA), right ventricle (RV) and pulmonary artery (PA).

Abnormalities of the cardiac contour

Enlargement of the left ventricle, which is most frequently due to hypertension, ischaemic heart disease, aortic valve disease and mitral regurgitation, produces depression and elongation of the cardiac apex (Fig. 5.3). Left ventricular enlargement is better seen in the lateral view. A normal left ventricle may be displaced posteriorly by an enlarged right ventricle.

Right ventricular enlargement, usually the consequence of pulmonary hypertension or pulmonary stenosis, produces an elevation of the cardiac apex in the postero-anterior view, and in the lateral views of the heart makes the normally straight anterior border of the heart bulge towards or impinge on the sternum.

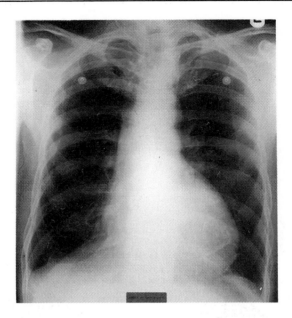

Fig. 5.3 Left ventricular enlargement. Depression and elongation of the cardiac apex in left ventricular enlargement.

The body of the *left atrium* enlarges posteriorly and to the right, but its appendage protrudes to the left. Thus, in the postero-anterior view, the left atrial appendage is seen on the left border of the heart between the pulmonary artery and the left ventricle (Fig. 5.4), whereas the main body of the left atrium forms a dense shadow within the right atrial border, or protrudes to the right above the right atrium on the right side of the heart. Left atrial enlargement is best diagnosed in the lateral view in which it can be seen displacing the barium-filled oesophagus posteriorly.

The *right atrium* enlarges mainly to the right and, in the postero-anterior view, makes the right border of the heart more prominent.

Enlargement of the *ascending aorta*, as from post-stenotic dilatation in aortic stenosis or from aneurysm of the ascending aorta, is seen as a projection to the right (Fig. 5.5). The sclerotic 'uncoiled' aorta of the elderly produces a loop above the heart shadow (Fig. 5.6).

A *pericardial effusion* causes generalized enlargement of the cardiac silhouette, with both lateral borders being smoothly convex (Fig. 5.7).

Calcification within the heart can sometimes be suspected on a plain radiograph (Fig. 5.8), but tomography and fluoroscopy are necessary for confirmation. Calcification in the mitral valve, which is usually rheumatic, is best visualized in the lateral view in which it is

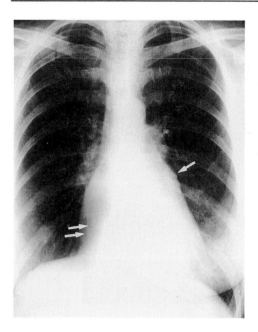

Fig. 5.4 Left atrial enlargement. The bulge produced by the left atrial appendage (arrowed) is seen on the left border of the heart between the positions of the pulmonary artery and left ventricle. This results in 'straightening' of the left heart border. Enlargement of the left atrium causes a double shadow to appear in the right heart border (arrows).

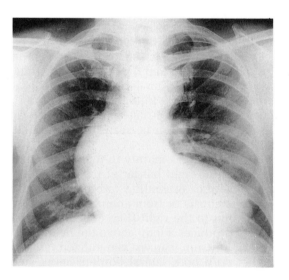

Fig. 5.5 Dilatation of the ascending aorta. Ascending aortic dilatation causes expansion of the upper right heart border. This example is due to the presence of a syphilitic aneurysm in the ascending aorta.

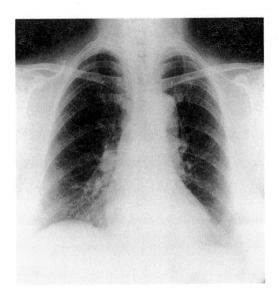

Fig. 5.6 Unfolded aorta.

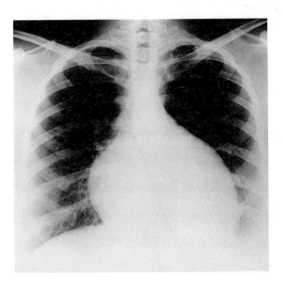

Fig. 5.7 Gross cardiac enlargement due to a pericardial effusion. Both lateral borders of the heart are smoothly convex.

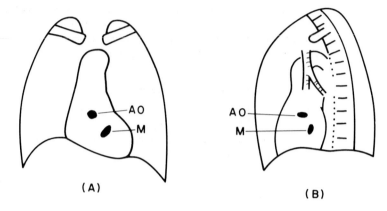

Fig. 5.8 The position of the aortic (AO) and mitral (M) valve calcification in the postero-anterior view (A) and lateral view (B).

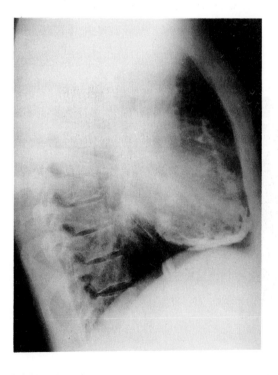

Fig. 5.9 Pericardial calcification. Lateral chest X-ray. A 'shell' of calcium is present outlining the inferior aspect of the ventricles.

seen in the posterior third of the cardiac mass. The aortic valve is located more in the centre of the heart; in the postero-anterior view it is situated just to the left of the spine. Calcification of the pericardium is best seen in a penetrated lateral view (Fig. 5.9).

Abnormalities of the pulmonary circulation

The plain chest radiograph is of great value in demonstrating abnormalities of the pulmonary circulation.

Pulmonary venous hypertension, as occurs in left ventricular failure and mitral stenosis, is revealed by:

- *dilatation of the pulmonary veins*, particularly those draining the upper zones (upper lobe venous diversion);
- *interstitial oedema* causing thin horizontal lines at the bases (Kerley's lines), due to fluid in the interlobular septa and distended lymphatics;
- *alveolar oedema* causing a fluffy opacification (Fig. 5.10) spreading out from the hilar region, often providing a 'butterfly' appearance. The oedema can occasionally be unilateral.

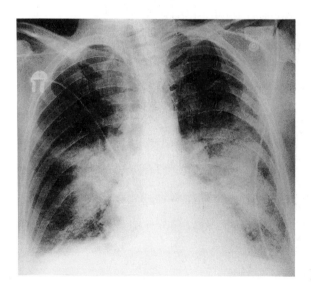

Fig. 5.10 Pulmonary oedema. Chest X-ray of a patient with severe pulmonary oedema following myocardial infarction. Widespread opacification is evident throughout the lung fields due to alveolar oedema.

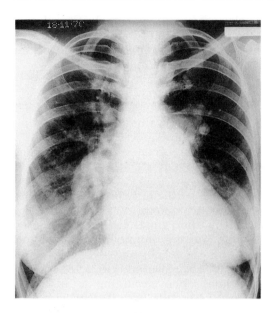

Fig. 5.11 Atrial septal defect. There is marked dilatation of the pulmonary conus and proximal pulmonary arteries. In this patient there is 'pruning' of the distal pulmonary markings due to the development of pulmonary hypertension.

In moderate pulmonary arterial hypertension, the main right and left pulmonary arteries are enlarged, although the more peripheral arteries may be normal. In severe pulmonary hypertension, the major pulmonary arteries, which are greatly dilated, contrast with narrowed peripheral pulmonary arteries; the major arteries appear to be 'cut off'.

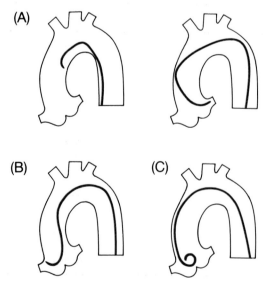

Fig. 5.12 Cardiac catheters. (A) A Judkins left coronary catheter advanced around the aortic arch to engage the left coronary artery. (B) Judkins right coronary catheter. (C) Pigtail catheter in aortic root.

When there is increased pulmonary blood flow, as in atrial septal defect, ventricular septal defect and persistent ductus arteriosus, both main and peripheral pulmonary arteries are dilated (Fig. 5.11). Fluoroscopy may show a vigorous pulsation (the 'hilar dance').

When the pulmonary blood flow is decreased, as in pulmonary stenosis, the pulmonary arteries are poorly seen. However, the main and left pulmonary arteries may be dilated by the jet of blood emerging from the stenosis.

Cardiac catheterization and angiocardiography

These techniques are undertaken in order to establish a precise diagnosis and to assess the severity of the disorders present.

Cardiac catheterization permits:

- the recording of pressures within the heart and great vessels (see Table 5.1) for normal pressures;
- the sampling of blood for blood gases;
- the injection of indicators for the measurement of cardiac output;
- the injection of radio-opaque substances which can delineate abnormalities of anatomy or function;
- the introduction of a balloon-tipped catheter for therapeutic purposes, e.g. the Rashkind procedure and coronary angioplasty;

Table 5.1 Normal cardiovascular pressures (mmHg)

	Mean	Range
Right atrium — mean	4	0–8
Right ventricle		
systolic	25	15–30
end diastolic	4	0–8
Pulmonary artery		
systolic	25	15–30
diastolic	10	5–15
mean	15	10–20
Pulmonary artery wedge — mean	10	5–14
Left atrium — mean	7	4–12
Left ventricle		
systolic	120	90–140
end diastolic	7	4–12
Aorta		
systolic	120	90–140
diastolic	70	60–90
mean	85	70–105

- the introduction of a bioptome, to obtain a sample of endocardium or myocardium.

A selection of cardiac catheters is illustrated in Fig. 5.12.

Right heart catheterization

Under local anaesthesia, a catheter is introduced percutaneously or by cutdown into a basilic, saphenous or femoral vein, and advanced to the right atrium. It is manoeuvred with fluoroscopic control through the tricuspid valve to the right ventricle, thence to the pulmonary artery and finally wedged in a distal pulmonary artery. The pulmonary arterial wedge (pulmonary capillary) tracing so obtained is an indirect measurement of pressure in the left atrium (Fig. 5.13).

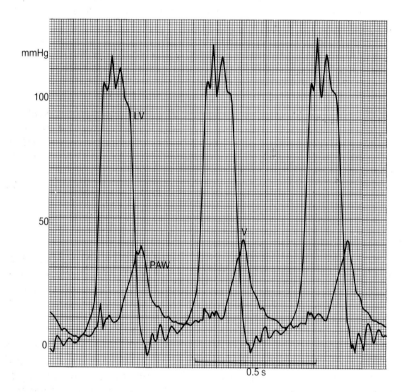

Fig. 5.13 Pulmonary artery wedge tracing. A pulmonary artery wedge tracing (PAW) is shown together with a left ventricular tracing (LV). There is a prominent V wave in the pulmonary wedge tracing due to mitral regurgitation.

If appropriate radiological facilities are not available, a (Swan–Ganz) catheter with a balloon close to its tip may be used. If the balloon is inflated when the right atrium is reached, the tip will 'float' into a pulmonary artery. If the balloon is impacted in the artery, a pulmonary artery wedge tracing is obtained.

If there is a septal defect, the catheter may be passed through this into the left side of the heart; if there is a persistent ductus arteriosus, this may be traversed.

As the catheter is withdrawn from the pulmonary artery, blood samples can be obtained from each vessel and chamber. When a left-to-right shunt is present, the blood is found to be more oxygenated in the affected chamber and beyond than it is in the great veins:

- *persistent ductus arteriosus*, the oxygen saturation in the left pulmonary artery exceeds that in the right ventricle;
- *ventricular septal defect*, the oxygen saturation in the right ventricle and pulmonary artery is greater than that in the right atrium;
- *atrial septal defect*, the oxygen saturation in the right atrium exceeds that in the superior and inferior venae cavae.

The presence of valve stenoses can be demonstrated:

- pulmonary stenosis can be confirmed by showing a systolic pressure difference between the pulmonary artery and right ventricle. This can be distinguished from infundibular stenosis in which the pressure gradient lies within the outflow tract of the right ventricle;
- tricuspid stenosis is present if the diastolic pressure in the right atrium is higher than that in the right ventricle.

Left heart catheterization

Under local anaesthesia, a catheter is introduced into the femoral or brachial artery and advanced retrogradely until it reaches the aortic valve. The catheter can then be manipulated across the valve and into the left ventricle. The catheter is used to measure pressures or to deliver contrast injections (angiography).

Pressure measurements. The severity of a stenotic lesion is best determined by measuring both the pressure difference and the blood flow across the valve. This requires the simultaneous recording of pressures on both sides of the valve and the estimation of cardiac output:

- *aortic stenosis* is assessed by pressure difference between the left ventricle and the aorta. This can be distinguished from cases of

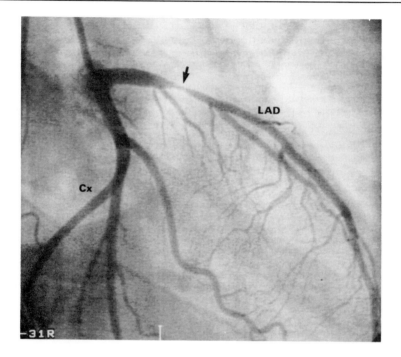

(A)

Fig. 5.14 Coronary angiography. Contrast medium has been injected into the left coronary artery. (A) Right anterior oblique projection. (B) Left anterior oblique projection. The left coronary artery divides into left anterior descending (LAD) and circumflex (Cx) branches. A stenosis in the proximal LAD is arrowed.

sub-aortic stenosis or hypertrophic cardiomyopathy, in which the pressure drop lies within the cavity of the left ventricle;
• *mitral stenosis* is assessed by the pressure difference between the pulmonary artery wedge and left ventricular pressures.

Angiocardiography. By the injection of contrast medium it is possible to demonstrate the anatomy of the chambers of the heart and the coronary arteries and the great arteries, and to observe the patterns of blood flow. Cine films are taken at 25–50 frames per second in one or two planes.

The contrast medium is injected at the site most appropriate for the delineation of the suspected abnormality. Therefore, in ventricular septal defect and mitral regurgitation, the injection is made into the left ventricle; in aortic regurgitation it is made into the aorta. When

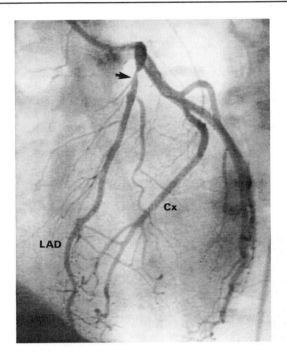

(B)

Fig. 5.14   continued.

coronary angiography is performed, selective injections are made into each of the two main coronary arteries (see Fig. 5.14 and p. 108).

Indications for and risks of cardiac catheterization and angiocardiography

Cardiac catheterization and angiocardiography are procedures which require considerable skill and experience on the part of the physician and entail some discomfort and hazard for the patient. The natural anxiety of patients prior to the procedure is best allayed by previous preparation and explanation, combined with the use of a sedative if necessary. Anaesthesia may have to be employed in children, but should be avoided if possible because of its effects on haemodynamics and blood gases.

Right heart catheterization entails little danger, although arrhythmias may be provoked when the catheter tip is in the right ventricle. Left heart catheterization imposes a slightly greater risk. The injection of radio-opaque contrast medium in angiocardiography often provokes transient ventricular arrhythmias and, occasionally, ventricular fibrillation. The mortality associated with routine coronary angiography is of the order of 1–2 per 1000 cases. There is also a morbidity due to complications which include dissection and thrombosis of the catheterized artery or vein, pulmonary and systemic embolism, haemorrhage from puncture sites and toxic reactions to the contrast medium.

These techniques are mainly used to evaluate the nature and extent of the heart disease prior to cardiac surgery, but they are also of value when doubt exists as to the nature of a murmur, or the cause of chest pain. In recent years, echocardiography and Doppler ultrasound have rendered cardiac catheterization unnecessary in many cases of congenital and valvar heart disease, but it is still required when these techniques provide an equivocal result or when coronary arteriography is also needed.

The measurement of cardiac output

The cardiac output can be measured by one of two techniques: the Fick principle and the indicator–dilution method.

The Fick principle. Fick pointed out that:

- the quantity of blood traversing the lungs in a given period of time equals the cardiac output;
- the change in oxygen (O_2) concentration between pulmonary arteries (PA) and pulmonary veins (PV) depends upon the O_2 uptake in the lungs, and the volume of blood into which it is absorbed, i.e. the cardiac output (CO).

Therefore,

$$PVO_2 - PAO_2 = \frac{O_2 \text{ uptake}}{CO} \text{ and } CO = \frac{O_2 \text{ uptake}}{PVO_2 - PAO_2}$$

Oxygen uptake is derived from the analysis of expired air. Blood samples are obtained by catheterization, arterial blood being used instead of pulmonary venous blood.

Indicator–dilution method. This is based on a similar principle, namely that the concentration of an injected substance in the blood is dependent upon the amount of that substance injected and the volume of blood in which it is diluted.

Currently, the most popular technique is to use cold saline and to measure the change in temperature with a thermistor attached to a catheter tip. An injection of cold saline, of known volume and temperature, is injected into a vein or the right atrium and the temperature is sampled in the pulmonary artery. Pulmonary flotation catheters, incorporating a right atrial port, pulmonary arterial port and thermistor are available for this purpose.

Radionuclide studies

Nuclear imaging is of value in two major contexts which particularly relate to ischaemic heart disease: the demonstration of abnormalities of myocardial perfusion and the evaluation of left ventricular function.

Myocardial perfusion studies

Certain radiopharmaceuticals, of which thallium-201 is the one most commonly used, are taken up into the myocardium in proportion to the regional blood flow. They therefore do not concentrate in areas of ischaemia or fibrosis. Thallium imaging has been found to be of greatest value in the detection of transient myocardial ischaemia in patients with suspected angina pectoris (Fig. 5.15). If the radio-isotope is injected intravenously during an exercise test at the time when the patient develops chest pain or ST depression, a 'cold spot' will be seen corresponding to the area of ischaemia, while the rest of the myocardium will take up the isotope. If nuclear imaging is repeated some 4 h later, when no ischaemia is present, the 'cold spot' will be seen to have disappeared. A reversible defect, therefore, provides evidence of impaired myocardial perfusion, raising the possibility that the patient might benefit from a revascularisation procedure, either coronary artery bypass grafting or angioplasty. An area of previous myocardial infarction will also appear as a perfusion defect on the initial exercise scan, but the perfusion defect is irreversible and is still present on the resting scan 4 h later.

Thallium scanning is relatively sensitive and specific. However, because of the cost of thallium, it is frequently reserved as a second line procedure to exercise testing. There are some situations in which a thallium scan is particularly useful:

- in patients with an equivocal exercise ECG. A thallium scan may clarify the diagnosis, without resort to coronary angiography;
- to localise the site of ischaemia. Electrocardiography provides only limited information as to which coronary territory may be ischaemic. The localization of a reversible defect on thallium scanning identifies which artery or arteries are functionally inadequate. This can be particularly useful in identifying target

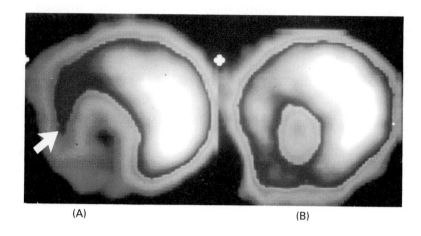

(A)　　　　　　　　　　　　　(B)

Fig. 5.15 Thallium scan. (A) Peak exercise. There is a defect in thallium uptake (arrowed), corresponding to an apical perfusion deficit. (B) After rest for 4 hours, uptake normalizes in this region. This reversible defect is indicative of ischaemia. A non-reversible, fixed defect would indicate infarction.

lesions for coronary angioplasty or in assessing inadequate graft function following coronary artery bypass grafting;

- *in patients incapable of performing an exercise stress test.* A dipyridamole thallium scan provides a useful assessment of ischaemia, in patients incapable of performing an exercise stress test. Patients with peripheral vascular disease, for example, may develop claudication on exercise testing, preventing achievement of a workload which enables their coronary status to be assessed. An injection of dypyridamole provides an alternative to stress testing. Dipyridamole is a coronary vasodilator, which causes greater dilatation in non-diseased than in diseased coronary vessels. As a result a 'coronary steal' phenomenon may occur, whereby blood-flow increases in the non-diseased coronary segments at the expense of the diseased. Just as for exercise testing, this will show up as a perfusion defect on thallium imaging.

Thallium imaging is relatively sensitive and specific, but unfortunately the cost of thallium and the degree of skill and experience necessary for optimal interpretation limit its application.

Radionuclide ventriculography

The most common technique for the imaging of left ventricular function involves the use of technetium-labelled red cells so that the pool of blood in the left ventricle can be detected. By using the ECG to 'gate' the images ('gated pool scan'), segments of the cardiac cycle from successive beats can be superimposed. By obtaining 20 or more exposures during each cardiac cycle, it is possible to record the radionuclide equivalent of a cine-angiogram. This technique allows the evaluation of several aspects of left ventricular function including contractility of the ventricle, end-systolic and end-diastolic volumes and the detection of regional wall abnormalities including ventricular aneurysms.

Echocardiography

When an ultrasonic beam encounters a boundary between structures of different acoustic densities, some of the waves are reflected. These can be detected and used to provide an electrical signal. The procedure of echocardiography exploits this principle to identify many cardiac structures and to study their movements (Figs. 5.16 and 5.17).

A piezo-electric crystal, which acts both as transmitter and receiver, is used to generate high-frequency pulses of very short duration. These travel through body tissues at known velocity: the 'echoes' which occur from interfaces are detected by the transducer, amplified and then displayed either on an oscilloscope or on a strip-chart recorder. Bone and lung both interfere with ultrasonic transmission, so that the views that can be obtained of the heart are limited.

The transducer is usually placed in the fourth left intercostal space close to the sternal edge. As can be seen in Figs 5.16 and 5.17, by rotating the probe a sweeping view of many of the intracardiac structures may be obtained.

In cross-sectional (two-dimensional, 2D) echocardiography, an ultrasonic beam is moved rapidly across the heart (or a series of ultrasonic elements are fired in sequence) to allow a real-time recording of changes in cardiac shape and movement, which are displayed on a videotape (Fig. 5.18).

M-mode and 2-D echocardiography are of great value in assessing a wide spectrum of valvular and myocardial disorders:

- valve stenoses;
- prosthetic heart valves;
- infective endocarditis;
- chamber dimensions;
- ventricular function;

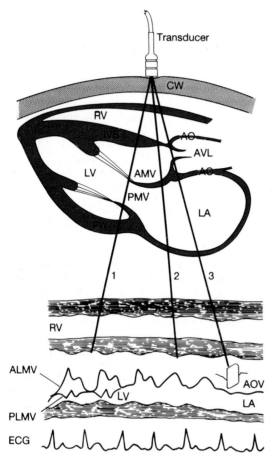

Fig. 5.16   The transducer is angled in different directions to permit study of the various cardiac structures. (1) The beam traverses the right ventricle (RV), interventricular septum (IVS), and anterior and posterior leaflets of the mitral valve (ALMV and PLMV). These leaflets separate abruptly as the blood flows rapidly from the left atrium to the left ventricle. As the flow decreases they approximate only to be separated again when atrial contraction propels more blood into the ventricle. (2) Provides good views of the RV, septum, ALMV and left atrium. (3) Shows separation of the aortic valve cusps in systole.

- ventricular hypertrophy;
- cardiomyopathies;
- atrial myxoma;
- aortic aneurysms;
- pericardial effusion and tamponade;
- congenital heart disease.

Echocardiography has proved particularly valuable in studying disorders of the mitral valve. In the normal valve, the cusps open rapidly in early diastole and return quickly towards the closed position, being further propelled downwards by atrial systole before finally moving upwards before closure. In mitral stenosis, the diastolic closure rate is slow and the posterior cusp, instead of moving away from the anterior cusp during diastole, moves forward with it (Fig. 5.19). Other abnormalities which may be detected are multiple echoes

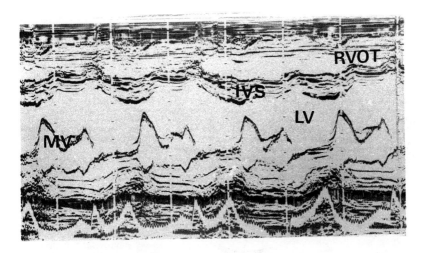

Fig. 5.17 Normal echocardiogram, corresponding to 12A, view (1), showing right ventricular outflow tract, interventricular septum, both cusps of the mitral valve, and the left ventricular cavity. RVOT = right ventricular outflow tract. IVS = interventricular septum. MV = mitral valve. LV = left ventricle.

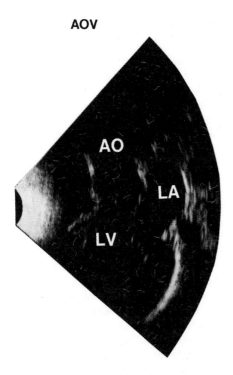

Fig. 5.18 Cross-sectional long axis parasternal view of a normal heart showing the aortic root, aortic valve, left ventricle and left atrium. LV = left ventricle, AO = aorta, LA = left atrium.

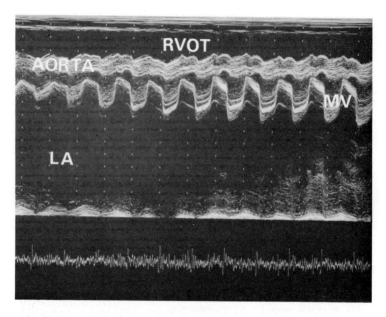

Fig. 5.19 Severe mitral stenosis — an M-mode parasternal echocardiogram. The left atrium (LA) is huge and the mitral valve shows the characteristic slow diastolic closure rate. RVOT = right ventricular outflow tract. MV = mitral valve.

suggesting calcification, and abnormal movements of the leaflets during systole, indicating prolapse of the cusps (Fig. 5.20).

Although calcification of the aortic valve may be readily demonstrated, other abnormalities of this valve are less diagnostic. However, a useful indicator of aortic regurgitation is the fluttering of the mitral valve which may be produced by the regurgitant jet during early diastole.

Doppler ultrasound

This technique makes use of the familiar phenomenon whereby the pitch of a sound appears to become higher as its source approaches us, and falls as it goes away. In the body, the blood corpuscles act as moving targets which reflect the ultrasound wave, and alter its pitch, depending upon the direction and velocity of blood flow. There are three forms of Doppler examination:

Pulsed Doppler. A single transducer is used, which first emits a brief ultrasound pulse, and then switches to receive the returning signal. Because ultrasound has a constant velocity in the body, the depth of the target can be determined by the interval between emission and return of the signal. The time interval and, therefore, the depth of the target area being examined can be varied as required, and

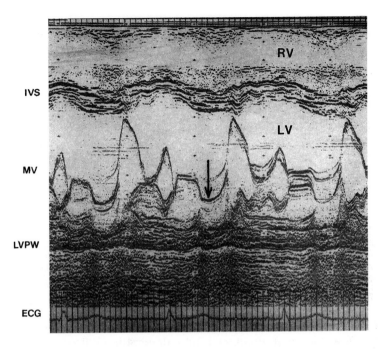

Fig. 5.20 Mitral valve prolapse. M-mode echocardiogram showing (arrow) 'hammock-ing' appearance of mitral cusp as it prolapses posteriorly during late systole.

can be correlated with a simultaneously recorded cross-sectional echocardiogram, thus locating precisely the site of the area being examined, Unfortunately, there is a limit to the rate at which pulses can be generated, because one wave may not have returned before the next is generated, leading to distortion (aliasing) of the signal. This prevents the recognition of high velocities. Pulsed Doppler, therefore, is used to sample blood velocities at specific sites within the heart, but cannot be used to measure the high velocities encountered with moderately or severely stenosed valves.

Continuous wave (CW) Doppler. This enables high velocities to be recorded. In this technique, one transducer continuously emits ultrasound, which is detected by a separate receiver. Although continuous wave Doppler can record high velocities, it cannot identify the depth at which the signal originated. The pressure gradient across a stenotic lesion can be calculated from the Bernoulli equation:

Pressure gradient $= 4 \times (\text{Velocity})^2$

Colour Doppler. Colour flow imaging is essentially a Doppler technique which enables the direction of blood flow through the heart

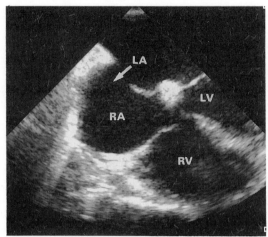

Fig. 5.21 Transoesophageal echo. The four chambers of the heart are shown. LA = left atrium, RA = right atrium, RV = right ventricle, LV = left ventricle. The patient has an atrial septal defect. The communication between the left atrium and right atrium is arrowed.

to be identified and displayed in colour. Blood flow towards the transducer is illustrated as red and away from the transducer as blue.

Doppler echocardiography has proved of great value in:

- valve gradient estimation to assess severity of stenoses. This is particularly useful in the case of the aortic valve;
- demonstration of valve regurgitation, although estimation of the severity of regurgitation is unreliable. Even mild physiological degrees of regurgitation may be detectable, particularly in the tricuspid area;
- evaluation of prosthetic valves;
- evaluation of congenital heart disease.

In many cases the combination of 2-D and Doppler echocardiographic investigations can obviate the need for invasive investigations.

Oesophageal echocardiography

In many patients, the technical quality of echocardiograms recorded via the conventional transthoracic route, with the ultrasound probe applied to the anterior chest wall, is limited. Oesophageal echocardiography provides an alternative means of imaging (Fig. 5.21). The oesophagus lies just posterior to the left atrium. Passage of a specialized oesophageal ultrasound probe provides uniformly high quality images, particularly of posterior structures within the heart.

Oesophageal echocardiography is proving particularly useful in diagnosing:

- vegetations in patients with bacterial endocarditis;
- dissection of the thoracic aorta;
- the demonstration of thrombi and masses within the left atrium.

Further reading

Feigenbaum, H. (1986) *Echocardiography*, 4th edn. Philadelphia: Lea & Febiger.

Gerson, M.C. (Ed.) (1987) *Cardiac Nuclear Medicine.* New York: McGraw Hill.

Grainger, R.G. & Allison, D.J. (Eds) (1986) *Diagnostic Radiology.* Edinburgh: Churchill Livingstone.

Jefferson, K. & Rees, S. (1980) *Clinical Cardiac Radiology,* 2nd edn. London: Butterworth.

Mendel, D. & Oldershaw, P. (1986) *Cardiac Catheterization,* 3rd edn. Oxford: Blackwell.

Popp, R.L. (1990) Echocardiography. *New England Journal of Medicine* **323**: 101, 165.

Task Force on Assessment of Cardiovascular Procedures (1986) Guidelines for clinical use of cardiac radionuclide imaging. *Circulation 74*: 1469A.

Diseases of the Coronary Arteries — Causes, Pathology and Prevention

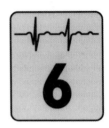

6

THE CORONARY CIRCULATION

There are two major coronary arteries — right and left (Fig. 6.1). The right coronary artery arises from the right coronary sinus of Valsalva and runs down in the groove between the right atrium and the right ventricle. In most hearts, its branches supply the sinus node, the atrioventricular node and bundle, the right ventricle and the inferior part of the left ventricle. The left coronary artery, which arises from the left coronary sinus of Valsalva, soon divides into two large branches: the anterior descending branch which runs down between the two ventricles anteriorly, and the left circumflex branch which passes around in the groove between the left atrium and the left ventricle. The anterior descending artery supplies the interventricular septum and the anterior wall of the left ventricle. The circumflex supplies the lateral and posterior aspects of the left ventricle. The major vessels traverse the external surface of the myocardium, sending branches perpendicularly into the muscle mass. There are normally many small anastomoses between the coronary arteries, but these are of no functional importance. When an area of the heart becomes ischaemic, the anastomoses enlarge and then provide a collateral blood supply to the affected muscle which is often vital for its survival.

The arteries divide to form arterioles and capillaries similar to those elsewhere in the body, and the venules and veins join to form larger venous channels. Virtually all the blood from the left coronary artery eventually drains into the coronary sinus; that from the right coronary artery drains mainly into the anterior cardiac veins. From these veins the blood passes into the right atrium.

The blood flow in the coronary arteries resembles that in other regions in being dependent on the blood pressure and on the vascular resistance of the arteries and arterioles. A distinctive feature of the coronary circulation is that the arteries are compressed by the contracting myocardium during systole so that the resistance to flow

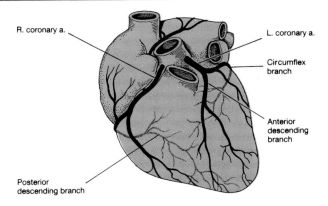

Fig. 6.1 The anatomy of the coronary arteries (see text).

at that time is sharply increased. Consequently, coronary blood flow occurs mainly during diastole. Flow is largely determined by the calibre of the small coronary arteries. Certainly, the aortic diastolic pressure is also a determinant of coronary flow; but according to Poiseuille's equation, flow is dependent directly on pressure differences but related to the fourth power of the radius. Therefore, a doubling of aortic diastolic pressure doubles coronary flow, whereas a doubling of the radius of the coronary arteries leads to a 16-fold increase in flow. In health, variations in coronary blood flow are mainly due to changes in impedance in the small coronary arteries; these dilate in response to a fall in tissue oxygen tension but they are also under the influence of the autonomic nervous system. Variations in tone also occur in the large coronary arteries but these affect blood flow only if these vessels are narrowed by disease or they are extreme (spasm).

In the normal resting heart, almost all the oxygen is extracted during its passage through the capillaries; coronary sinus blood is therefore almost completely desaturated. Unlike other organs, the heart cannot call upon a venous oxygen reserve when faced by increased demands, and is largely dependent upon the ability of the coronary arteries to increase their diameter.

CORONARY ARTERY DISEASE

Coronary artery disease is the commonest cause of heart disease and the most important single cause of death in the affluent countries of the world. In the overwhelming majority of cases, disease of the coronary arteries is due to:

- atherosclerosis. ✓

However, the coronary arteries may also be involved in other disorders:

- congenital abnormalities such as arteriovenous fistulae and anomalous origin from the pulmonary artery;
- coronary embolism associated with thrombosis arising in the left atrium or ventricle or from mitral or aortic valve prostheses, or from infective endocarditis;
- syphilitic aortitis involving the coronary ostia (p. 331);
- occlusion of a coronary artery due to dissecting aneurysm (p. 312);
- polyarteritis (p. 339) and other connective tissue diseases;
- coronary artery spasm which may affect both diseased and otherwise normal vessels (p. 93).

Definitions

Atherosclerosis has been defined (by a WHO study group) as 'a variable combination of changes of the intima of arteries (as distinguished from arterioles) consisting of a focal accumulation of lipids, complex carbohydrates, blood and blood products, fibrous tissue and calcium deposits, and associated with medial changes'. It is synonymous with *atheroma* but not with *arteriosclerosis*, which is a less specific term used to describe hardening of arteries and arterioles.

Coronary artery disease. This term is used to describe coronary arteries which are affected by a pathological process. Coronary artery disease usually exists for many years before a disorder of myocardial function develops. It is, therefore, not synonymous with coronary (or ischaemic) *heart* disease.

Ischaemic heart disease is cardiac disease resulting from myocardial ischaemia. Although myocardial ischaemia also occurs in such conditions as aortic stenosis, the term 'ischaemic heart disease' is generally applied only to cases of atherosclerotic origin.

Coronary heart disease and *atherosclerotic heart disease* are synonymous with ischaemic heart disease.

Coronary thrombosis refers to occlusion of a coronary artery by thrombus. This may or may not lead to myocardial infarction.

Coronary occlusion. This term is used to describe occlusion of the coronary artery by any cause. Again, this may or may not cause myocardial infarction.

Myocardial infarction is necrosis of a portion of heart muscle as a result of inadequate blood supply.

Silent ischaemia is ischaemia in the absence of symptoms. The term is applied particularly to episodes of ST elevation or depression unaccompanied by pain.

VASOSPASTIC ANGINA (PRINZMETAL'S ANGINA)

This term is used to describe a syndrome of which the essential features are angina pectoris due to an increase in coronary vasomotor tone and ST elevation in the ECG. The angina is attributable not, as in classical angina, to an increase in myocardial oxygen demand, but to a transient reduction in coronary blood flow. The disorder may occur either in otherwise apparently normal coronary arteries, or in atherosclerotic vessels. In the former case, the increase in tone must be extreme (spasm), but in severely stenotic arteries, even physiological changes in tone can produce a critical reduction in blood flow. The mechanism for coronary spasm is unknown, but it may be provoked by certain drugs, notably ergometrine.

The clinical picture is typically one of anginal pain occurring at rest, particularly in the early morning. The attacks are usually self-limiting, but the pain may be severe; they very seldom lead on to myocardial infarction. Nitrates and calcium antagonists are effective both in the treatment of individual episodes and when used prophylactically.

Coronary atherosclerosis

Pathology of coronary atherosclerosis and its complications

The atherosclerotic process probably starts with the 'fatty streak'. Fatty streaks are a common finding in the intima of young people; macroscopically, they appear as yellow patches within the arterial wall. They are mainly composed of lipid-laden foam cells which are derived from macrophages and, to a lesser extent, from smooth-muscle cells. Depending upon their location and the presence of the relevant risk factors, the fatty streak may progress to the characteristic lesion of atherosclerosis — the fibro-lipid plaque (Fig 6.2). The major components of the plaque are lipid and arterial smooth muscle cells and their products, such as fibrous proteins and complex carbohydrates. Plaques vary from one another in their composition. At one extreme are fatty plaques, containing a large pool of cholesterol and its esters, separated from the lumen by a thin fibrous cap. At the other extreme are solid plaques, consisting of smooth muscle cells and connective tissue. Calcification may be superimposed. These deposits are focal and are most commonly located at the bends and bifurcations of arteries.

The atheromatous plaque, which is produced by this process, may itself narrow the lumen of the artery. The fibrous cap is prone to fracture, allowing the necrotic core to ulcerate and trigger off platelet aggregation and fibrin deposition. This is a repetitive process and leads to further narrowing, which may proceed to complete occlusion.

Necropsies on patients who have experienced *angina pectoris*

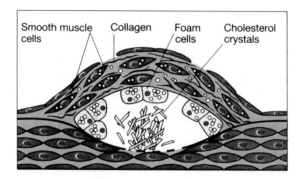

Fig. 6.2 A diagrammatic representation of an atheromatous plaque showing outer cap containing collagen and smooth muscle cells, and inner core showing foam cells and extracellular cholesterol crystals. (With permission from G.R. Thompson, *A Handbook of Hyperlipidaemia*, Current Science, 1989.)

usually reveal widespread but patchy coronary atherosclerosis and myocardial fibrosis. Evidence of old coronary occlusion and myocardial infarction is common. The basic pathological cause for the angina is the coronary arterial narrowing which has reduced the lumen of at least one of the three main coronary arteries by 75%. In most cases, two or all three of these arteries are affected.

Sudden death is often attributed to coronary artery disease when widespread coronary atherosclerosis is present. Recent coronary occlusion or myocardial infarction can be demonstrated in only a minority of cases but plaque rupture and non-occlusive thrombus are common. In most instances, it is probable that acute myocardial ischaemia has provoked fatal ventricular fibrillation.

The essential pathological feature of *acute myocardial infarction* is myocardial necrosis. This is usually, but not always, the consequence of total occlusion of a coronary artery. Plaque rupture is commonly found at necropsy; plaques which rupture are typically rich in lipid and have only a thin cap. There is often evidence of an inflammatory state with many macrophages and T lymphocytes within the plaque. Disruption of the cap allows blood to enter the lipid pool; collagen, crystalline cholesterol and oxidized low-density lipoproteins trigger the formation of a platelet-rich thrombus within the intima. A fibrin-rich thrombus may become superimposed and project into the lumen. It may further expand as many red cells infiltrate the network of fibrin to cause total occlusion. The thrombus will usually lyse spontaneously in the days after infarction but the process can be greatly accelerated by thrombolytic drugs.

If death occurs soon after the onset of myocardial infarction, there may be no gross changes in the myocardium, but enzyme-staining reactions and electron microscopy will reveal evidence of damage. Later, the infarcted area appears pale and is surrounded by a reddish area due to hyperaemia. Microscopically, the muscle cells lose their nuclei and, subsequently, necrotic changes take place in adjacent connective tissue and blood vessel walls. Leucocytic infiltration occurs at the edges of the infarct. The removal of necrotic muscle starts about the third day and continues for about 2 weeks. At the same time, granulation tissue containing blood vessels and fibroblasts invades the necrotic area. Finally, the infarct zone is replaced by scar tissue over a period lasting between 2 and 8 weeks. If the infarction involves the endocardial surface, a mural thrombus may develop; if it affects the epicardium, there may be pericarditis.

The location and size of a myocardial infarction depend upon the artery that is occluded and the collateral blood supply. In some cases, the infarct extends from the endocardium to the epicardium (transmural infarction); in others, only the subendocardial territory is involved. If the left anterior descending artery is occluded, the infarction involves the anterior wall of the left ventricle and may involve the septum. If the left circumflex is occluded, the infarction affects the lateral or posterior walls of the left ventricle. If the right coronary artery is occluded, the infarction chiefly affects the inferior (diaphragmatic) surface of the left ventricle but also the septum and right ventricle. Coronary artery occlusion may not lead to myocardial infarction if the area supplied by the occluded artery has an adequate collateral supply from adjacent arteries.

The infarcted tissue may thin and stretch in the days after infarction, particularly if this has been anterior. It is due to a combination of stretching of the tissues and the sliding of muscle bundles over each other. This process, known as infarct expansion, has adverse effects on left ventricular shape and contractile ability and is probably an important component of subsequent cardiac failure. It may be preventable if the load on the left ventricle is minimized in the early post-infarction period, as by the use of ACE inhibitors (see p. 384).

The pathogenesis of atherosclerosis

Atherosclerosis results from interactions between the arterial wall and the constituents of the blood. A number of elements play important roles:

- the endothelium;
- monocytes/macrophages;
- smooth muscle cells;
- platelets;
- blood lipids.

The endothelium is composed of a single layer of cells that acts as a barrier, albeit a highly selective one, between the components of the blood and the arterial wall. Endothelial cells are also metabolically active, generate vasoactive substances, and present a non-thrombogenic surface (because they can form prostacyclin and because they have a coating of heparan sulphate). They can form the mitogen (i.e. growth factor) platelet-derived growth factor (PDGF) and produce endothelium-derived relaxant factor (EDRF) which causes relaxation of the underlying smooth muscle. The loss of integrity of the endothelium is of critical importance in the development of atherosclerosis. Very often the endothelium is denuded over plaques. Even when it is not, there is endothelial dysfunction.

Macrophages, which are derived from circulating monocytes, secrete several biologically important substances, including a number of growth factors (such as PDGF) and toxic oxygen metabolites. They also have receptors for oxidized low-density lipoprotein (LDL), which they ingest and degrade. They are the major source of foam cells in the fatty streak and the fibro-lipid plaque, and play a key role in the connective tissue proliferation.

Smooth muscle cells, derived originally from the media, change their characteristics when they migrate to the intima. Instead of being primarily contractile, they take on many secretory functions. They also become responsive to growth factors (such as PDGF) and are then able to proliferate. They are an essential component of advanced atherosclerotic lesions, in which they accumulate lipid and form foam cells.

Platelets are crucially involved in the complication of thrombosis but also play a major role in the development of atherosclerosis. When activated, they release vasoconstrictor substances and growth factors which can stimulate virtually all the cell types found in the tissues.

Lipids are important components of most plaques, and affect the function of the endothelium, smooth muscle cells and macrophages. They contribute to the formation of foam cells, but there is also a considerable amount of free cholesterol in the tissues of many lesions. Much of the lipid that is taken up is in chemically altered form, having been modified by oxidation or acetylation. Modified LDL is a powerful chemoattractant for monocytes, and macrophages take up LDL avidly in the modified but not in the unmodified form.

'Response to injury' hypothesis

There is still much to be learned about the genesis of atherosclerosis, but current thinking is best integrated under the 'response to injury' hypothesis. This proposes that the initial lesion is one in which the endothelium is 'injured' in some way, although the term 'injury' is used to cover functional disorders as well as physical disruption. Chronic hyperlipidaemia, with an increase in circulating low-density lipoprotein, leads to changes in the function of monocytes and platelets, as well as in the endothelial cells. The monocytes adhere to the endothelium, and are attracted to migrate into the subendothelial layer, where they become macrophages and take up lipid. These macrophages may secrete free oxygen radicals that further damage the endothelium; they also secrete growth factors that stimulate the migration and proliferation of smooth muscle cells. Damage to the intima may lead to exposure of platelets to the underlying connective tissue and foam cells, with consequent adherence, aggregation and thrombus formation. Mural thrombi may become incorporated into the plaque and contribute to progression of the atherosclerotic process.

Incidence and prevalence of ischaemic heart disease

The incidence of ischaemic heart disease varies greatly between countries and within them, but in all, the mortality from this cause rises rapidly with age. Few females, however, suffer from coronary disease under the age of 45; indeed under the age of 65, more than three times as many men die from coronary disease as do women. In the older age groups the incidence is approximately equal in the two sexes.

Myocardial infarction was seldom recorded as a cause of death until the 1920s, but subsequently the number of deaths attributed to it rose rapidly in Western countries, particularly after the Second World War. It peaked in the United States and Australia in the 1960s; subsequently the mortality in these countries has virtually halved (Fig 6.3). Mortality from the disease rose until the 1970s in the UK since when there has been a modest fall of about 20% for men and 15% for women. Within the UK, at least twice as many people die from coronary heart disease in parts of south-west Scotland as in south-east England. South Asians living in the UK have substantially higher rates than the UK population as a whole.

The reasons for the differences in incidence and the remarkably changing mortality rates are not well understood, but probably relate mainly to diet and smoking behaviour.

Risk factors for ischaemic heart disease and their control

Much remains to be learned about the causes of ischaemic heart disease, but epidemiological studies and clinical trials have provided valuable information about the risk factors associated with the development of coronary disease and the ways in which the risk of the disease can be reduced.

Lipid disorders. There is much circumstantial evidence to incriminate lipid abnormalities in the genesis of atheroma:

- deposition of lipid in the arterial wall occurs at an early, if not at

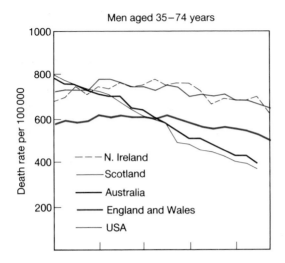

Men aged 35–74 years

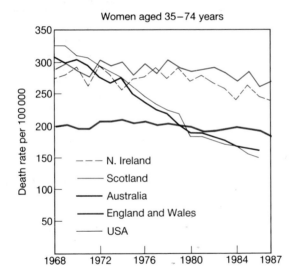

Women aged 35–74 years

Fig. 6.3 The changing mortalities in different countries. (With permission from Julian and Marley, *Coronary Heart Disease: The Facts*, Oxford: Oxford University Press, 1991.)

the initial, stage of the process;
- atheroma can be induced in animals by cholesterol feeding and other means of raising plasma cholesterol levels. However, the lesions differ from those in the human in not being associated with thrombosis;
- there is a high incidence of ischaemic (atherosclerotic) heart disease in individuals with elevated plasma lipid levels, particularly if they have familial hyperlipoproteinaemia;
- there is increasing epidemiological evidence that high levels of high density lipoproteins (HDL) are protective against ischaemic

heart disease in contrast to the adverse effects of high levels of low density lipoproteins.

Hyperlipoproteinaemias are subdivided into several types, based on whether cholesterol, triglycerides or chylomicrons are increased (see Table 6.1). Only types II and III are clearly associated with coronary atherosclerosis, although a relationship to type IV seems probable. Of particular interest from the genetic point of view is familial hypercholesterolaemia. Homozygotes, who have been found to have absent low density lipoprotein (LDL) receptors, develop coronary disease in childhood or adolescence. Heterozygotes have a reduced number of LDL receptors, and often develop coronary disease as young adults.

Table 6.1   Hyperlipoproteinaemias

Types	Chylomicrons	Cholesterol	Triglycerides	Clinical aspects
I	+++	↑	↑	Rare, Familial. Childhood hepatospleno-megaly. Xanthomata. No definite association with coronary disease
IIa	—	↑	—	Often familial. Tendinous and tuberous xanthomata
IIb	—	↑	↑	associated with early atherosclerosis
III	—	↑		Orange and yellow palmar creases. Xanthomata. Peripheral and coronary artery disease
IV	—	——	↑	Familial or dietary. Also oral contraceptives. Probable association with atherosclerosis
V	++	↑	↑	Rare. Abdominal pain. Pancreatitis. Not definitely associated with atherosclerosis

Certain other types of disorder which disturb lipid metabolism are associated with a high incidence of coronary disease. These include hypothyroidism and diabetes mellitus. Women who have had bilateral oophorectomy are liable to develop hypercholesterolaemia and premature coronary disease.

Even when these specific disease processes are excluded, there is a strong relationship between high levels of LDL and low levels of HDL and the risk of developing coronary disease at a relatively early age. Thus, in countries such as the United States and the UK, in which the average plasma cholesterol level of the community is relatively high, there is a much higher incidence of coronary artery disease than in those countries in which hypercholesterolaemia is rare. In long-term studies of whole populations, it has been shown that the higher the level of plasma cholesterol, the greater is the individual's risk of developing coronary artery disease. The cause of the high cholesterol levels is not yet fully established, although it seems likely that it is related in part to dietary factors. A high content of saturated fat (mainly of animal origin) in the diet is particularly suspect but a relative deficiency of polyunsaturated fats may also be important.

The *detection* of hyperlipidaemia depends upon blood sampling. Cholesterol estimations can be undertaken in the non-fasting state, but some other lipid measurements, such as triglyceride, require that the subject is fasting. Single measurements may be misleading both because of inaccuracy of the method and because of variability in the cholesterol level from time to time. Therefore, if a high level is suspected a repeat measurement should be obtained and, particularly if drug treatment is contemplated, a full lipid profile (to include high-density lipoproteins) obtained.

The significance of a particular cholesterol level depends upon many factors, such as age, gender and the presence of other risk factors such as cigarette smoking and hypertension. Thus a cholesterol level of 6.0 mmol/litre without other risk factors is associated with a very good prognosis, while a much lower figure would be associated with a higher risk of disease if the subject smoked and had a high blood pressure. Thus, the decision of how to treat an individual therefore does not depend on the lipid level alone. A figure of 7.8 mmol/litre has been suggested as a level where vigorous intervention is required, using drugs only if diet fails.

Blood lipids should be measured in anyone with known ischaemic heart disease, diabetes or hypertension requiring drug treatment, or with a family history of hyperlipidaemia of coronary disease at a relatively young age (e.g. under the age of 55). In other individuals, cholesterol testing is not of great value, and may cause unnecessary anxiety.

Treatment of hyperlipidaemia should start with dietary measures. Weight reduction alone substantially reduces hypertriglyceridaemia;

alcohol restriction reinforces this. For hypercholesterolaemia, total fat should be reduced to 25–30% of food energy, polyunsaturated fatty acids, especially linoleic acid, providing 7–10%.

Several types of drug are used to correct hyperlipidaemia:

- *bile-acid sequestrants* are anion-exchange resins, which are not absorbed. Cholestyramine 8–12 g twice daily is effective in hypercholesterolaemia, but is unpleasant to take, and may cause dyspepsia and constipation. A large trial with this drug showed a reduction in myocardial infarction but no effect on total mortality;
- *nicotinic acid* reduces triglycerides and, to a lesser extent, cholesterol. The most troublesome side-effect is flushing, which can be diminished by aspirin. Treatment should start with 100 mg three times daily, and rise slowly to 1–2 g three times daily;
- *fibrates* reduce triglycerides, and to a lesser extent, cholesterol. Trials with fibrates have shown a reduction in coronary events, including myocardial infarction and death, but not in overall death rate;
- *HMG CoA reductase inhibitors* ('Statins) block cholesterol synthesis in the liver by inhibiting the enzyme 3-hydroxy-3-methylglutaryl coenzyme A reductase. They reduce plasma cholesterol by 25% or more. At present their use is confined to patients with a cholesterol level in excess of 7.8 mmol/litre which is unresponsive to other therapy.

Dietary fat and ischaemic heart disease. Major differences in lipid levels in different communities can be largely accounted for by diet. The low-density lipoprotein (LDL) cholesterol level in the blood is determined chiefly by the intake of saturated fat, which is converted into cholesterol by the liver. There is relatively little cholesterol in the diet, so that the control of saturated fat is more important than limiting cholesterol intake. Polyunsaturates lower LDL cholesterol; monounsaturates also do so if they are substituted for saturates. The ratio of polyunsaturated fat to saturated fat in the diet is known as the P:S ratio; there are wide variations between P:S ratios in different countries, being high — about 1.0 — in Japan and about 0.37 in the UK. Most of the saturated fat is derived from dairy products and fatty meat; a substantial impact on the P:S ratio can be made by substituting skimmed or semi-skimmed milk for the full fat form, a polyunsaturated margarine for butter, olive or polyunsaturated oil for saturated oils, and lean meat, chicken or fish for fatty meat.

Hypertension. The higher the blood pressure, whether systolic or diastolic, the greater is the risk of developing ischaemic heart disease. Hypertension may contribute to its development in two ways: by accelerating the development of arterial disease and by increasing the work load of the left ventricle. Evidence from clinical trials suggests that antihypertensive agents lower coronary mortality only moderately — less than one might have anticipated. This may be because the trials have been short-lived, or because the agents used have had adverse effects that counteracted the benefit of lowering blood pressure (see Chapter 14 and p. 305).

Obesity is common in patients with ischaemic heart disease, but is often associated with other risk factors such as diabetes, hyperlipidaemia, and hypertension. It is probably an independent risk factor, particularly in women. A high waist-to-hip ratio (common in South Asian men) has been linked to coronary disease. Weight loss is to be encouraged as a way of diminishing risk.

Family history. Coronary artery disease often occurs in several members of the same family. While this may indicate a genetic factor, a shared environment (e.g. diet and smoking) may partially explain it. but it is likely that both genetic and environmental factors are involved. The inherited tendency is usually mediated through hyperlipidaemia (see p. 99) or hypertension. Although nothing can be done to correct the family history, it is important to recognize that those with familial disorders are very susceptible to environmental influences. The other risk factors should be attended to particularly diligently.

Cigarette smoking. Heavy consumption of cigarettes is associated with a high incidence of myocardial infarction and sudden death. The association is particularly striking in the younger age groups, but applies at all ages. Giving up smoking reduces the risk, but the full effect may take some years to achieve. The avoidance of smoking is perhaps the most important single preventive measure in Western countries.

Physical activity. Physical exercise appears to have a protective effect. Its mechanism is not clear, but it may increase high density lipoprotein, reduce blood clotting and, perhaps, encourage the enlargement of the coronary arteries and their anastomoses. Everyone who can do so should exercise regularly. Simple forms of physical activity such as brisk walking, cycling and swimming are adequate if performed for at least 20 min three times a week. The middle-aged, if unfit, should take up exercise gradually and should avoid the most vigorous competitive games such as squash.

Mental stress. It is widely believed that stress contributes to the development of coronary disease. This may well be so, but convincing evidence is not, as yet, available, perhaps because it is a very difficult area to study. There is no doubt, however, that stress can aggravate the symptoms of those with heart disease.

Diabetes. Ischaemic heart disease develops more frequently and at an earlier age in those with diabetes.

Insulin resistance. Many individuals with ischaemic heart disease who are not frankly diabetic are insulin resistant, i.e. they require a higher insulin level than others to maintain a normal blood glucose. Obesity and physical inactivity seem to be important factors in its occurrence.

Haemostatic factors. It has recently been shown that individuals with high levels of factor VII activity and fibrinogen have an enhanced risk of coronary events.

Alcohol and coffee. Alcohol in moderation (e.g. 1–2 glasses of wine a day) is associated with a reduced incidence of ischaemic heart disease, but heavier drinking leads to hypertension and an increased risk. The consumption of more than six cups of coffee has also been linked to a higher risk.

Public health approaches to prevention of ischaemic heart disease

Changes in lifestyle are clearly important in the prevention of coronary disease, and these to a large extent are the responsibility of the individual. However, health professionals and the Government also play an important role.

Two strategies have been suggested to prevent coronary disease — a 'high-risk' strategy, involving the identification and treatment of those at high risk, e.g. hyperlipidaemic individuals, or a 'population' strategy, aimed at reducing risk factors in the community at large. The two approaches are not incompatible and both should be pursued, because whilst the high-risk patients are those most likely to benefit, they are relatively few in number and constitute only a small proportion of those who develop coronary disease.

Those at high risk can be identified on the basis of a family history of hyperlipidaemia or of coronary disease at a young age, or by a combination of risk factors such as hypertension, smoking, and diabetes. Such individuals should have their lipids checked; they require skilled advice on the control of their risk factors. The population at large need advice about a healthy diet and not smoking, the need for exercise and for having their blood pressure taken at least every 5 years. Both doctors and the Government need to be involved in providing such information; national food and taxation policies can strongly influence behaviour.

Further reading

Fuster, F., Badimon, L., Badimon, J. J. & Chesebro, J. H. (1992) The pathogenesis of coronary artery disease and the acute coronary syndromes. *New England Journal of Medicine* **326**: 242 and 310.
Leaf, A. & Ryan, T.J. (1990) Prevention of coronary artery disease. *New England Journal of Medicine* **323**: 1416.

Coronary Heart Disease — Clinical Manifestations

7

ANGINA PECTORIS

Definition

Angina pectoris is a discomfort in the chest and adjacent areas due to a transient inadequate blood supply to the heart. As originally described by Heberden, it was only a symptom complex; there was no implied association with the heart. Today, the term is still used to describe a symptom, but its relationship to myocardial ischaemia is an essential component of the definition. As discussed on p. 91, there are many causes but coronary atherosclerosis is much the commonest. Almost invariably, at least one of the major coronary arteries has a reduction in luminal diameter of 70% or more; frequently two or three major arteries are involved. In most patients, there is a clear relationship to exercise, but the threshold for this may vary, presumably due to changes in coronary vasomotor tone.

Characteristics of angina pectoris

Anginal pain has four major characteristics:

- its location;
- its character;
- its relation to exercise;
- its duration.

The location of angina pectoris. Angina pectoris is most often felt behind the middle or upper third of the sternum. Even when the discomfort may be more obvious in another area, the sternal region is usually involved to some extent. Angina may also be felt in the lower sternal or xiphisternal region, over both sides of the chest, more commonly the left, in the neck and lower jaw and in both arms, again particularly the left. It may affect only the upper arm, but often reaches the elbow, the wrist or the fingers. In some patients the elbow region escapes and the patient is aware of discomfort in the upper arm and a tingling feeling in the fingers. Rarely, it may radiate through to the left scapular region. It is very unusual for the pain to be located predominantly under the left nipple and virtually never is it confined to this area.

The character of angina pectoris. Angina pectoris is most frequently likened to a pressing feeling, a tight band, or a heavy weight. Many patients deny actual pain and refer only to a sense of discomfort. It is not usually severe but can cause much anxiety and distress. It is not stabbing in quality, but the terms 'sharp' (meaning intense rather the knife-like) and 'burning' are sometimes used. The sensations in other areas are often different in character. In the neck, it is frequently described as 'choking'; in the lower jaw it may 'like toothache'. The feeling in the arms is usually one of numbness, heaviness or tingling.

The relationship of angina pectoris to exercise and other provoking factors. Angina pectoris is usually provoked by exertion, nearly always that of walking, particularly uphill. The amount of exercise required to produce angina varies from time to time in any individual, but it is more readily provoked after a heavy meal or in cold weather. Emotion is also an important provoking factor; it may be readily induced by anger and irritation. Angina often develops during sexual intercourse.

Some patients experience nocturnal angina, which wakes them up. In some cases this may be due to dreams, but it is probable that increased coronary artery tone, which is maximal in the early morning, is often responsible.

Angina pectoris may be provoked by several different types of tachycardia, particularly paroxysmal tachycardia associated with very rapid ventricular rates. Anaemia also contributes to its development, although it is unusual for it to do so in the absence of coronary atherosclerosis.

The duration of the attack. Most attacks last 1–3 min. Their duration is seldom less than 30 s or more than 15 min, although a vague sensation of discomfort may persist after the pain has stopped.

Other symptoms and signs in angina pectoris. Some patients complain of breathlessness accompanying the anginal pain. Other symptoms include flatulence, feelings of faintness, and acute anxiety. Tachycardia and a rise in blood pressure may be noted during an attack but there are usually no abnormal signs.

The electrocardiogram

In between attacks of angina pectoris, the ECG is usually normal. There may, however, be evidence of old myocardial infarction, or non-specific changes such as flattening or inversion of T waves, or signs of bundle branch block or left ventricular hypertrophy. If the patient is seen during an attack there are usually well-marked abnormalities which take the form of a horizontal or downward sloping depression of the ST segment (Fig. 7.1). Similar changes may be provoked by an exercise test (see below).

Diagnosis

By definition, angina is a symptom complex with a pathophysiological basis of myocardial ischaemia. The diagnosis must, therefore, depend on the history, combined with evidence of inadequate coronary blood flow.

There is usually no problem in determining the location of the pain and the factors that provoke it, but patients often find it difficult to find the words to describe the sensation they experience and estimates of the duration of the attack are often inaccurate. Most weight must therefore be placed on the first two elements. If the pain is located solely in the left sub-mammary region, or if it lasts for only a few seconds, it is almost certainly not ischaemic. Angina is seldom associated with tenderness of the chest wall, although it may occasionally be so. It is usually, but not always, relieved by glyceryl trinitrate. Angina pectoris is unlikely if walking is not a provoking factor, but some patients take so little exercise that the symptom arises only on emotion or at night.

Physical examination is of comparatively little value except for the exclusion of such causes as aortic stenosis and cardiomyopathy. However, because angina pectoris is often associated with hyperten-

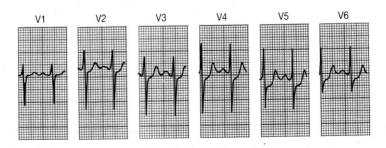

Fig. 7.1 ST depression during myocardial ischaemia. The chest leads are shown during an episode of angina. Extensive ST depression is evident, most marked in leads V5 and V6.

sion, with diabetes and with aortic valve disease, the characteristic findings of these conditions may be observed.

Evidence of myocardial ischaemia is provided by the presence of characteristic ST segment changes during an attack. As spontaneous attacks are seldom witnessed, it may be necessary to carry out an exercise test. The patient may be made to exercise on a bicycle ergometer or a treadmill, preferably until the chest discomfort is provoked. Standard and chest lead ECGs should be obtained during exercise and during the first 10 min of rest (see Fig. 2.20). A positive exercise test is one which shows a horizontal downward sloping ST depression of 1 mm or more. ST segments which slope upwards from the J point should not be regarded as evidence of ischaemia as they are often seen in normal individuals with tachycardia.

Unfortunately, even after careful history-taking and ECG examination, the diagnosis may remain uncertain. Radionuclide studies with thallium-201 may be helpful, but in some cases it is necessary to resort to coronary arteriography to establish the presence of coronary arterial disease (see Fig. 5.14). This potentially hazardous procedure is seldom justified for diagnostic purposes alone, but it is essential in patients being considered for coronary artery surgery or angioplasty. It involves the introduction of specially designed catheters into the brachial or femoral arteries. The left and right coronary arteries are entered and radio-opaque medium is injected. Cineangiographic records are obtained in various positions to ensure a good visualization of all the major vessels. Left ventriculography is also undertaken to assess myocardial function. Deaths from coronary angiography may result from coronary occlusion and dissection. Ventricular fibrillation may occur also, but is usually corrected without difficulty. The mortality of this investigation is about 0.1%.

Differential diagnosis

Although the diagnosis of angina can usually be established on the basis of the history and ECG, there are a number of other conditions which have to be considered in the differential diagnosis. Perhaps the most common difficulty arises with musculoskeletal pains in the chest wall. Frequently no cause is found for such pains which are often associated with tenderness and usually located on one side of the chest rather than centrally. These pains are most likely to be provoked by such actions as lifting and pulling, which produce tension of the muscles attached to the ribs. Amongst identifiable musculoskeletal conditions may be included Tietze's syndrome (in which there is an inflammation of one or more costochondral junctions), a slipping rib cartilage, fractured ribs, or metastatic lesions in ribs. In these conditions, unlike angina, there is tenderness and the symptoms may be aggravated by inspiration. The pain of cervical spondylosis is sometimes most severe in the upper chest region and accompanied by discomfort in the shoulders and arms.

Stabbing pains under the left breast and persistent aches in the same region are common and are most unlikely to be due to ischaemic heart disease. It is often not possible to establish their cause, but these symptoms are very common in those with anxiety neurosis.

Disorders of the gastrointestinal tract may be difficult to differentiate from angina pectoris. Oesophageal reflux, often associated with hiatus hernia, gives rise to a central chest pain, but this seldom radiates to the arms, is of a more burning or bursting character, and is more readily provoked by stooping or lying flat, although it may be produced by exercise. The pain of peptic ulcer is usually situated in the epigastric region, and is associated with tenderness. It is related to food rather than to exertion and is usually relieved by alkalis or milk and not be glyceryl trinitrate. Cholecystitis and cholelithiasis may give rise to pain in the lower sternal region, but there is usually tenderness either in the epigastrium or in the right subcostal area; there is frequently associated nausea, and the pain is not related to exertion. It is important to recognize that these gastrointestinal conditions, particularly hiatus hernia and cholecystitis, are common in patients with ischaemic heart disease, and the presence of one of these disorders does not preclude the coexistence of angina pectoris.

Prognosis

Most patients who develop angina pectoris live a normal or nearly normal life for many years. Symptoms are liable to vary from time to time, becoming worse in winter and improving the subsequent summer. They may disappear altogether for months or years.

It is difficult to give an accurate prognosis for any individual, but the outlook is relatively unfavourable if there is associated hypertension, advanced age, cardiac failure or preceding myocardial infarction. Coronary angiographic studies have shown that the prognosis is good if disease is confined to one artery. By contrast, severe narrowing of the left main coronary artery and diffuse lesions of all three arteries are associated with a high risk of early death.

Most patients live for 5 years and about one-third live for 10 years or more. The risk of sudden death or acute myocardial infarction is always present; before such events occur, there is frequently an exacerbation of the angina.

Treatment

The general management of angina pectoris is of great importance. The anxiety that the diagnosis arouses may cause incapacity, and it is important to emphasize the relatively good prognosis. Intense cold, walking into a wind or unnecessarily uphill should be avoided if they provoke the pain, as should taking large meals. Usually, the patient can continue his or her occupation, but should attempt to avoid unnecessary stresses, and learn how to relax. Physical exercise is to be encouraged provided it does not induce discomfort as it increases the threshold at which angina develops, but sudden strenuous effort should not be undertaken. Blood lipids should be estimated and high levels should be treated by diet, if possible, and by drugs if this proves ineffective. Obesity must be corrected. Cigarette smoking should be strongly discouraged.

Drug therapy

Nitrates. Nitrates have been in use in the management of angina for more than 100 years, but they remain first line treatment.

The major pharmacological effect of nitrates is the relaxation of smooth muscle, which seems to result from an increase in intracellular cyclic guanosine monophosphate (cGMP). Dilatation occurs in the coronary arteries, and in the peripheral arteries and veins. The former action leads directly to an increase in coronary blood flow, arterial dilatation leads to a fall in afterload, and a reduction in venous tone causes pooling, with a diminished venous return and preload. The relative importance of these different effects varies from one patient to another. Thus, the coronary vasodilator action is of particular value when an increase in coronary artery tone is an important component of angina, whereas it may have little influence in an artery with a fixed stenosis. In the latter situation, it is probably the venodilator action that is most relevant.

Most nitrates undergo extensive first pass metabolism in the liver; this may be overcome by administering large doses, but the effects are rather unpredictable. Alternatives are to use *isosorbide mononitrate* which does not undergo first pass metabolism, or to bypass the gut by sublingual, buccal, or transdermal administration.

Nitrates have relatively minor side-effects, but headache is very common. This tends to diminish with continued use, but some patients find it even more distressing than the angina. Nitrates (particularly glyceryl trinitrate) may cause hypotension and syncope; patients should be advised to take at least their first dose sitting down.

A problem with continuous nitrate therapy is the development of tolerance. This can be avoided by a regimen that ensures a period in the day with little or no nitrate in the blood.

Glyceryl trinitrate (nitroglycerin, trinitrin) is standard therapy in angina pectoris. It is given sublingually in a dose of 0.2–0.5 mg. It will stop an attack of angina in about 2 min, but is particularly effective if given prophylactically. Patients should, therefore, be encouraged to take a tablet when they anticipate an attack; they should also be advised that the drug is not addictive, as many fear that they will become drug dependent.

Long-acting oral nitrates are effective if given in sufficient dosage, but headache is a common problem, and the regimen should ensure a nitrate-free period. The same considerations apply to transdermal patches.

Intravenous nitrates are of considerable value in unstable angina and in cardiac failure. Nitrates should be diluted before use. Glass bottles are preferable; with nitroglycerin, intravenous tubing that minimally absorbs the drug is necessary. Nitroglycerin should be given initially in a dosage of 5 µg per minute; the dose may be increased each 5 min by 5 µg, and later, 10 µg per minute, as necessary, with very careful observation of the blood pressure. Isosorbide dinitrate therapy may be started at 20 µg a minute, and increased by steps of 20 µg.

Beta-adrenoceptor blocking drugs. These are now given routinely to all but the mildest case, unless there are contraindications to their use. They block the action of catecholamines in increasing heart rate, blood pressure and cardiac contractility and thereby limit the myocardial oxygen needs on exercise or psychological stress. Unfortunately, they can exacerbate cardiac failure and may cause bronchospasm in those with obstructive airways disease. When given to patients free of heart failure or a history of asthma or bronchitis, beta-blocking drugs seldom give rise to serious side-effects but minor ones are quite common. These include fatigue, unpleasant dreams and nausea.

In general, the choice of a particular beta-blocker is not of importance, but it is preferable to use a cardioselective drug for patients with suspected obstructive airways disease or insulin-dependent diabetes. Compliance is more likely to be achieved if one uses a preparation which need be given only once or twice a day, such as atenolol, sotalol or nadolol or the long-acting formulations of propranolol and metoprolol. A lower dosage of a beta-blocker may be effective when it is combined with a longacting nitrate or calcium antagonist.

Calcium antagonists. Calcium has an essential role in both the electrical and mechanical functions of the heart. It is also involved in the contraction of coronary and peripheral arteries. As described on p. 9, the entry of calcium ions into the cell is an important component in the generation of the action potential, being partially responsible for depolarization and for the plateau phase. The slow calcium current is largely responsible for depolarization of the atrioventricular node. Calcium in the cell binds to troponin, which leads to actin–myosin crossbridge formation (p. 1). In the resting phase, calcium is bound to a number of structures within the cell including the nucleus, mitochondria, sarcolemma, the T system and the sarcoplasmic reticulum. The small quantity of calcium that enters the cell during depolarization is not sufficient by itself to initiate contraction but appears to stimulate the release of the ion from the sarcoplasmic reticulum and this in turn binds to troponin and stimulates the actin–myosin contraction. The process is reversed during relaxation. The rate of development of tension in the myocardium and the total tension developed depends on the rate at which calcium becomes available and the amount which becomes available, respectively.

The five main calcium antagonists currently available are verapamil, diltiazem, nicardipine, nifedipine and amlodipine (see Appendix, p. 381). Verapamil and diltiazem have potent electrophysiological effects, depressing the action potential in the atrioventricular node specifically. They may lead to bradycardia. They are used for the treatment of supraventricular tachycardias involving the atrioventricular node. Their value in angina pectoris is probably due to a combination of peripheral and coronary vasodilatation and a reduction of the tachycardia which occurs on exertion. A dosage of 120 mg verapamil three times daily is usually required to control angina; the commonest side-effect is constipation. Diltiazem is relatively free from side-effects; the customary dosage is 60 mg three times daily. Nifedipine has little effect on the atrioventricular node; it exerts its main pharmacological effect on the peripheral and coronary arteries. The peripheral vasodilatation it induces leads to a reflex tachycardia and may also lead to hypotension. Although effective in exercise-induced angina, it may aggravate it because of tachycardia. It has been found particularly helpful in the management of coronary artery spasm but when used in exercise-induced angina is better combined with a beta-blocking drug. It is also being used in the management of hypertension in association with other antihypertensive drugs. The usual dosage is 10–20 mg thrice daily. Many patients suffer from side-effects with nifedipine but they are seldom serious. Some 20–30% have peripheral oedema as a result of vasodilatation. Others complain of headaches, gastrointestinal disturbances, flushing, dizziness and syncope. Nicardipine is similar to nifedipine. The dosage is 5–30 mg three times a day.

Calcium antagonists can worsen cardiac performance in those with poor left ventricular function, and generally should be avoided in patients with cardiac failure.

Coronary artery bypass surgery.   The narrowed segments of coronary arteries can be bypassed by using a saphenous vein or internal mammary (thoracic) artery. In the former case, one end of the vein is attached to the ascending aorta and the other to the affected artery beyond the most distal obstruction as demonstrated by coronary arteriography (Fig. 7.2). If an arterial graft is used, the proximal end of the vessel is not detached, but the distal end is sectioned and inserted into the coronary artery.

Grafts may, if necessary, be inserted into all the three major arteries, and into their larger branches. Provided left ventricular function is not severely impaired, the mortality of the operation is less

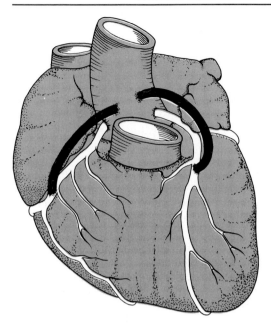

Fig. 7.2 Two saphenous vein bypass grafts, from the aorta to the anterior descending and right coronary arteries, respectively. (With permission from Julian and Marley, *Coronary Heart Disease: The Facts*, Oxford: Oxford University Press, 1991.)

than 2% in most centres. A small proportion of vein grafts close shortly after insertion, but most stay open for at least 5 years; following this, there is an increasing tendency to closure, particularly in patients with hyperlipidaemia. It has been found that antiplatelet therapy (e.g. aspirin 300mg daily) is helpful in maintaining patency, and a lipid-lowering regimen should be given to those with hyperlipidaemia.

The results of surgery are usually very satisfactory, at least for 5–10 years. Angina is abolished in at least 50% of cases, and greatly improved in a further 30–40%. As well as relieving angina, coronary artery surgery benefits the prognosis of patients with disease of the left main coronary artery, and also those who have disease of the three major vessels, together with left ventricular dysfunction, provided this is not too severe. Late deterioration may be due to graft closure, or to progression of the disease in the ungrafted vessels.

Surgery is indicated for those whose angina is not adequately relieved by full medical treatment, but it should also be considered as a measure to improve prognosis, even in the absence of severe symptoms, in the younger patient with advanced coronary disease.

Percutaneous transluminal coronary angioplasty (PTCA). A nonelastic balloon mounted close to the tip of a specially designed catheter can be passed to the site of a coronary stenosis and inflated there (Fig. 7.3). This process produces clefts in the atheromatous lesion, compression and redistribution of its contents, endothelial

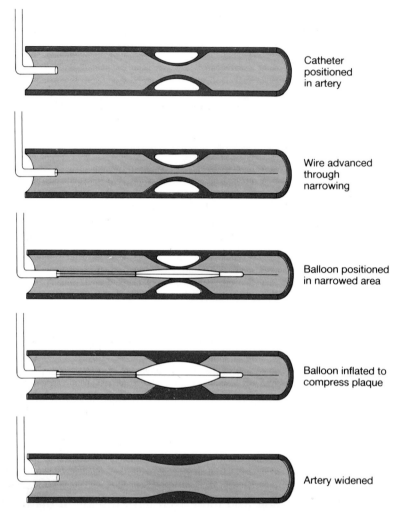

Catheter
positioned
in artery

Wire advanced
through
narrowing

Balloon positioned
in narrowed area

Balloon inflated to
compress plaque

Artery widened

Fig. 7.3 Percutaneous transluminal coronary angioplasty. (With permission from Julian and Marley, *Coronary Heart Disease: The Facts*, Oxford: Oxford University Press, 1991.)

desquamation, and stretching of the media. In most cases, this results in a substantial increase in the arterial lumen. Initially, angioplasty was used for proximal lesions occurring in patients with disease of only one coronary artery. With greater experience and with improved apparatus, experts in the technique can now successfully dilate lesions in several arteries, even if these are relatively distal. Angioplasty should not be attempted if the left main coronary artery is involved, and it is not likely to be successful if the lesion is long or if the vessel is occluded (although recently occluded vessels may sometimes be reopened). Some 80–90% of apparently suitable stenoses can be dilated; dilatation usually succeeds in relieving symptoms. However, the procedure may be complicated by acute coronary occlusion due to dissection, spasm or thrombosis, which may require emergency coronary bypass surgery. Angioplasty has a mortality of about 1% and a risk of myocardial infarction of approximately 3%. Restenosis occurs within 6 months in about 25% of cases, but this may not result in the recurrence of symptoms. If it does, repeat angioplasty is often successful.

The main indication for the procedure is angina unresponsive to medical treatment, whether this is stable or unstable.

Angioplasty is carried out under local anaesthesia. Patients can usually be mobilized the following day and be discharged 1 or 2 days thereafter. Because of the risks of thrombosis and coronary artery spasm after angioplasty, patients are often kept on calcium antagonists and antiplatelet agents (such as aspirin) for weeks or months after the procedure.

Unstable angina

Angina is regarded as being unstable if it has developed for the first time recently, or if pre-existing angina has worsened for no apparent reason. Several mechanisms may be involved, which include rupture of an atheromatous plaque, with or without superimposed thrombosis, and coronary spasm. The clinical picture is very variable, ranging from relatively mild attacks of pain on exertion to recurrent attacks of severe pain at rest which are unresponsive to full medical treatment. During the episodes of pain, there are usually transient ECG changes, such as ST depression or elevation, or T wave abnormalities. The chief concern in unstable angina is the substantial risk of progression to myocardial infarction in the ensuing days or weeks. This outcome affects 10–20% of the patients, but particularly those who do not respond promptly to medical treatment.

It is difficult to be sure of the mechanisms involved in any particular case, and it is probably best to combine beta-blockers and calcium antagonists, if neither are contraindicated. Nitrates should be taken orally as necessary, and if other forms of drug therapy have failed, the addition of intravenous nitrates is often effective (see p. 110). Heparin has been found to reduce the risk of a myocardial infarction, as has aspirin. The latter should be given in a dosage of 150–300 mg a day, and continued indefinitely.

If a prompt response to rest and medical treatment is not achieved, it is best to proceed without delay to coronary arteriography, and then to angioplasty or coronary artery bypass surgery if these seem indicated.

MYOCARDIAL INFARCTION

Definition

Myocardial infarction is the term applied to myocardial necrosis secondary to an acute interruption of the coronary blood supply. Its pathology is described in Chapter 6 (p. 94).

Clinical features

The common presenting symptom of myocardial infarction is severe chest pain. This is predominantly in the sternal region, but may radiate to both sides of the chest, to the jaw, to the shoulders and to one or both arms. It is usually described as tight, pressing, heavy or constricting. Sometimes the patient may deny 'pain' and describe a discomfort, not amounting to pain, in the centre of the chest. Although it can be brief, the pain usually lasts for more than half an hour and may continue for several hours. Unlike the pain of angina, it is seldom associated with exertion and it is not relieved by rest or glyceryl trinitrate. The pain may be maximal at the onset, but often increases in intensity for a period of minutes or hours and then remains constant until it gradually recedes. Frequently, the patient gives a history of the recent onset of angina or the exacerbation of pre-existing angina in the preceding days or weeks.

The pain may be overshadowed by other symptoms, such as breathlessness or syncope. Occasionally, it is obscured because the infarction develops during anaesthesia or at the time of a cerebrovascular accident. Rarely, infarction may be truly pain-free.

Once the pain has been controlled, the patient may remain free of symptoms and make an uninterrupted recovery. However, complications develop in a substantial proportion of cases. The most important of these are:

- arrhythmias;
- cardiogenic shock;
- left ventricular failure.

These complications, which will be considered in detail later, are the common causes of death and are responsible for many of the abnormal physical signs which may be observed.

Physical signs

During the earliest stages of the attack, patients are obviously distressed, and may be sweaty and cold. The general appearance improves when the pain is controlled and often, within a few hours, they look well.

The pulse may be normal in volume and rate, but in severe attacks it is small and fast. Arrhythmias or bradycardia are also common.

The blood pressure usually falls progressively over a period of hours and days, reaching its minimum some time during the first week, and returning towards normal slowly over the next 2–3 weeks. There may be, however, a sharp fall in blood pressure at the onset of the infarction, which may progress to the severe hypotension of cardiogenic shock, or may resolve. Transient hypertension, perhaps resulting from intense pain, is sometimes observed.

The jugular venous pressure is usually normal or slightly elevated early in the course of acute myocardial infarction; it is seldom markedly elevated due to right-sided heart failure.

The apex beat, which is often difficult to feel, may be displaced outwards. Between the apex and the left sternal edge a systolic pulsation may be detectable, due to a protrusion of the infarcted anterior wall of the heart.

The first and second heart sounds are often soft. A fourth (or atrial) sound can be heard in most cases; a third heart sound is common when there is heart failure or shock.

A soft pansystolic murmur at the apex is not uncommon and is caused by mitral regurgitation either as a result of papillary muscle malfunction or secondary to dilatation of the left ventricle. Rarely, a loud systolic murmur may develop at the left sternal edge, due to a rupture of the ventricular septum, or at the apex, due to rupture of a papillary muscle. A transient pericardial rub occurs in perhaps 20% of patients, usually on the second or third day.

Pulmonary crepitations are common but of little importance unless they are widespread and numerous because of pulmonary oedema.

Most of the abnormal physical signs described disappear within a few days of the onset of infarction, except in the most severely affected patients.

A fever, seldom exceeding 38°C (101°F), usually commences within the first 24 h and subsides in under a week. There is often a slight leucocytosis and an increase in the erythrocyte sedimentation rate. The pyrexia, leucocytosis and raised ESR represent a reaction to myocardial necrosis.

Early complications

Disturbances of rate, rhythm and conduction.   These occur in 95% of patients with acute myocardial infarction. In about half of these, they are severe enough to be of clinical importance.

Sinus tachycardia is common and is an index of severity. Sinus bradycardia frequently occurs at the onset of infarction, being sometimes part of the vasovagal syndrome. It is particularly associated

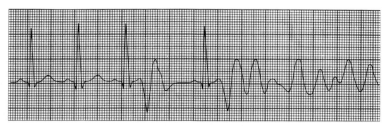

Fig. 7.4 Ventricular ectopic beats interrupting the T wave of preceding beats (R-on-T phenomenon). The second such beat initiates ventricular fibrillation.

with inferior myocardial infarction, but may be provoked by morphine and digitalis. It is usually benign, but can cause hypotension or encourage the development of ectopic rhythms.

The atrial tachycardias, including atrial fibrillation, which occur in about 15% of patients, may precipitate cardiac failure or shock. Atrial fibrillation is usually transient and seldom lasts for more than a few days.

Ventricular ectopic beats are almost invariable; they are usually of no consequence, but those of the R-on-T variety (Fig. 7.4) may be precursors of ventricular fibrillation.

Ventricular tachycardia is dangerous both because it can cause shock and cardiac failure and because it may progress to ventricular fibrillation.

Ventricular fibrillation is the most important single cause of death in acute myocardial infarction and occurs in 8–10% of hospitalized patients. In about half of these cases, there has been no preceding shock or cardiac failure and the ventricular fibrillation is 'primary'. In the remainder, it can be regarded as being secondary to these complications.

Heart block occurs in about 5% of patients with acute myocardial infarction. It is particularly common when the inferior surface of the heart is affected because the right coronary artery supplies both this aspect of the myocardium and the junctional tissues. First degree block (prolonged PR interval) is of little significance except as a precursor of more advanced block. Second degree block, usually of the Wenckebach type, is potentially dangerous because bradycardia may be poorly tolerated and because of the risk of progression to complete heart block and ventricular asystole. In spite of the risk, most patients tolerate these conduction defects well but need to be observed closely for the development of hypotension, cardiac failure or asystole. Normal AV conduction is almost always restored if the patient survives the acute attack..

When heart block complicates anterior infarction, it carries a very high mortality. The block results from damage to both bundle branches and is almost invariably accompanied by widespread myocardial damage. The patients usually have cardiac failure and have a bad prognosis even if their heart block is successfully treated.

Cardiogenic shock. As mentioned, the patient at the onset of infarction is often pale, distressed and hypotensive. This situation, which is often transient, may be attributed to pain and should not be described as cardiogenic shock. This term should be restricted to those patients who have the clinical picture of hypotension, with cold cyanosed extremities, sweating, and mental torpor, which lasts at least half an hour, or who deteriorate rapidly until the blood pressure can no longer be recorded. There is a low cardiac output and a peripheral resistance insufficient to compensate for this, together with oliguria, hypoxia, and acidosis. Arrhythmias and cardiac failure are frequently associated and the mortality is 80–90% irrespective of treatment. Shock is largely the result of severe myocardial damage with more than 40% of the ventricular wall being infarcted. Occasionally, the shock picture is accounted for by arrhythmias such as ventricular tachycardia or complete heart block, in which case correction of the arrhythmia may result in recovery. In a few patients, particularly those who have been receiving diuretics, hypovolaemia may be a factor. In others, it is the consequence of right ventricular infarction. Rarely, a surgically correctable disorder, such as a ruptured papillary muscle or a ventricular septal defect may be responsible.

Left ventricular failure. This is seldom present at the onset, but develops within 48 h in perhaps two-thirds of patients with acute myocardial infarction. It can be suspected from tachycardia, a third heart sound, widespread pulmonary crepitations and pulmonary venous congestion or oedema on the chest radiograph. Catheterization using a Swan–Ganz or similar catheter, will show a pulmonary wedge pressure in excess of 20 mmHg.

Right ventricular failure. A slight elevation of the jugular venous pressure is common in the first days after acute infarction. Infarction of the right ventricle, which is almost always associated with inferior wall infarction, may cause a high venous pressure and, rarely, the shock syndrome, even in the presence of good left ventricular function. The classical features of failure of the right side of heart — peripheral oedema and hepatomegaly — are rare and usually take several days to develop even in the patient with severe myocardial damage.

Pulmonary embolism and infarction. Twenty or more years ago, pulmonary embolism caused death in about 3% of all patients admitted to hospital with acute myocardial infarction. It has become relatively rare, presumably because patients are now mobilized much earlier than they were. It is usually preceded by deep vein thrombosis in the legs, but this may not be clinically evident. Pulmonary embolism should be suspected if hypotension or right heart failure develop some days after the onset of myocardial infarction, and also when there is a pleural type of chest pain with or without haemoptysis.

Systemic arterial embolism. Embolism may occur from mural thrombi situated in the left ventricle or left atrium. Hemiplegia is the most common result, but there may be occlusion of any artery.

Cerebrovascular accidents. Cerebrovascular accidents may precede, accompany or follow acute myocardial infarction. As mentioned, cerebral embolism is one cause, but cerebral infarction may develop, as may cerebral haemorrhage, particularly when thrombolytic drugs are used.

Cardiac rupture. Rupture through the wall of the left ventricle is responsible for about 10% of all deaths and particularly affects the elderly and the hypertensive. It is most likely to occur during the first few days and usually causes the clinical picture of cardiac arrest, but the electrocardiogram shows continuing electrical activity (so-called 'electromechanical dissociation'). Occasionally, the picture may be that of cardiac tamponade.

Rupture through the interventricular septum occurs in about one in every 200 patients with acute myocardial infarction. This produces the sudden onset of severe heart failure, accompanied by a systolic thrill and murmur at the left sternal edge. The patient deteriorates rapidly over a period of a few days; survival for more than a few weeks is unusual.

Papillary muscle rupture and malfunction. When a papillary muscle ruptures, a loud apical pansystolic murmur appears in association with the sudden development of left ventricular failure. Death usually occurs within a few hours or days. Partial rupture may produce the features of mitral regurgitation with or without left-sided heart failure.

The electrocardiogram

The ECG is virtually always transiently or permanently abnormal after acute myocardial infarction. Because the ECG diagnosis of infarction depends upon the observation of a sequence of changes with time, serial records are vital.

The characteristic abnormalities (Fig. 7.5) are:

- pathological Q waves;
- ST segment elevation;
- T wave inversion.

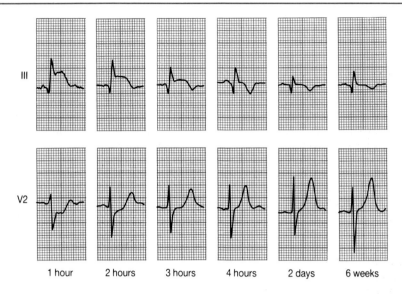

III

V2

1 hour   2 hours   3 hours   4 hours   2 days   6 weeks

Fig. 7.5   Progression of ECG changes in myocardial infarction. The progression of ECG changes during and after an inferior infarct is shown. Lead III (upper series) faces the area of infarction. V2 (lower series) demonstrates reciprocal changes. The time of each ECG from onset of symptoms is shown. The patient received thrombolytic therapy on initial presentation at 1 hour. In lead III, early ST elevation rapidly resolves, to be succeeded by a biphasic T wave and subsequently by T wave inversion. A Q wave develops over several hours. In the remote lead, V2, there is initial ST depression. This resolves with the disappearance of ST elevation in lead III.

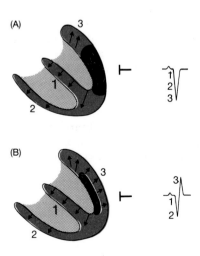

Fig. 7.6   (A) The appearances recorded from an electrode over the left ventricle in extensive left ventricular infarction. The initial vector is directed, as usual, away from the left ventricle due to depolarization of the septum, and is followed by that of depolarization of the right ventricle and non-infarcted areas of the left ventricle in a direction away from the infarction. A totally negative deflection (QS) is obtained. (B) The appearances obtained from an electrode placed over the left ventricle when the infarction is less extensive. The initial vector is, as usual, directed from left to right across the septum, and provides the first component of the Q wave. Subsequently, the right ventricle and the non-infarcted areas of the endocardium of the left ventricle are depolarized, continuing the Q wave. Finally, depolarization reaches the epicardium superficial to the infarcted area, producing a terminal R wave.

Although the precise mechanisms responsible for these ECG changes are not yet determined, it is probable that the Q wave changes are the result of muscle death, that the ST abnormalities are due to muscle injury, and that the T wave abnormalities are due to ischaemia.

Dead tissue, which is unpolarized, takes no part in electrical activation, but can transmit changes in the electrical potential in other tissues. In Fig. 7.6 can be seen the effect of infarcted tissue on depolarization of the heart. With the electrode situated facing the left ventricle, depolarization commences, as usual, from the left side of the septum to the right (vector 1). Subsequently depolarization spreads to affect the right ventricle and those parts of the left ventricle away from the infarct. Vector 2 is therefore directed away from the electrode and produces a deepening of the Q wave. Finally, the muscle around the area of the infarct may become activated and produce a terminal R wave (vector 3). Sometimes, Q wave infarctions are described as 'transmural'; this is an undesirable term, as they do not necessarily involve the full thickness of the myocardium.

In the injured zone, the cells remain polarized, but the transmembrane potential is less than normal, because of loss of cellular potassium. Repolarization of the injured tissue occurs more quickly than normal and a voltage gradient develops between the normal and injured tissue. This is reflected in ST elevation over the area of injury.

The T wave abnormalities are believed to be due to changes in the direction of repolarization in ischaemic tissue.

Q waves. Q waves may take several hours to develop after the onset of infarction. They usually persist indefinitely because the scar tissue which replaces the infarcted muscle is similarly uninvolved in electrical activation. Normally, Q waves in leads facing the left ventricle do not exceed 2 mm in depth or 0.03 s in width. Q waves and QS waves are normal in aVR, and are commonly found in V1 and V2. Deep Q waves are often also seen normally in lead III. The Q wave in lead III should only be considered definitely abnormal if it exceeds 0.03 sec in duration, and if it is accompanied by Q waves in either lead II or aVF. The 'normal' Q wave in lead III usually diminishes or disappears on deep inspiration, whereas the 'pathological' Q wave persists.

ST elevation. ST segment elevation often commences within minutes of the onset of myocardial infarction but may be delayed for many hours. In the earliest stage, the elevated ST segment may retain the normal upward concavity, but before long it becomes convex and 'coves' downwards to the T wave. ST elevation is confined to those leads facing the infarct. In leads distant from the infarct, so-called 'reciprocal' ST depression is often seen (Fig. 7.5). The ST segment usually returns to the iso-electric line within 48–72 h. Persistent elevation suggests a ventricular aneurysm.

T wave inversion. T wave inversion occurs slightly later than ST

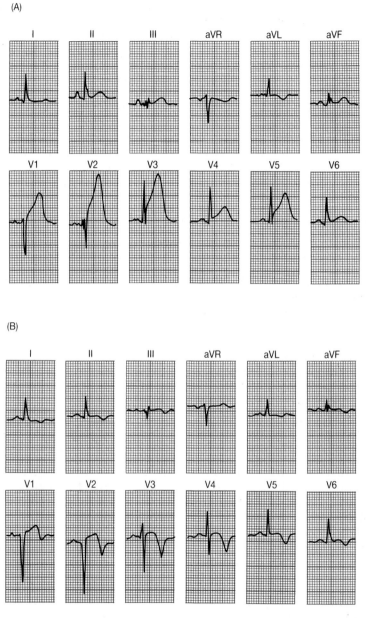

Fig. 7.7 Anteroseptal myocardial infarction. (A) 12-lead ECG recorded within one hour of onset of symptoms. Hyperacute changes are evident with marked ST elevation across the anterior chest lead. Tall peaked T waves are present in lead V2 and V3. (B) 12 hours later the acute ST changes have largely resolved, and have been succeeded by T wave inversion. A deep Q wave is present in lead V2.

elevation during the course of myocardial infarction; there is a stage when this ST segment is returning towards the iso-electric line whilst the T wave is becoming inverted. Later, the ST segment becomes isoelectric and the T wave becomes symmetrically, often deeply, inverted. As healing takes place, the T wave usually becomes less inverted and eventually upright and normal, but the inversion sometimes persists.

Q waves are often absent in small myocardial infarctions, but ST and T wave changes are almost invariable. The recognition of myocardial infarction on the ECG can be difficult if there has been previous infarction which has resulted in persistent Q waves, ST elevation or T wave inversion.

Left bundle branch block may also obscure the changes of infarction, because in this disorder the septum is depolarized from right to left; this produces an initial R wave in left ventricular leads, preventing the appearance of a Q wave. The diagnosis can sometimes be made from ST and T wave changes.

The leads in which the infarct patterns are seen depend upon its location:

- *Anteroseptal* infarction produces changes in one or more of the leads V1 to V4 (Fig 7.7).
- *Anterolateral* infarction produces changes from V4 to V6, and lead I and aVL.
- *Anterior* infarction is indicated by more widespread changes including most of the leads from V1 to V6, as well as leads I and II and aVL.

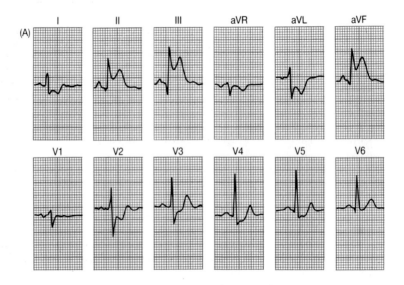

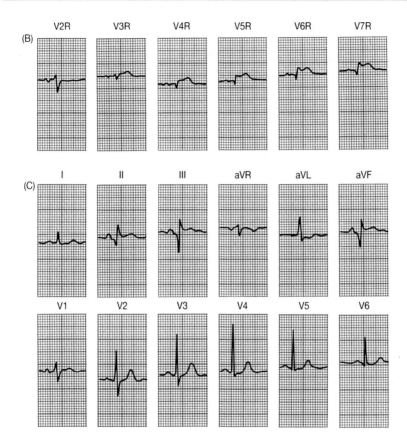

Fig. 7.8 Inferior myocardial infarction. (A) Conventional 12-lead ECG recorded one hour after the onset of symptoms showing ST elevation in leads II, III and aVF. There is reciprocal ST depression across the anterior chest leads, extending into leads I and aVL. (B) Right-sided chest leads recorded simultaneously. ST-elevation is apparent in leads V3R to V7R, indicating right ventricular infarction. (C) Conventional 12-lead ECG recorded 12 hours later. The acute ST segment changes have largely resolved. There are now deep Q waves in leads II, III and aVF.

- Inferior (or diaphragmatic) infarction is registered by changes in leads II, III and aVF (Fig. 7.8).
- Strictly posterior myocardial infarction does not produce Q waves in the standard 12 leads. However, the loss of electrical activity from the posterior part of the left ventricle, leads to a tall R in V1, because the forces depolarizing the right ventricle are unopposed (Fig. 7.9).
- Right ventricular infarction (which is almost always associated with inferior infarction) produces transient ST elevation in V4R (Fig. 7.8B).

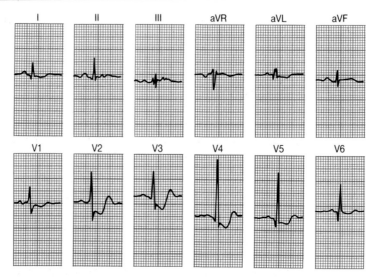

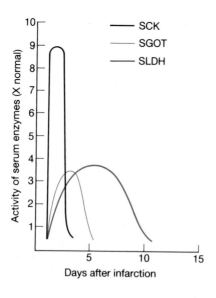

Fig. 7.9 Posterior myocardial infarction. Tall R waves are present in leads V1 and V2 accompanied by deep ST depression. These are reciprocal changes arising from a posterior infarction.

Fig. 7.10 Changes in serum enzyme activity following myocardial infarction. Serum creatine phosphokinase (SCK) increases earlier and to a relatively greater extent than SGOT and SLDH (see text).

Further leads may be required for infarcts in unusual sites, V7 and V8 being helpful in lateral infarcts, and leads in the second or third intercostal spaces for high anterior and lateral infarcts.

Serum enzymes (Fig. 7.10)

Certain enzymes, present in high concentration in cardiac tissue, are released by necrosis of the myocardium. Their activity in the serum, therefore, rises and falls after myocardial infarction. The amount of enzyme released roughly parallels the severity of myocardial damage.

Serum creatine phosphokinase (SCK). Creatine phosphokinase, which occurs in heart, skeletal muscle and brain, rises within 6 h of the onset of infarction, reaching a peak in 18–24 h. It may become normal after 72 h. Apart from myocardial infarction, abnormally high levels occur in muscle diseases, in cerebrovascular damage, after muscular exercise and with intramuscular injections.

The MB isoenzyme of CK is virtually specific for cardiac muscle and is now widely used in the diagnosis of myocardial infarction.

Serum glutamic oxalo-acetic transaminase (SGOT). This enzyme, also called aspartate transaminase (ASAT), is found particularly in the heart, skeletal muscle, brain, liver and kidney. After infarction, the SGOT rises in about 12 h and reaches its peak in 24–36 h, returning to normal from the third to the fifth day.

Serum lactate dehydrogenase (SLDH). This enzyme is found in the heart, but also in red cells. It rises relatively late after infarction, reach its peak 24–48 h afterwards, and may remain abnormal from 1 to 3 weeks. Unfortunately, even slight haemolysis raises its level. Isoenzymes are more specific.

Diagnostic levels for these enzymes have not been quoted as they vary considerably from one laboratory to another.

Radionuclide and echocardiographic investigations

Perfusion defects can be demonstrated using thallium-201 in most patients within the first few hours, but may disappear later. Technetium pyrophosphate concentrates in the infarcted area producing a 'hot spot', several hours after the onset; this is not, however, a very specific or sensitive test.

Echocardiography shows loss of the normal systolic thinning of the ventricular wall in the region of the infarction.

Diagnosis

In most cases, the diagnosis is suspected from the character, location and duration of the chest pain. The persistence of the pain beyond 15 min, its lack of relationship to exercise and the failure of glyceryl trinitrate to relieve it usually serve to differentiate it from angina pectoris. The development of abnormal physical signs, and more particularly, the appearance of arrhythmias, shock and failure also suggest that infarction has occurred. Fever, leucocytosis and raised ESR indicate necrosis rather than ischaemia. The definitive diagnosis depends upon the recognition of the ECG changes, supported by abnormal serum enzyme levels. Infarction is virtually certain if Q waves appear during the course of the illness, or if sequential ST and T wave changes are accompanied by transient but significant elevations of serum enzyme levels. Difficulties in diagnosis arise when the ECG or enzyme level changes are equivocal, or if serial ECG records or enzyme estimations are not made at appropriate times.

It is exceedingly difficult to differentiate some cases of acute myocardial infarction from unstable angina. This syndrome is characterized by attacks of ischaemic pain which are more prolonged and less related to exertion than are those of typical effort-induced angina pectoris, but there is no necrosis, nor are there the enzyme abnormalities of myocardial infarction. There may be ST elevation or depression but Q waves are not a feature.

The differentiation of myocardial infarction from massive pulmonary embolism may be difficult, but the chest pain of myocardial infarction is usually more severe and the breathlessness less marked. In pulmonary embolism, the ECG may be normal, or there may be characteristic abnormalities (see p. 320) and although there may be changes in SLDH and SGOT, SCK (and, more specifically MB–CK) is usually not raised. In cases of doubt, pulmonary angiography or radio-isotope scanning of the chest are helpful. Pulmonary infarction can be recognized by the location and pleural character of the pain and the radiographic appearances.

Acute pericarditis may produce symptoms and signs similar to those of an acute myocardial infarction (see p. 207). In many cases, the pericarditis is preceded by an upper respiratory infection and cough. The chest pain is more aching or stabbing in character, and is made worse by deep inspiration, movement or lying flat. Pyrexia often precedes the pain, whereas the temperature rise of myocardial infarction usually takes at least 12 h to develop. Although pericarditis may produce ST elevation and T wave inversion, the ST elevation is concave upwards (see Fig. 10.1) and is widespread rather than focal. Abnormal Q waves do not occur and enzyme changes occur only if there is accompanying myocarditis.

Dissecting aneurysm can cause severe central chest pain similar to that of acute myocardial infarction (see p. 312). The pain usually has a tearing quality, and tends to move into the upper dorsal spinal region and into the abdomen. The ECG does not show the changes of myocardial infarction, except when the dissection involves the origin of a coronary artery. In cases of doubt, the arterial pulses should be repeatedly checked, and a chest radiograph obtained to determine whether there is mediastinal widening. Echocardiography, computed tomography, and magnetic resonance imaging are of diagnostic value.

Prognosis

In about one-quarter of all episodes of acute myocardial infarction, death occurs suddenly within minutes of the onset. Such cases are seldom seen by a physician. The remainder of this discussion is concerned with the prognosis of those who survive this immediate period.

The overall natural mortality, excluding the very early deaths, is approximately 15–30%, but this has been greatly reduced by treatment so that the in-hospital mortality now averages about 10%. The risk of death depends upon many factors, including the age of the patient, previous myocardial infarction and the presence of other diseases, as well as the extent of the infarction.

The mortality of the acute attack rises sharply with age. Today the death rate is probably less than 5% in those under 50 years of age,but may rise to 20–30% in the elderly. Mortality is higher in women than in men, but this is largely accounted for by the fact that infarction occurs relatively uncommonly in the younger female. The mortality is greater in recurrent compared with first infarction, particularly when there has been preceding cardiac failure.

The risk of dying is highest in the first few hours and decreases rapidly thereafter. Some 60% or more of all deaths within 4 weeks occur within the first 2 days. During this time, prognostication is difficult because dangerous arrhythmias may develop unpredictably. At the end of 48 h, the assessment of the prognosis for the rest of the 4-week period is reasonably accurate if the blood pressure, the signs of cardiac failure and the occurrence of serious arrhythmias are taken into account. Cardiogenic shock carries a mortality of 80–90%. Persistent tachycardia, continuing gallop rhythm and the development of right-sided heart failure are unfavourable features. Ventricular tachycardia, bundle branch block and atrial fibrillation are associated with a high mortality. Death may occur unexpectedly, late in the course of acute myocardial infarction, from further myocardial infarction, rupture and pulmonary embolism.

The ECG provides little information of prognostic value, except that, in general, patients with Q waves do worse than those without. High serum enzyme levels, indicating extensive necrosis, are unfavourable.

In those patients who have survived acute myocardial infarction, the outlook is better than is often appreciated. The prognosis is best in those who are free of hypertension, angina and cardiac failure. Overall, between 80 and 90% of patients survive at least 1 year, approximately 75% survive 5 years, 50% 10 years and 25% 20 years. The risk of further infarction and sudden death persists but diminishes as time elapses.

Treatment

Immediate treatment. The management of the early phase of myocardial infarction is critical; resuscitation from cardiac arrest is most often required at this time and interventions to limit infarct size should be administered as soon as possible. It is, therefore, of great importance that resuscitation and other relevant facilities should be available outside hospital. Depending upon local circumstances, these can be provided by suitably trained and equipped doctors or by paramedical personnel.

Usually, the most urgent measure is the relief of pain. When this is severe, opiates such as intravenous morphine sulphate (10 mg) or diamorphine (5 mg) are required and may have to be repeated. Unfortunately, these drugs may produce bradycardia, hypotension and respiratory depression, and it is advisable to combine them with atropine 0.5 mg, if there is bradycardia, or a drug such as perchlorperazine if there is not. The inhalation of nitrous oxide 50% and oxygen 50% is useful if other analgesic measures are unavailable or have failed. Intravenous beta-blockers may help to relieve pain. Oxygen should be given if the patient is breathless or distressed.

In recent years, it has become usual to admit all those with suspected myocardial infarction to hospital. The main purpose of this is to ensure that intensive care is available in the first few unpredictable hours. There is, however, a case for leaving at home those patients whose circumstances are good if the clinical state is satisfactory several hours after the onset, particularly if they are elderly or live a long distance from the nearest coronary care unit.

General management. The patient must be confined to bed immediately, but the degree of restriction depends upon the severity of the infarction. If this has been mild and there is no evidence of cardiogenic shock or cardiac failure, patients should be allowed to feed themselves, use a commode, and gently exercise their legs from the outset. Within 1–2 days it may be possible for them to sit out of bed. The mildest cases may be permitted to walk a few steps shortly after this and may be ready for discharge from hospital after 5–10 days, at which time they should be able to walk up a few stairs. If, however, during the first days there is evidence of a severe infarction, or if there have been dangerous arrhythmias, the patient requires strict bed rest which may have to be continued until the complication has been brought satisfactorily under control. The subsequent progress of those with more severe infarction is necessarily slow, but in most cases discharge from hospital is possible in 3–4 weeks.

One of the greatest dangers after a myocardial infarction is the development of an unwarranted anxiety. This can be prevented by encouragement and explanation from the onset; the patient must understand that there is a good chance of recovery and return to near normal activity. At every stage an optimistic attitude should prevail, and it should be apparent that the physician expects his patient to recover.

Intensive care. For the first few days after the onset of acute myocardial infarction, the risk of sudden and unexpected death is high. This is largely due to arrhythmias, which can be treated or prevented by appropriate therapy. Because of the close observation required at this time, and the need to have appropriate equipment and skills immediately available, intensive care of a special kind is required.

'Coronary Care' of patients with myocardial infarction has three essential components:

- the concentration of patients at maximal risk in special areas;
- their care by nurses and doctors with specialized training;
- the immediate availability of apparatus for monitoring the ECG and for resuscitation.

Coronary care units should reduce anxiety; the patient should initially be reassured by the constant observation and the excellence of the medical and nursing care. Subsequently, when the most acute stage is over, he should be encouraged that close supervision is no longer necessary.

Thrombolytic therapy and aspirin. Thrombolytic agents can dissolve recently formed clots in the coronary arteries. Large clinical trials have shown that the mortality of acute myocardial infarction can be reduced by 25–50% by these drugs, the effect being greatest when they are given in the first 4 h after the onset of symptoms. Most experience has been obtained with streptokinase, 1 500 000 units being infused intravenously over 1 h. This agent may occasionally cause allergic reactions and anaphylaxis, and it can be hypotensive, particularly if administered too rapidly. Another thrombolytic, anistreplase, resembles streptokinase in its side-effects, but has the advantage that it can be given by an intravenous injection over 2–5 min. Another agent, alteplase (rt-PA), is genetically engineered and does not induce allergic reactions or hypotension. It has to be infused over 3 h. Because they cause antibody production, streptokinase and anistreplase should not be readministered within a 1-year period; if further thrombolytic treatment is necessary within this time period, alteplase should be used. Anistreplase and alteplase are much more expensive than streptokinase.

The main risk of all thrombolytic agents is bleeding, and they should be avoided either when there is serious doubt as to the diagnosis or if there is a particular danger of haemorrhage, as after surgery, trauma, stroke or with an active peptic ulcer. With these provisos, thrombolytic therapy should be regarded as routine for patients seen within the first few hours from the onset of suspected myocardial infarction.

Clinical trials have also established that aspirin in a dosage of 160 mg daily reduces mortality after acute myocardial infarction by some 20–25%, possibly by the prevention of further infarction. It, too, should be regarded as routine in the absence of contraindications.

Anticoagulant therapy. Anticoagulants may be used for several different purposes in myocardial infarction:

- to prevent the progression or recurrence of thrombosis in the coronary arteries. Heparin should be administered if alteplase is being given because of an otherwise high risk of reocclusion. It is uncertain whether it is necessary with the other thrombolytics;
- to prevent or treat deep vein thrombosis and pulmonary embolism. Early mobilization has made these complications less common than they used to be; however, they remain a substantial risk in those with large infarctions, particularly if complicated by heart failure;
- to prevent or treat thrombo-embolism from the left side of the heart; this complication is most likely to occur in those with large anterior infarctions, atrial fibrillation or ventricular aneurysms.

Low-dose heparin (e.g. 5000 units 8-hourly subcutaneously) can prevent the development of deep vein thrombosis, but is inadequate once thrombosis has occurred. Intravenous heparin is then required. Preferably this should be given continuously in a dosage which maintains the activated partial thromboplastin time (APTT) between 1.5 and 2 times the pre-heparin control value. Alternatively, if APTT monitoring is not available, heparin may be given intravenously, 5000 units every 4 h.

In general, heparin should be administered for at least 5–7 days, even if warfarin is being given concurrently. The only common unwanted effect is haemorrhage, which can be rapidly counteracted by protamine sulphate. Rarely, there may be thrombocytopenia or anaphylaxis.

When longer-term treatment is needed, oral anticoagulant drugs should be given. Warfarin is the most commonly used of the drugs. It may be administered initially as 10 mg daily for 3 days, and the dosage subsequently adjusted depending upon the prothrombin ratio. Prothrombin ratios are now usually expressed in terms of the International Normalized Ratio (INR). This should be kept between 2.0 and 4.5, the higher end of the range being aimed for in higher risk patients (e.g. those with recurrent thrombosis and pulmonary embolism).

If warfarin therapy is undertaken, the possibility of interactions with other drugs must be borne in mind. Antagonists include barbiturates and cholestyramine; potentiators include amiodarone, aspirin, cimetidine and phenylbutazone.

Bleeding is quite common with warfarin. If it is mild, all that is required is an adjustment in dosage. Severe bleeding calls for the use of vitamin K, or concentrated factor replacement (the former should not be used if clotting would be particularly hazardous, e.g. in the presence of a prosthetic valve).

There is some evidence that anticoagulant therapy prevents further myocardial infarction. Long-term treatment should be undertaken only if the patient is known to be co-operative, if the doctor is prepared to supervise the patient and his anticoagulant control carefully, and if a reliable laboratory is available.

Management of rhythm and conduction disorders. Ventricular fibrillation is best treated by immediate d.c. shock of 200 J, without prior closed-chest cardiac massage or artificial ventilation (see pp. 181, 364). If a defibrillator is not immediately available, external resuscitation must be initiated and continued until the apparatus arrives. The prognosis of patients with ventricular fibrillation depends upon their condition prior to the onset of this arrhythmia. If free of shock or cardiac failure, and if d.c. shock is immediately available, 90% have a chance of being alive 1 month later. If either of these complications has been present, the chances are approximately 25%.

Ventricular fibrillation is frequently preceded by other ventricular arrhythmias, notably ventricular tachycardia and ventricular ectopic beats of the R-on-T variety. When these arrhythmias appear, lignocaine or other anti-arrhythmic drugs should be given (p. 179).

Atrial flutter and fibrillation, should be treated with digitalis glycosides if the ventricular rate is high. Digoxin may be given in a dosage of 0.5 mg intravenously (if digitalis has not been administered during the preceding week). Subsequently, digoxin may be given orally. If the heart rate is not brought under control quickly, sinus rhythm should be restored by synchronized d.c. shock. Supraventricular tachycardias may be treated similarly, if carotid sinus pressure is ineffective.

Asystole responds poorly to therapy, but an attempt should be made to restore electrical activity by a blow on the chest, closed chest cardiac resuscitation or electrical pacemaking. First-degree heart block requires no treatment but should be closely observed for progression. Bradycardia due to more advanced block is common during the early hours and can often be corrected by atropine. If the bradycardia is persistent, especially if associated with hypotension, an endocardial electrode should be placed in the right ventricle and attached to an external pacemaker. If pacemaking facilities are not available, a slow intravenous infusion of isoprenaline may be given (1–5 mg in 500 ml 5% laevulose) taking care to avoid sinus tachycardia and ventricular arrhythmias.

Sinus bradycardia is usually relatively harmless, but if it is producing hypotension or is associated with ventricular ectopic activity, atropine in a dosage of 0.3 mg should be given intravenously, and repeated if necessary, taking care not to induce tachycardia.

Management of cardiac failure and shock. More than 60% of patients with myocardial infarction have some evidence of cardiac failure, as shown by chest radiography, but in many of these it is transient and asymptomatic and requires no treatment. If, on the other hand, there is dyspnoea, or pulmonary oedema, or a gallop rhythm, or prolonged or profound hypotension, the prognosis is poor. In such cases, every effort must be made to determine the factors that have led to cardiac failure, to evaluate carefully the haemodynamic status, and to institute appropriate treatment.

The most important single factor is the extent of myocardial damage sustained in the current and previous myocardial infarctions. Others, which are more amenable to correction, are:

- arrhythmias and conduction disorders;
- hypovolaemia, sometimes the consequence of previous treatment with diuretics, antihypertensives and pressor drugs;
- right ventricular infarction, which may produce a clinical picture of high venous pressure, with low systemic arterial and pulmonary wedge pressures;
- previous treatment with beta-adrenoceptor drugs;
- lesions such as a ventricular septal defect which are surgically correctable.

If possible patients with cardiac failure or shock should be categorized using the data available from intravascular monitoring with a Swan–Ganz catheter. Three major groups can be identified:

- those with 'backward' failure, i.e. with a cardiac index $>2.2 \text{l}/\text{min}/\text{m}^2$ and pulmonary wedge pressure $>18 \text{ mmHg}$. Such patients maintain their blood pressure but have pulmonary oedema. Appropriate treatment includes diuretics and vasodilators (e.g. nitrates) and, possibly, digitalis;
- those with 'forward' failure, i.e. with a cardiac index $< 2.2 \text{l}/\text{min}/\text{m}^2$ and pulmonary artery wedge pressure $<12 \text{ mmHg}$. Such patients usually respond to the administration of plasma expanders;
- those with both pulmonary oedema and hypotension (cardiac output $<2.2 \text{l}/\text{min}/\text{m}^2$ and pulmonary artery wedge pressure $>18 \text{ mmHg}$). The mortality in this group is very high, but an attempt should be made to improve left ventricular function by reducing afterload (with vasodilators) and increasing contractility with inotropic drugs (see also Chapter 8).

It is important neither to overload the circulation nor to lower the filling pressure of the left ventricle excessively. One should aim to keep the pulmonary artery wedge pressure between 15 and 20 mmHg.

The intra-aortic balloon pump (see p. 361) can cause temporary clinical improvement, but this is not maintained unless some major factor can be corrected, e.g. the surgical closure of a ventricular septal defect.

Surgical treatment and angioplasty

Surgery has little part to play in the acute phase of myocardial infarction except for the few patients who develop a ventricular septal defect; these require early repair. Other surgically treatable complications include ventricular aneurysm and papillary muscle rupture; operation is preferably delayed for 6 weeks. If a patient develops these lesions at a time when corrective surgery would be inappropriate, an intra-aortic balloon pump may be invaluable in supporting the circulation for 1–2 weeks.

Angioplasty is now commonly performed during the convalescent period of 1–6 weeks after infarction. It is mainly indicated for angina not responding to medical treatment.

Late complications in acute myocardial infarction

The major risks of infarction occur during the first few days, but complications can arise over a period of several weeks. These include further infarction, the recurrence of serious arrhythmias, and sudden death. Amongst other complications are ventricular aneurysm formation, the post-myocardial infarction syndrome and the shoulder-hand syndrome.

Ventricular aneurysm formation occurs in 10–20% of patients. Although the prognosis in those affected is reasonably good, the area of paradoxically moving non-contractile myocardium leads to extra work for the remaining heart muscle. In some cases this contributes to cardiac failure, and there is also a risk of embolism from mural thrombi. The presence of an aneurysm is suggested by a systolic pulsation of the anterior chest wall lasting more than 3 weeks after the infarction. Other evidence includes persistent QS waves and ST elevation in the affected leads, an abnormal rounded protrusion from the left ventricular wall on the chest radiograph (Fig. 7.11), and paradoxical movement on fluoroscopy. These features are not always present. The aneurysm may be demonstrated by echocardiography, radionuclide studies and left ventriculography. If it is causing heart failure or serious arrhythmias, surgical removal of the aneurysm may be necessary. Anticoagulants reduce the risk of thrombo-embolism.

The post-myocardial infarction syndrome ('Dressler's') is charac-

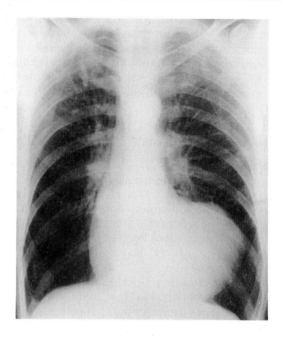

Fig. 7.11   Left ventricular aneurysm. An abnormal, rounded protrusion of the left heart border is apparent.

terized by pericardial pain, accompanied by pericardial rub, fever, pleurisy and a leucocytosis. It may occur at any time in the weeks or months after an infarction, and has been attributed to an immune reaction to necrotic cardiac muscle. It usually responds well to aspirin and, if necessary, a short course of prednisolone.

The shoulder–hand syndrome afflicts a small percentage of patients some weeks after infarction, particularly if there has been prolonged immobilization. There is a limitation of movement of the shoulder joint, associated with tenderness and pain, and there may be swelling of the hands and fingers with nodules on the palms.

Rehabilitation and secondary prevention after myocardial infarction

Although many patients make an initially satisfactory recovery following myocardial infarction, the longer term outcome in terms of return to normal activities, including work, and freedom from recurrences is often disappointing.

Failure to return to a normal life may be due to physical factors, but it is often the result of anxiety or inadequate instruction and rehabilitation. It is helpful if, in the milder case, a limited exercise tolerance test is carried out 1–2 weeks after the infarction in which the patient exercises until a heart rate of 120–130 is achieved. If such a heart rate can be attained without cardiac symptoms or ST depression on the ECG, the outlook is very good and the patient can be encouraged to return quickly to a near normal life. For example, 4–8 weeks after discharge, the individual should be walking out of doors and up hills and stairs, be able to return to car driving and sexual activity, and should go back to work, provided this is not physically strenuous, shortly thereafter. Patients whose exercise tolerance is less good require slower convalescence and more careful observation. If angina pectoris or dyspnoea are major symptoms, careful attention to drug therapy and consideration of angioplasty or surgery is necessary.

Many patients find a formal rehabilitation programme helpful in restoring confidence and physical well-being. The patient usually attends two or three out-patient sessions a week for a period of 3–6 months. A graduated exercise programme, tailored to the individual patient, is accompanied by counselling on lifestyle, and advice on preventive measures and relaxation techniques.

The long-term use of beta-adrenoceptor blocking drugs after myocardial infarction reduces mortality in the succeeding years. They appear to be particularly beneficial in those whose acute episode was complicated by serious arrhythmias or cardiac failure; it is recommended that they are given on a long-term basis to such patients, unless there are contraindications (such as uncontrolled heart failure). They are also indicated for hypertension and angina pectoris.

The stopping of smoking and the control of hyperlipidaemia, hypertension and diabetes are all important in the survivor of myocardial infarction.

Drugs, such as mexiletine, disopyramide and amiodarone, are indicated for patients with recurrent serious ventricular arrhythmias, but their effectiveness and safety in the individual patient must be established.

CARDIAC FAILURE (see also Chapter 8)

In a small proportion of patients with ischaemic heart disease, the initial manifestation is cardiac failure, which may be either left-sided or right-sided. The clinical picture is that of a dilated cardio-myopathy. The ECG may or may not provide conclusive evidence of coronary disease. Echocardiography and radionuclide imaging usually demonstrate regional, as opposed to global, dysfunction and may show an aneurysm. Except in the latter case, surgery (other than transplantation) is not indicated.

SUDDEN DEATH

Death often occurs suddenly in patients with coronary atherosclerosis. In about 50% of cases, the subject is known to have suffered from angina pectoris, or to have had a previous myocardial infarction. In a proportion of the remainder, it is possible to obtain a history from relatives that an attack of pain had preceded the fatal event, but in quite a substantial number death occurs without any warning whatsoever.

When sudden death occurs under circumstances in which the patient is observed, ventricular fibrillation is frequently the cause. Occasionally ventricular asystole is responsible; in the elderly ventricular rupture is not uncommon.

Prompt defibrillation is frequently effective in restoring life in those who appear to die suddenly. As most cases occur outside hospital, success depends upon there being someone trained in cardiopulmonary resuscitation at hand and the ready availability of personnel equipped with the necessary apparatus. Those who have been successfully resuscitated require careful observation and evaluation because of the risk of 'recurrent sudden death'. They should be investigated for arrhythmias by dynamic electrocardiography (Holter monitoring) and, probably, by electrophysiological testing to determine whether antiarrhythmic therapy is needed and, if so, which drug is the most suitable. In some cases, it is appropriate to insert an implantable defibrillator (p. 197) whilst in others surgery can be used to remove the area of myocardium responsible for the arrhythmia.

Further reading

Baim, D.S. (1992) Coronary angioplasty as a treatment of coronary artery disease. *New England Journal of Medicine* **326:** 56.

Fuster, V., Cohen, M. & Halpern, J. (1989) Aspirin in the prevention of coronary disease. *New England Journal of Medicine* **321:** 183.

Guidelines and indications for coronary bypass graft surgery. (1991) *Journal of the American College of Cardiology* **17:** 543.

Hirsh, J. (1991) Heparin. *New England Journal of Medicine* **324:** 1565.

Hirsh, J. (1991) Oral anticoagulant drugs. *New England Journal of Medicine* **324:** 1865.

ISIS-2 Collaborative Group. (1988) Randomized trial of intravenous streptokinase, oral aspirin, both, or neither among 17 187 cases of suspected acute myocardial infarction. *Lancet* **ii:** 349.

Julian, D.G. (Ed.) (1985) *Angina Pectoris*, 2nd edn. Edinburgh: Churchill Livingstone.

Kent, K.M. (1987) Coronary angioplasty. *New England Journal of Medicine* **316:** 1148.

Parker, J.O. (1987) Nitrate therapy in stable angina pectoris. *New England Journal of Medicine* **316:** 1635.

Roussouw, J.E., Lewis, B. & Rifkind, B.M. (1990) The value of lowering cholesterol after myocardial infarction. *New England Journal of Medicine* **323:** 1112.

Wenger, N.K. (1986) Rehabilitation of the coronary patient. *Progress in Cardiovascular Diseases* **29:** 181.

Wheatley, D.J. (Ed.) (1986) *Surgery of Coronary Artery Disease*. London: Chapman & Hall.

Heart Failure

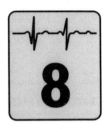

Failure in anything implies expectations unfulfilled, and one's definition of heart failure depends upon what one expects of the heart. No single definition suffices because the clinical and physiological criteria necessarily differ.

The clinician regards his patient as having heart failure when there are symptoms or physical signs attributable to inadequate cardiac performance. The physiologist regards the heart as failing when the contractility of the ventricles or the cardiac output falls outside the statistically defined normal range. There is no clear distinction between normality and abnormality; values in the 'abnormal' range may be found in normal hearts in the face of extreme demand, and 'normal' values may be encountered in diseased hearts when the demands are slight. None the less, if one is aware of the shortcomings, some definitions of heart failure may be accepted.

To Sir Thomas Lewis, heart failure was 'an inability of the heart to discharge its contents adequately'; to Paul Wood it was 'a state in which the heart fails to maintain an adequate circulation for the needs of the body despite a satisfactory venous filling pressure' (thereby excluding from consideration inadequate cardiac output due to insufficient venous return).

Cardiac failure, as it is understood in clinical practice, denotes the presence of one of the complexes of symptoms and signs associated with the 'congestion' of tissues and organs or attributable to the inadequate perfusion of tissues and organs:

- *pulmonary venous congestion* results from disordered function of the left ventricle or left atrium;
- *systemic venous congestion* is similarly due to disorders of the right ventricle and atrium, but is often the end-result of left-sided heart failure. The clinical features derive, in the main, from engorgement of the systemic veins and capillaries.

The heart has also failed when it cannot maintain an adequate blood pressure in spite of a peripheral vascular resistance that is normal or high but, by convention, this type of cardiac failure is referred to as acute circulatory failure or cardiogenic shock rather than heart failure.

THE PATHOPHYSIOLOGY OF HEART FAILURE

The causes of heart failure

The heart fails either because it is subjected to an overwhelming load, or because the heart muscle is disordered (Fig. 8.1):

- *a volume load* is imposed by disorders which demand that the ventricle expels more blood per minute than is normal. Examples include thyrotoxicosis and anaemia, in which the total cardiac output is increased; and mitral regurgitation and aortic regurgitation, in which the left ventricle has to expel not only the normal

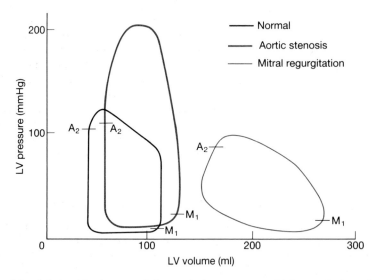

Fig. 8.1   Relationships between left ventricular pressure and left ventricular volume in the normal heart, in aortic stenosis and in mitral regurgitation. In the normal heart, following the closure of the mitral valve (M_1), there is a rapid rise in pressure without any change in volume until the aortic valve opens. Pressure then rises more slowly as the left ventricle ejects blood; in later systole, there is a fall-off in pressure, though ejection continues until the aortic valve closes (A_2). The phase of isovolumetric relaxation then occurs followed by diastolic filling with little change in pressure. The salient feature of aortic stenosis is the pressure load; mitral regurgitation is associated with a volume load leading to an increase in ventricular volume at the end of both systole and diastole.

forward flow into the aorta but also the large volume of regurgitated blood as well;

- a pressure *load* is imposed by disorders which increase resistance to outflow from the ventricles (typified by systemic hypertension due to increased impedance of the peripheral arterioles, and by aortic stenosis in which there is narrowing of the outflow orifice of the left ventricle);
- disorders *of myocardial* function result not only from diminished contractility but also from loss of contractile tissue, as occurs in myocardial infarction. An additional factor in this condition is a paradoxical movement of infarcted muscle which further increases the work of the remaining myocardium.

In many cases, a combination of mechanisms contribute to failure. For example in patients with rheumatic heart disease, myocardial damage, valve narrowing and regurgitation may all be contributory.

Cardiac and circulatory responses in heart failure

The heart at first responds to pressure and volume overloads in much the same way as it does to normal increases in demand, such as those imposed by exercise. As the disorder progresses, more cardiac and circulatory adjustments take place which, for a time, may maintain an adequate circulation but many of the so called 'compensatory' mechanisms are inappropriate. During evolution the circulatory system has had to evolve methods of combating blood loss and trauma rather than, for example, myocardial infarction, and the responses invoked are relevant to the former stresses rather than the latter. Indeed, the clinical manifestations of heart failure are largely the effects of 'compensatory' mechanisms which eventually embarrass the circulation.

Dilatation of the heart — increase in end-diastolic volume

In response to a volume load, the heart dilates, i.e. the ventricular volume is increased. Up to a point, dilatation is a normal and efficient response but it is abnormal when it cannot be wholly ascribed to the volume load. Pathological dilatation of this kind occurs when there is myocardial disease, when, because of decreased contractility, the ventricle must be stretched to a greater extent for a given stroke volume. Even in those cases in which dilatation may at first be regarded as a physiological response, it eventually becomes disadvantageous because, as the ventricle increases in size, greater tension is required in the myocardium to expel a given volume of blood. This is in accordance with the law of Laplace which indicates that the tension in the myocardium (T) is proportional to the intraventricular pressure (P) multiplied by the radius (R) of the ventricular chamber ($T \propto PR$). The greater tension results in increased oxygen requirements and eventually leads to hypertrophy.

Hypertrophy of the heart

When the ventricle has to face a chronic increase of pressure load, such as that imposed by arterial hypertension, aortic stenosis or pulmonary hypertension, the myocardium hypertrophies, i.e. it increases in weight as a result of an enlargement of individual muscle fibres. The process affects only those chambers upon which there are increased demands. The mechanism responsible for the development of cardiac hypertrophy is uncertain but it seems likely that it is a response to increased stretching or tension in muscle fibres which result from a raised diastolic volume or pressure. Hypertrophy may be regarded as a normal compensatory mechanism which permits the heart to cope with the increased demands, but becomes self-defeating when it is excessive. The thickening of the fibres increases the distance by which oxygen has to diffuse from the capillaries; eventually this leads to impaired oxygenation of the centre of the fibre. It is probable that this hypoxia is an important factor in the fibrosis which frequently develops in hypertrophied muscle.

Impaired myocardial contractility

In many types of heart disease, the major defect lies in the myocardium itself. This is the case in ischaemic heart disease, myocarditis and cardiomyopathy, and myocardial involvement is often considerable in rheumatic heart disease. Even when the primary disturbance is that of a volume or pressure overload, intrinsic myocardial function may be eventually affected adversely by dilatation and hypertrophy. Why the impaired myocardial contractility develops is uncertain, but it has been attributed by some to overstretching of the sarcomeres (see p. 3). There may be a slowing up in the conversion of chemical energy into muscular work as a result of depression in the activity of ATPase, the enzyme responsible for the release of energy from ATP. Other possible contributory factors include depletion of noradrenaline (norepinephrine) stores in the myocardium.

The cardiac output in heart failure

By definition cardiac failure is present when the cardiac output is insufficient for the needs of the body, but some patients with an output in the normal range manifest the clinical features of cardiac failure, whereas other patients with low outputs are free of symptoms and signs. However, in cardiac failure, even if the cardiac output is

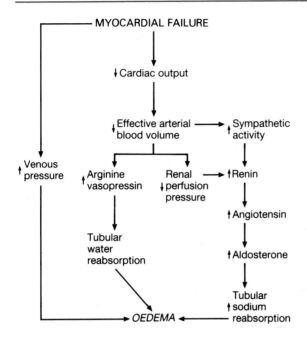

Fig. 8.2   Some of the neuroendocrine and renal responses to cardiac failure.

normal at rest it usually responds inadequately to exercise. In conditions such as beri-beri and thyrotoxicosis, in which the cardiac output is abnormally high, it is still insufficient for the exceptional metabolic demands.

Neuroendocrine response to heart failure

Cardiac failure activates several components of the neuroendocrine system, which play an important intermediary role in its clinical manifestations (Fig. 8.2).

Sympathetic nervous system.   Activation of the sympathetic nervous system results in an increase in myocardial contractility, heart rate, and vasoconstriction of arteries and veins. Although this may be beneficial in maintaining blood pressure, it is adverse in so far as it increases preload, afterload, and myocardial oxygen requirement. There is also an increased plasma noradrenaline, but myocardial catecholamines are reduced.

Renin–angiotensin–aldosterone systems.   Both the fall in cardiac output itself and the increase in sympathetic tone reduce effective blood flow to the kidney and, consequently, increase renin secretion.

Salt restriction and diuretic therapy also augment this. As a result, there is a rise in angiotensin II levels, which leads directly to vasoconstriction and indirectly, by stimulating aldosterone secretion, to sodium retention and the expansion of blood volume. This is advantageous in so far as increasing preload helps to maintain stroke volume by the Starling mechanism, but it does so at the expense of circulatory congestion.

Arginine vasopressin (antidiuretic hormone).   The reduced effective blood volume of heart failure stimulates the release of arginine vasopressin, leading to water retention. This is a feature of late, rather than early, cardiac failure.

Atrial natriuretic peptide.   Distension of the atria leads to the release of this peptide which has natriuretic and vasodilator properties. Its role in cardiac failure is still unclear.

The regional circulations in cardiac failure

There is a redistribution of blood flow to different organs and tissues in cardiac failure, as there is on exercise. This redistribution is mediated through vasoconstriction in certain areas, notably the renal arterioles. The renal blood flow falls disproportionately, and may be reduced to one-quarter of normal. There is little reduction in the coronary or cerebral blood flow, but there is vasoconstriction of the skin and splanchnic vessels.

Salt and water retention

An almost invariable feature of cardiac failure is the retention of sodium and water. This leads to a substantial increase in extracellular and plasma volume and plays a large part in the production of the clinical features of cardiac failure. Some of the factors responsible for the fluid and salt retention are discussed above, but undoubtedly there are still undiscovered mechanisms.

   Diminished glomerular filtration. Glomerular filtration is reduced in cardiac failure, although to a lesser extent than is renal blood flow. Diminished glomerular filtration may play some part in sodium retention, but it is probably not an important factor except when the failure is severe.

   Increased tubular reabsorption. There is abundant experimental evidence that tubular reabsorption of sodium is increased in cardiac failure. There is no doubt that, in certain patients, there is increased aldosterone secretion, and that this hormone, by its action on the distal tubule, promotes the reabsorption of sodium whilst increasing the excretion of potassium and hydrogen. However, evidence of hyperaldosteronism is confined to advanced failure; aldosterone antagonists are relatively ineffective in the treatment of sodium retention in early failure. The enhanced tubular reabsorption of sodium found in cardiac failure seems to be mediated through some mechanism as yet undiscovered.

As mentioned, water retention in heart failure is usually secondary to sodium retention. In some patients with advanced cardiac failure, however, there is a disproportionate retention of water. In these patients, the kidneys can no longer excrete solute-free water and the serum sodium concentration falls as a result of dilution ('dilutional hyponatraemia').

Raised venous pressure in cardiac failure

When the left ventricle fails the pulmonary venous pressure rises, and when the right ventricle fails the pressure rises in the systemic veins. This can be largely explained by the inability of the failing ventricle to discharge the blood presented to it effectively. The increased blood volume resulting from sodium and water retention contributes to the venous return and is thus a factor in producing the raised venous pressure, as is venoconstriction.

The effect of left ventricular failure on the lungs

As explained above, when the left ventricle fails, the diastolic pressure in the left ventricle rises and with it the left atrial pressure. Since the pulmonary veins and capillaries are in continuity with the left atrium, the pressures in these vessels rise concomitantly. In mild left ventricular failure, the pressures in the left atrium and pulmonary veins are within normal limits at rest but rise on exercise. As failure advances, the left atrial pressure progressively increases from its normal level of 5–10 mmHg to one of 25–30 mmHg. The hydrostatic pressure in the capillaries is then close to that needed to overcome the osmotic pressure exerted by the plasma proteins and may lead to an exudation of fluid from the capillaries into the alveolar walls and alveoli. If the pressure in the atrium rises rapidly, there may be a sudden exudation of fluid into the alveoli. If this process takes place slowly, exudation may proceed gradually with a slow build up of tissue tension occurring in the alveolar wall. This restricts further exudation of fluid and limits the risk to the alveoli. In response to this process, some fibrosis may take place in the alveolar wall. The pulmonary congestion caused by the high pulmonary venous pressure and by the changes in the alveolar walls makes the lung more rigid (less compliant). As a result of this, more work must be done by the respiratory muscles to move a given volume of air.

Arrhythmias in heart failure

Patients with heart failure have a high incidence of sudden death. The majority of deaths are thought to be due to ventricular tachycardia or ventricular fibrillation.

A number of factors contribute to the occurrence of ventricular tachyarrhythmias in patients with heart failure. These include:

- high circulating catecholamine levels;
- electrolyte disturbance, particularly diuretic-induced hypo-kalaemia;
- proarrhythmic effects of inotropic drugs (p. 151);
- stretch on the myocardium may result in arrhythmias through the process of 'contraction-excitation feedback'.

Arrhythmia prevention in patients with heart failure is a particular problem. The efficacy of antiarrhythmic drugs is reduced and there is, moreover, an increased incidence of proarrhythmic side-effects. In addition, most antiarrhythmic drugs have negative inotropic effects.

Although vasodilator treatment with ACE inhibitors has been shown to reduce mortality due to progression of heart failure (p. 156), it has not reduced mortality from sudden death, and this remains a major unsolved problem.

CLINICAL SYNDROMES OF HEART FAILURE

Left heart failure

Aetiology

The features of left heart failure develop when there is a major obstruction to outflow from the left atrium (e.g. mitral stenosis) or when the left ventricle can no longer cope with the demands upon it. The common causes of left ventricular failure are:

- myocardial infarction;
- systemic hypertension;
- aortic valve disease;
- mitral regurgitation;
- cardiomyopathy.

Clinical features

The clinical features of left-side cardiac failure are largely the consequence of pulmonary congestion. The symptoms are:

- dyspnoea on exertion;
- orthopnoea and paroxysmal nocturnal dyspnoea;
- acute pulmonary oedema.

The physical signs of left ventricular failure may include:

- pulmonary crepitations;
- third heart sound;
- pleural effusion;
- pulsus alternans – alternative large and low volume pulse — this is an indication of severe left ventricular failure.

Investigations.   The chest radiograph shows:

- pulmonary venous congestion particularly of the upper lobe;
- interstitial oedema;
- alveolar oedema.

Some of these features are illustrated in Fig. 5.10.

The electrocardiogram may be of value although it does not provide direct evidence of left heart failure. For example, it is unusual for hypertension or aortic valve disease to lead to the symptoms of left heart failure without producing ECG evidence of left ventricular hypertrophy first. Again, it is unusual for coronary artery disease to lead to left heart failure if the ECG is normal. This is not, however, true of mitral regurgitation.

Differential diagnosis.   The diagnosis of left heart failure is usually not difficult when there is progressive dyspnoea coupled with clinical evidence of advanced left-sided heart disease. However, this evidence may not always be unequivocal and there may be difficulty in distinguishing the symptoms of heart failure from those of pulmonary disease. The dyspnoea of left heart failure is more likely to be provoked by lying down flat. Patients with dyspnoea due to pulmonary disease usually have a history of asthmatic attacks or of chronic cough and sputum.

Paroxysmal nocturnal dyspnoea and acute pulmonary oedema may be difficult to differentiate from acute respiratory attacks. The latter are commonly associated with bronchospasm and purulent sputum. In contrast, the patient with acute pulmonary oedema is usually free of pulmonary infection, has fine crepitations rather than rhonchi and is liable to cough up pink frothy sputum. Furthermore, examination usually reveals the signs of left-sided heart disease. Correct diagnosis is of great importance because the therapy of the two conditions is different. For example, morphine may be lethal in respiratory failure, but invaluable in acute pulmonary oedema. Similarly, high concentrations of oxygen are useful in acute pulmonary oedema but may be dangerous in respiratory failure. The chest radiograph is also helpful in showing signs of oedema or infection. In cases of doubt, estimation of the arterial CO_2 tension is of value because this is usually low in acute pulmonary oedema and high in respiratory failure.

Right heart failure

Aetiology

Failure of the right side of the heart occurs when the right ventricle can no longer cope with the demands upon it, or when there is tricuspid stenosis. Common causes of right ventricular failure include:

- left ventricular failure with its consequent effects upon the pulmonary circulation;
- right ventricular infarction;
- pulmonary disease, particularly chronic bronchitis and emphysema;
- pulmonary hypertension (see p. 322);
- pulmonary valve disease;
- tricuspid regurgitation.

Clinical features

The characteristic features of right heart failure are:

- *elevated jugular venous pressure*. In the normal individual, the venous pressure in the internal jugular veins does not exceed 2 cm vertically above the sternal angle when the patient is reclining at 45°. In right heart failure this figure is exceeded. Even if normal at rest, it rises on exercise;
- *hepatomegaly*. If chronic, this may result in cirrhosis;
- *oedema*. This is of the dependent type and usually most evident in the pretibial and ankle regions;
- *ascites*. This may occasionally occur in patients with severe right heart failure.

Other clinical features of cardiac failure

There are a number of common but less specific features of cardiac failure. Fatigue is a frequent symptom which is difficult to evaluate.

The nutrition of patients with cardiac failure is often good in the early stages, but cachexia sets in as disability increases. In the very advanced case, cerebral symptoms may develop with dulling of consciousness, confusion or changes in personality. Patients with cardiac failure are prone to develop venous thrombosis and pulmonary emboli are common. Mild jaundice, due to hepatic congestion or cirrhosis, is quite frequent in right-sided heart failure. Proteinuria due to renal congestion is often present.

THE MANAGEMENT OF CARDIAC FAILURE

Ideally, the treatment of cardiac failure is the correction of the cause, but for a variety of reasons this may not be possible, at least initially. In some conditions, such as ischaemic heart disease and the cardiomyopathies, no currently available methods of treatment affect the underlying lesions. In other disorders, the radical treatment necessary for cure, such as major surgery, cannot be safely undertaken until cardiac failure has been corrected.

The principles of treating cardiac failure may be enumerated as follows:

- the correction or amelioration of the underlying disease;
- the control of precipitating factors;
- the reduction of demands on the heart by weight loss and the restriction of physical activity;
- the improvement of myocardial function by the administration of inotropic drugs such as the digitalis glycosides;
- the correction of sodium and water retention;
- reduction of preload and/or afterload by vasodilator drugs.

The correction or amelioration of the underlying cause

When heart disease is due to such causes as thyrotoxicosis or hypertension, corrective treatment can be started immediately. In congenital and rheumatic heart disease, surgical management is usually required, but this may have to be deferred until the maximum benefit has been achieved from medical treatment.

In the case of ischaemic heart disease, the cause of heart failure is generally previous myocardial infarction rather than ongoing ischaemia. Coronary revascularization procedures cannot ameliorate the damage caused by previous infarction and for this reason play little part in the management of heart failure.

The control of complicating factors

Cardiac failure is often precipitated or exacerbated by factors superimposed on the underlying heart disease. Amongst these are:

- arrhythmias;
- infections;
- pulmonary embolism;
- anaemia;
- excessive sodium intake;
- over-exertion.

The recognition of precipitating factors is of great importance in the management of heart failure, because the correction of these complicating conditions will often result in the abolition of symptoms.

Restriction of activity

Rest reduces the demands on the heart and leads to a fall in venous pressure and a reduction in pulmonary congestion. It allows a relative increase in renal blood flow and often leads to a diuresis. However, bed rest also encourages the development of venous thrombosis and pulmonary embolism.

The degree of physical restriction necessary depends upon the severity of the cardiac failure. When there is severe pulmonary congestion or peripheral oedema, a period of complete rest may be required. At this time, the patient is usually most comfortable propped up by two or more pillows in bed or in an armchair. Complete bed rest is seldom necessary for more than a few days, after which a gradual increase in activity should be encouraged, depending upon the response. In patients with lesser degrees of cardiac failure, moderate exercise should be encouraged as this leads to a gradual improvement in exercise capacity.

Drug therapy

Drugs used in the management of patients with heart failure are summarized in Table 8.1.

Table 8.1   Drugs used in the management of heart failure

General category	Specific examples
Ionotropic drugs	
Digitalis glycosides	Digoxin
Sympathomimetic drugs	Dopamine, dobutamine
Phosphodiesterase inhibitors	Enoximone, milrinone
Diuretics	
Loop diuretics	Frusemide, bumetanide
Thiazide diuretics	Bendrofluazide, hydrochlorothiazide
Potassium-sparing diuretics	Amiloride, triamterene, spironolactone
Vasodilators	
ACE inhibitors	Captopril, enalapril, lisinopril
Arterial dilators	Hydralazine
Venous dilators	Nitrates
Mixed arterial and venous dilators	Prazosin, nitroprusside

THERAPY WITH INOTROPIC DRUGS

Drugs which increase myocardial contractility (positive inotropic agents) can augment cardiac output and relieve cardiac failure, but may also increase myocardial oxygen requirement. There is no doubt that in acute myocardial failure such drugs may be beneficial, but their long-term effectiveness is disputed and there are concerns that they may adversely influence survival through an increase in ventricular arrhythmias.

There are three main groups of inotropic drugs:

- digitalis glycosides;
- sympathomimetic agents;
- phosphodiesterase inhibitors.

Digitalis glycosides

These have, for many years, been regarded as standard therapy for cardiac failure and are the only inotropic agents widely used in the long-term oral management of patients with heart failure. They are of undoubted value in the control of atrial fibrillation and if this is of importance in the genesis of cardiac failure, they will quickly relieve it. Their role in cardiac failure in sinus rhythm remains controversial.

Mechanisms of action. The inotropic action of digitalis is mediated through the sodium/potassium–ATPase (sodium) pump, to which it binds. The inhibition of this pump leads to an accumulation of intracellular sodium; because of the sodium–calcium exchange system, this results in an increase in the amount of calcium available to activate contraction. Digitalis also has sympathomimetic and parasympathetic (vagal) effects. The latter is clinically important, in that it causes slowing of the sinus rate and delays conduction through the atrioventricular node. Digitalis reduces the refractory period of atrial and ventricular muscle and, therefore, enhances the risk of ectopic rhythms.

Administration. Digoxin is the most commonly used digitalis preparation. Because oral therapy is safest, this route should be used if possible. The intravenous route should be employed only in cases of urgency and should always be avoided if a digitalis preparation has been administered within the previous week.

Intravenous digoxin produces an effect within 15 min and has peak activity in about 2 h. When given by mouth, the effects start in about 1 h and are maximal at about 6 h.

Digoxin is excreted in an unchanged form by the kidneys. This is normally complete in 4–5 days, but is delayed in the presence of renal failure. For this reason digoxin dosage should be reduced in patients with impaired renal function

Drug interactions. Digitalis glycosides may be involved in important drug interactions. Quinidine increases the plasma concentrations of digoxin, probably by displacing it from tissue sites. Amiodarone and verapamil have similar effects. When any of these drugs is added the dosage of digoxin should be reduced. Because hypokalaemia enhances digitalis toxicity, concomitant treatment with potassium losing diuretics must be cautious.

Toxicity. The commonest toxic effects of digitalis therapy are malaise, anorexia, nausea and, later, vomiting. In some patients, there is excessive salivation, yellow vision or diarrhoea.

More serious than these symptoms are the many different types of conduction and rhythm disturbance that may occur:

- *ventricular ectopics.* These are generally well tolerated, but are an indication for reducing digitalis dosage;
- *ventricular tachycardia and ventricular fibrillation* may occur in cases of serious toxicity;
- *supraventricular rhythm disturbances* may be provoked, of which the most important is atrial tachycardia with block (p. 172);
- *atrioventricular dissociation* (p. 186) and junctional rhythms (p. 168) may occur. In more severe cases, complete heart block can develop.

Potassium depletion promotes the development of digitalis-induced disturbances of rhythm and conduction, and should be assumed to be present when these occur, in spite of a normal serum potassium. Digitalis should be discontinued immediately and potassium depletion corrected. It is important never to use d.c. shock therapy in the treatment of digitalis-induced arrhythmias.

Toxicity can usually be corrected by withholding the drug and, if indicated, giving potassium. Pacing may be required for heart block, and antiarrhythmic drugs for arrhythmias. In severe cases of digitalis poisoning, fragments of antidigoxin antibodies (Digibind) may be used to bind digoxin and rapidly reverse toxic effects.

Plasma digoxin levels. Plasma digoxin levels are of limited value in assessing toxicity. Therapeutic and toxic ranges overlap and consequently a digoxin level which is therapeutic in one patient may be toxic in another. As a generalization, provided the serum potassium is normal, toxicity is unlikely with digoxin concentrations below 2µg/litre and very likely with values greater than 4 µg/litre.

Digoxin estimation should only be undertaken when there is a definite indication. The mere fact that a patient is taking digoxin is not an indication for an assay, in the absence of other clinical indications. Appropriate indications include:

- suspected toxicity;

- changing renal function;
- subtherapeutic clinical response;
- potential drug interactions;
- suspected poor compliance.

It is essential that samples should be timed correctly — at least 6 h should elapse between the time of dosing and the time of sampling.

Indications.   Digitalis is indicated in cardiac failure for the control of atrial arrhythmias. Its role in cardiac failure in sinus rhythm remains controversial. It is most likely to be efficacious if there is cardiomegaly with a dilated ventricle and a third heart sound. It is unlikely to be helpful in cases of constrictive pericarditis or in mitral stenosis without atrial fibrillation. It is potentially dangerous in hypertrophic cardiomyopathy (p. 220).

It is relatively easy to assess the therapeutic effectiveness of digitalis therapy in patients with tachycardia due to an arrhythmia. When there is atrial fibrillation, a satisfactory result is usually obtained when the heart rate has been slowed to 70/min at rest. If such a rate is difficult to achieve, it suggests some complicating factor, such as infection, pulmonary infarction or thyrotoxicosis. Bradycardia should be avoided. It may be difficult to assess the effectiveness of digitalis therapy in the patient in regular sinus rhythm. However, improvement in symptoms and the disappearance of the tachycardia and gallop rhythm of cardiac failure suggest that an adequate dose is being given.

Sympathomimetic agents

Drugs such as dopamine and dobutamine are used intravenously for acute heart failure and are discussed on p. 158.

Phosphodiesterase inhibitors

These drugs are of value when used intravenously for acute heart failure. Drugs include milrinone and enoximone. Some phosphodiesterase inhibitors can also be used orally, for the longterm management of heart failure, but there is evidence to suggest that this may in fact increase mortality, due to an increased incidence of arrhythmias.

THE MANAGEMENT OF SODIUM AND WATER RETENTION

Low salt diets effectively counteract cardiac failure. However, with the availability of potent diuretic drugs, no extreme limitation of sodium intake is usually necessary. Nevertheless, some restriction is desirable and inability to control cardiac failure is quite often due to the patient not reducing sodium intake sufficiently. All patients should be advised not to add salt at meals and to avoid obviously salty foods. Occasionally, a strict salt restriction must be applied. It is seldom necessary to practise water restriction, but in cases of dilutional hyponatraemia, a limitation of 1 litre/day may be helpful. These may be identified by a lack of response to conventional treatment for cardiac failure in association with a low serum sodium concentration.

Diuretics are valuable in the treatment of symptomatic heart failure. All the commonly used diuretics act by promoting sodium excretion, with enhanced water excretion as a secondary effect.

The loop diuretics: frusemide, bumetanide

These drugs prevent reabsorption at multiple sites including the proximal and distal tubules and the ascending limb of the loop of Henle. They produce a profound diuresis with the excretion of large quantities of sodium and chloride. When given by mouth, action commences in about 1 hour and is complete in 6–8 hours. If given intravenously, the onset of action is almost immediate.

Thiazide diuretics

The many drugs in this group are essentially similar except in their potency and duration of action. Most of the thiazide diuretics act for 12–24 h whereas polythiazide and chlorthalidone exert their effect for 48 h or more. They may have several sites of action, but the main mechanism is the inhibition of sodium reabsorption in the distal convoluted tubule.

These diuretics are less potent than the loop diuretics, but are rather more likely to produce hypokalaemia. If the serum potassium is low, or if the drugs are being given more than once a week, supplements of slow release potassium chloride should be used.

These drugs sometimes cause hyperglycaemia and hyper-uricaemia, and may precipitate diabetes and clinical gout. Other occasional undesirable effects include agranulocytosis, thrombocytopenia, nausea, abdominal discomfort, impotence and skin rashes.

Thiazide and loop diuretic combinations. Combination of a thiazide and loop diuretic is of value in patients with refractory oedema. A particularly vigorous diuresis may ensue, and it is advisable to reduce the dose of both drugs to guard against intravascular volume depletion, severe hypokalaemia and deterioration in renal function. Close supervision of such combination therapy is essential.

Potassium sparing diuretics

This group comprises two classes of agent:

- *spironolactone*. This drug is an aldosterone antagonist;
- *amiloride and triamterene*. These drugs inhibit the collecting duct sodium conductance.

Potassium-sparing diuretics are relatively ineffective when used singly. Their chief value in the treatment of heart failure is in combination with either a loop or a thiazide diuretic, to reduce the potassium losses associated with these agents.

Hyperkalaemia is a potential complication, particularly in patients with impaired renal function.

VASODILATOR THERAPY

Constriction of the arterioles and veins is a characteristic feature of cardiac failure. In early cardiac failure, the reduction in vascular bed may be beneficial in ensuring an adequate venous return and maintaining the blood pressure, but frequently, particularly in more advanced failure, the arteriolar constriction imposes an excessive afterload and a venoconstriction too high a preload. Depending upon the pathophysiology of the individual case, it may be desirable to reduce preload or afterload or both.

Generally, in cardiac failure, it has been found that the optimal filling (or end-diastolic) pressure of the left ventricle is between 15 and 20 mmHg. If the pressure is higher than this, pulmonary congestion will result. The administration of a venodilator will cause the filling pressure to fall, but the cardiac output either stays the same or increases. Ideally, before using a venodilator, the left ventricular end-diastolic pressure should be measured indirectly from a pulmonary wedge pressure recording. Venodilator drugs should not be given to patients with filling pressures of less than 15 mmHg; the administration of venodilating drugs should be discontinued when such a pressure has been achieved.

The increased arteriolar resistance that results in excessive afterload imposes a burden on the heart which leads to a fall in cardiac output with or without a rise in end-diastolic pressure. Arteriolar vasodilators usually result in a brisk rise in cardiac output.

Vasodilators differ in their predominant site of action:

- *nitrates* act predominantly as venodilators;
- *hydralazine* acts predominantly as an arterial dilator;
- *prazosin* provides a combination of arterial and veno-dilation.

Angiotensin converting enzyme (ACE) inhibitors

ACE inhibitors such as captopril and enalapril, have a unique mechanism in that they block the enhanced activity of the renin–angiotensin system (see p. 143), but have additional vasodilator properties. They seem to be superior to other orally administered vasodilators in their effectiveness and, at low dosages, in their lack of side-effects.

Two problems limit the use of ACE inhibitors in patients with heart failure, hypotension and renal impairment. As many patients with congestive heart failure have a low blood pressure, this restricts the use of these agents. The problem of hypotension is particularly marked after the first dose. First dose hypotension can be minimised by reducing the dose of the ACE inhibitor on commencing therapy (see Appendix) and omitting diuretics for 1–2 days beforehand.

ACE inhibitors occasionally cause deterioration of renal function. They are contraindicated in patients with an initial creatinine level greater than 200 μmol/litre.

Cough is a potentially troublesome side-effect, occurring in up to 10% of patients. The problem can frequently be overcome by a reduction in dosage.

DRUG TREATMENT AND PROGNOSIS

Although digoxin and diuretics are widely used in the symptomatic management of heart failure, only vasodilator therapy has been shown to improve prognosis:

- *an ACE inhibitor* (enalapril) has been shown to reduce mortality in patients with clinical features of failure;
- *a hydralazine/isosorbide dinitrate* combination has also been shown to reduce mortality;
- direct comparison of enalapril and the combination of hydralazine/isosorbide dinitrate has shown a greater reduction in mortality with enalapril.

In view of these mortality benefits, ACE inhibitors should be prescribed, unless contraindicated, in all patients with clinical evidence of left ventricular failure.

ACUTE CIRCULATORY FAILURE (SHOCK)

The terms acute circulatory failure, low output state, and shock are used to describe a syndrome comprising arterial hypotension, cold, moist and cyanosed extremities, a rapid weak pulse, a low urine output and a diminished level of consciousness. This clinical pattern is common to a number of disorders such as severe blood or gastrointestinal fluid loss, burns and acute myocardial infarction. As yet, physiological studies have not clearly defined the nature of the changes responsible for the clinical syndrome, but a common factor is a sudden fall in cardiac output associated with tissue hypoxia.

Causes of shock

There are a number of causes of shock:

- hypovolaemic shock. This is exemplified by haemorrhage and loss of fluid from burns, vomiting and diarrhoea;
- septicaemic shock;
- anaphylactic shock;
- acute pancreatitis;
- cardiogenic shock. Shock is described as cardiogenic when it is clearly cardiac in origin. This may be due to many different causes, including myocardial infarction, massive pulmonary embolism, dissecting aneurysm, pericardial tamponade, rupture of a valve cusp, and arrhythmias. In cardiogenic shock, the central venous pressure is usually raised, in contrast to hypovolaemic shock, in which it is characteristically low.

Although the fall in cardiac output and blood pressure is an essential feature of shock, these abnormalities are insufficient to account for the syndrome. Falls of the same magnitude may be seen in some patients in whom the clinical features of shock are not seen and in whom the prognosis is good. In the first stage of shock, there is a fall in cardiac output and blood pressure, due to either a diminution in venous return or to an inability of the myocardium to expel an adequate stroke volume. As a consequence of the hypotension, there is a fall in renal blood flow, with oliguria. Reflex tachycardia takes place. Compensatory mechanisms follow, with arteriolar constriction affecting particularly the kidneys, abdominal viscera, muscle and skin. Vasodilatation of the cerebral and coronary vessels permits the maintenance of a relatively good blood flow in these territories. If the vasoconstriction is sufficiently great, the blood pressure may be kept at or close to normal levels but at the expense of producing tissue hypoxia with consequent acidosis. If the underlying process can be corrected quickly, recovery may ensue, but if shock persists untreated for many hours, the stage of irreversibility may be reached. At this time, the correction of the original cause fails to prevent death. The nature of irreversible shock remains undetermined, but has been attributed to the production of endotoxins, and to irreparable cellular changes as a result of hypoxia in the liver, kidney, heart or brain.

Aetiological diagnosis

Although the condition responsible for shock is often obvious, there is sometimes no evident cause. In such cases, no effort must be spared in identifying it quickly, for successful therapy depends upon this.

Cardiac causes, provided they are thought of, can usually be recognized by a combination of clinical examination, ECG, X-ray and echocardiography. The cause of hypovolaemic shock may be difficult to establish; this applies particularly to intra-abdominal haemorrhage and to occult infection.

Treatment

General management

If the patient is in severe pain or distress, opiates should be given intravenously (provided there is no contraindication) and high-flow oxygen administered, preferably by a tight-fitting face mask making use of the Venturi principle, or by mechanical ventilation. Unless there is pulmonary oedema, the patient should be laid flat, with the legs slightly raised. A catheter should be introduced to measure urinary output. Arterial blood gases and pH should be monitored. Although central venous monitoring may be adequate for the less severe cases of traumatic shock, a Swan–Ganz balloon-tip catheter should be used to obtain pulmonary artery and 'pulmonary capillary wedge' pressures, particularly if a cardiac or pulmonary cause is known or suspected. As measurement of blood pressure by a sphygmomanometer is unreliable in severe shock, direct arterial pressure monitoring should be undertaken, when possible.

Correction of hypovolaemia

This is essential in shock which is not cardiogenic, but may also be of importance in myocardial infarction when prior diuretic therapy has caused fluid depletion, or in right ventricular infarction. One should aim to raise the central venous pressure to between 10 and 15 mmHg, and keep the pulmonary wedge (or pulmonary artery diastolic) pressure between 15 and 20 mmHg. Immediate replacement may be with saline; subsequently, the amount and nature of the fluid infused should be determined by estimates of that lost.

Inotropic agents

These drugs enhance myocardial contractility, but at the expense of increased oxygen consumption. The sympathomimetic drugs iso-prenaline and noradrenaline were much used in the past, but they have been largely superseded by dopamine and dobutamine.

The effects of dopamine, a natural precursor of noradrenaline, depend upon the dose. Administered intravenously in a dosage of 2–5 µg/kg/min, it causes dilatation of renal and mesenteric vessels; at doses of 5–10 µg/kg/min, it increases myocardial contractility and cardiac output. At higher doses, it causes vasoconstriction (it should not be infused directly into a peripheral vein as leakage may cause local necrosis). Dopamine may induce nausea and vomiting, and can lead to an excessive tachycardia and arrhythmias.

Dobutamine is a synthetic sympathomimetic agent whose predominant action is one of stimulating beta$_1$ activity. It is less likely to cause vasoconstriction or tachycardia than dopamine. It is given by intravenous infusion at a rate of 2.5–10 µg/kg/min.

Both these drugs need to be given with careful monitoring of intravascular pressures.

Vasodilator therapy

Vasodilator drugs are contraindicated in the presence of hypotension. However, when pulmonary oedema complicates shock, they may be combined with inotropic drugs, if the latter succeed in maintaining the blood pressure at a viable level. Intravenous glyceryl trinitrate or isosorbide dinitrate are commonly used and can be titrated against hypotensive response.

Mechanical support

The intra-aortic balloon pump is of value in acute myocardial infarction if shock has been caused by a surgically correctable lesion, such as a ventricular septal defect or papillary muscle rupture (see also p. 361).

CARDIAC TRANSPLANTATION

Cardiac transplantation is now well established in the management of refractory heart failure, not amenable to other forms of treatment. The prognosis of transplant recipients has dramatically improved, since the introduction of cyclosporin for immunosuppression. One-year survival is now approaching 90%, with a 5-year survival in excess of 60%.

In the majority of transplant recipients, the cause of heart failure is either cardiomyopathy or end-stage ischaemic heart disease. In both cases, the indication for treatment is severe symptoms, refractory to medical therapy and not amenable to other forms of surgery. Such patients have a very limited life expectancy, which is dramatically improved by transplantation.

The timing of transplantation is difficult. On the one hand, the patient must have severe enough impairment of left ventricular function to warrant a transplant. On the other, if the operation is undertaken at a stage when the patient has end-stage heart failure, causing failure of other organ systems, the success of transplantation decreases dramatically. For this reason, patients are best referred for transplant assessment sooner rather than later.

Immunosuppression

Immunosuppression is achieved by a combination of:

- cyclosporin;
- corticosteroids;
- azathioprine.

Using multiple therapy, successful immunosuppression can be achieved with lower doses of each agent. This minimises the side-effects of each. The degree of immunosuppression needs to be greatest in the earlier stages after transplantation, but can subsequently be reduced to a low maintenance level. Patients remain susceptible to episodes of rejection, but these can be managed by increasing immunosuppressive therapy when they occur.

Rejection

The recognition of episodes of rejection is important in transplant patients. The patient is generally non-specifically unwell. Clinical features may include the development of a third heart sound and atrial arrhythmias. The ECG may show reduction in QRS voltages, but this is a relatively late finding.

Diagnosis is based upon cardiac biopsy and this should be undertaken on suspicion of rejection. This is a simple procedure performed under local anaesthetic using either rigid biopsy forceps introduced into the jugular vein in the neck or using a biopsy catheter introduced into the femoral vein.

Complications

In addition to rejection, heart transplant recipients are subject to a number of other problems.

Infection. This remains a major cause of death in transplant recipients. Viral infections, such as cytomegalovirus and Herpes zoster, which produce relatively trivial infections in normal individuals, can be life-threatening in immunosuppressed patients. It is important that even minor symptoms should be investigated to detect and treat any infective illness early.

Accelerated atherosclerosis. Heart transplant patients develop accelerated atherosclerosis. This occurs both in patients whose pre-operative diagnosis was cardiomyopathy and in those with pre-operative ischaemic heart disease. It is important that any contributory factor to atherosclerosis, such as hypercholesterolaemia, should be adequately controlled. Patients should also undergo regular assessment with coronary angiography.

Cyclosporin nephrotoxicity. Patients should be regularly reviewed with a check of their renal function and cyclosporin levels, to minimize the risk of nephrotoxicity.

Cushingoid features. The features of Cushing disease are, in general, less troublesome with the advent of cyclosporin and reduction in steroid dosage.

Malignancy. It is well recognized that there is an increased incidence of malignant disease, particularly lymphoproliferative disorders, in immunosuppressed patients.

Despite these difficulties, cardiac transplantation is a highly successful procedure, in patients fortunate enough to receive a transplant. The main limitation in the growth of transplantation continues to be availability of donor hearts.

Heart/lung transplantation

Heart/lung transplantation is still much less common than simple heart transplantation. Conditions requiring heart/lung transplantation include primary pulmonary hypertension and congenital cardiac abnormalities which have resulted in Eisenmenger's syndrome. These indications have now grown to include patients with end-stage pulmonary disease, particularly patients with cystic fibrosis.

The success rate for heart/lung transplantation is not yet as good as that for heart transplantation, with 1-year survival figures reported of approximately 70%.

Further reading

Braunwald, E. (1992) Pathophysiology of heart failure. In Braunwald, E. (Ed.) *Heart Disease.* Philadelphia: Saunders.

Chatterjee, K. & Parmley, W.W. (1983) Vasodilator therapy for acute myocardial infarction and chronic congestive heart failure. *Journal of the American College of Cardiology* **1**: 133.

Dollery, C.T. & Corr, L. (1985) Drug treatment of heart failure. *British Heart Journal* **54**: 234.

Editorial (1992) The prevention of heart failure. *New England Journal of Medicine* **327**: 725.

Harris, P. (1983) Evolution and the cardiac patient. *Cardiovascular Research* **17**: 313, 373, 437.

Julian, D.G. & Wenger, N.K. (Eds) (1986) *Management of Heart Failure.* London: Butterworths.

Lant, A. (1985) Diuretics: clinical pharmacology and therapeutics. *Drugs* **29**: Part I: 57; Part II: 162.

Maclean, D. & Tudhope, G.R. (1983) Modern diuretic treatment. *British Medical Journal* **286**: 1419.

Packer, M. (1987) Do vasodilators prolong life in heart failure? *New England Journal of Medicine* **316**: 1471.

Parmley, W.W. (1989) Pathophysiology and current therapy of congestive heart failure. *Journal of the American College of Cardiology* **13**: 771.

Smith, T.W. (1988) Digitalis: mechanisms of action and chemical use. *New England Journal of Medicine* **318**: 358.

Disorders of Rate, Rhythm and Conduction

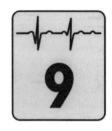

9

MECHANISMS OF ARRHYTHMIAS

As is discussed in more detail in Chapter 2, there are electrically two types of cell in the myocardium — the automatic and the non-automatic — the automatic cells having the capacity of self excitation. The group of automatic cells with the most rapid rate of spontaneous depolarization dominates the heart as the pacemaker. This is normally the sinus node, which is under the control both of the vagus and of the sympathetic nervous system. Ectopic rhythms, in which the heart is activated from a pacemaker other than the sinus node, arise from a variety of mechanisms:

- escape of lower centres;
- increased automaticity of other zones;
- re-entry.

Escape of lower centres

An increase in vagal activity reduces the rate of spontaneous depolarization of the sinus node and thereby slows the heart; another group of automatic cells may then exhibit a rate faster than that of the sinus node and become the pacemaker.

Increased automaticity of other zones

Increased sympathetic activity increases the rate of discharge not only of the sinus node, but also of other areas, including the ventricles. Ischaemia, digitalis intoxication and electrolyte disorders also enhance ventricular automaticity.

Re-entry

Re-entry arrhythmias arise due to a self-perpetuating 'circus' move-

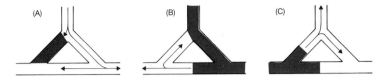

Fig. 9.1 The re-entry phenomenon. In (A) the impulse cannot enter a zone which is still in the refractory phase. In (B) this zone has become receptive as adjacent muscle becomes refractory. In (C) the impulse leaves the newly activated zone and re-enters the same tissue as was activated in (A) which has now recovered. The refractory zone is shown in red.

ment of the cardiac impulse. There are two requirements for re-entry:

- non-uniform refractoriness;
- slow conduction.

Non-uniform recovery of refractoriness is necessary to create an area of unidirectional conduction block (Fig. 9.1). Slow conduction is necessary to fulfil the fundamental requirement that conduction time over the re-entry circuit should exceed the longest refractory period of any point in the circuit.

For most re-entrant arrhythmias, the re-entrant conduction pathway cannot be defined anatomically. Re-entry occurs in small areas of atrial or ventricular muscle (micro re-entry). In some instances, however, the anatomical components of the re-entry circuit can be defined. The best example of such a macro re-entry pathway is the Wolff–Parkinson–White syndrome, in which a slender bundle of myocardium forms a bridge between the atria and the ventricles, bypassing the atrioventricular node (Fig. 9.2). Re-entry tachycardias commonly arise by conduction of the cardiac impulse from atrium to ventricle through the AV node and from ventricle to atrium over the accessory pathway. Slow conduction through the AV node ensures that conduction time over the re-entry circuit exceeds the maximum refractory period in the pathway.

In most re-entrant arrhythmias, however, the pathways are less clearly defined.

DISTURBANCES OF RATE AND RHYTHM

Sinus node abnormalities

Sinus tachycardia

Sinus tachycardia is sinus rhythm at a rate faster than is normal (Fig. 9.3). In adults, this is commonly defined as being greater than 100/

(A)   Sinus rhythm   (B)   Re-entry tachycardia

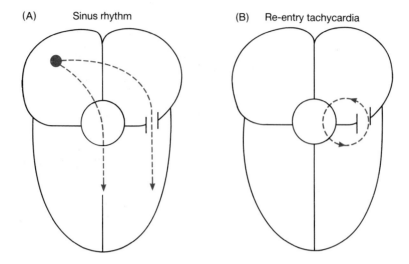

Fig. 9.2   Re-entry mechanisms: Wolff–Parkinson–White syndrome. (A) In sinus rhythm the ventricles are activated over two pathways, via the AV node and via an accessory pathway. (B) During the common form of re-entry tachycardia a reentrant loop is established conducting antegradely via the AV node and retrogradely via the accessory pathway.

min. In children the heart rate, even at rest, frequently exceeds 100 / min, and in infants may exceed 150/min. Amongst factors associated with disease which cause sinus tachycardia are:

- anaemia;
- hyperthyroidism;
- fever;
- blood loss and hypovolaemia;
- heart failure;
- drugs such as adrenaline, isoprenaline, ephedrine, propantheline, atropine and thyroxine.

Sinus tachycardia is seldom harmful and may be a compensatory mechanism.

The patient with sinus tachycardia may complain of palpitation which is of gradual and explicable onset, unlike the abrupt and unexpected appearance of the symptom in paroxysmal tachycardia. The diagnosis is usually obvious when there is a regular pulse at a rate of more than 100/min. Frequently, the tachycardia subsides during the examination as anxiety diminishes. Carotid sinus pressure causes little slowing in contrast to its usually dramatic effect in atrial

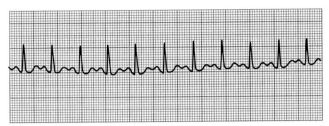

Fig. 9.3 Sinus tachycardia.

tachycardia or atrial flutter. The ECG shows P waves having a normal relationship to QRS complexes. The J point may be depressed; the ST then slopes upward.

Sinus tachycardia does not of itself require treatment although the underlying cause of tachycardia should be sought and, where necessary, treated.

Sinus bradycardia

Sinus bradycardia describes a slow heart in sinus rhythm (Fig. 9.4). This term is commonly applied to heart rates of less than 60/min, although such rates are frequently seen in healthy elderly people; in the highly trained athlete the heart rate may be less than 40/min. Amongst factors causing sinus bradycardia are:

- increased vagal tone (e.g. during carotid sinus massage);
- myxoedema;
- hypothermia;
- raised intracranial pressure;
- drugs including digitalis and the beta-adrenergic blocking agents such as propranolol.

Sinus bradycardia seldom gives rise to symptoms or undesirable haemodynamic effects but, occasionally, in the elderly and in acute

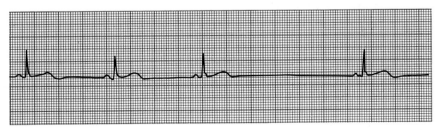

Fig. 9.4 Sinus bradycardia. A marked sinus bradycardia of 40 beats per minute is followed by a 2.7 second pause before the next sinus beat.

myocardial infarction, cardiac failure or hypotension may develop if the stroke output cannot be increased to compensate adequately for the slow rate. The heart can be accelerated by atropine 0.6 mg subcutaneously or intravenously. Oral sympathomimetics, such as long-acting isoprenaline, can also be used to treat sinus bradycardia, but in general pacing is preferable.

Sick sinus syndrome

Sinus bradycardia is a component of the sick sinus syndrome, a relatively common condition amongst the elderly. The bradycardia may be complicated by paroxysms of atrial tachyarrhythmias (tachycardia, flutter or fibrillation), the so-called bradycardia–tachycardia syndrome (Fig. 9.5). Syncope may result either from too slow or too fast a heart rate.

Sick sinus syndrome is seldom life-threatening, but frequently causes distressing symptoms of palpitations, dizziness or syncope. These can be treated by implantation of a pacemaker. Tachyarrhythmias may require antiarrhythmic drug therapy combined with a pacemaker to guard against bradycardia

Sinus arrhythmia (Fig. 9.6)

Normally, the sinus node does not discharge with absolute regularity owing to variations in vagal tone. These variations are related to

(A)

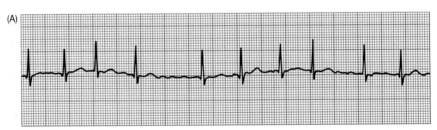

(B)

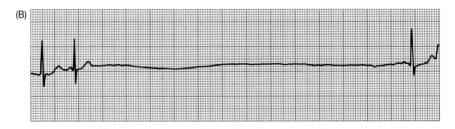

Fig. 9.5   Sick sinus syndrome with bradycardia and tachycardia. (A) Tachycardia due to atrial fibrillation. (B) Termination of atrial fibrillation is followed by a prolonged asystolic pause, eventually terminated by a sinus beat.

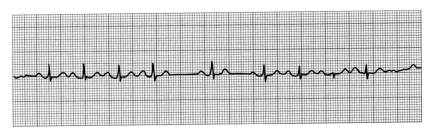

Fig. 9.6 Sinus arrhythmia. Acceleration of the sinus rate is evident during inspiration and slowing during expiration.

respiration, and it is characteristic in the young to find acceleration of the heart during inspiration with slowing during expiration. This phasic change in the rhythm of the heart is known as sinus arrhythmia. It is seldom clinically obvious in adults, but is occasionally seen in the healthy old person. It is of no clinical importance, but it must be differentiated from the other types of arrhythmia. Its relationship to respiration usually makes this easy.

Supraventricular arrhythmias

A variety of rhythm disturbances can arise in the atria and AV junctional area (that is, the AV node and adjacent specialized tissues). These may result from either increased automaticity or re-entry.

Atrial ectopic beats (atrial extrasystoles, atrial premature beats)

Atrial ectopic beats are common in normal individuals, but seldom give rise to symptoms, apart from an awareness of heart irregularity from time to time. They cause an occasional irregularity in an otherwise normal pulse, and are usually abolished by exercise. The diagnosis is readily confirmed from the ECG (Fig. 9.7) which shows a premature beat occurring earlier than the next anticipated sinus beat. The P wave differs in configuration from that of a sinus beat, because

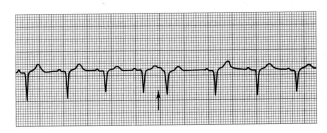

Fig. 9.7 Atrial ectopic beat. A premature P wave (arrowed) is followed by a QRS complex of normal appearance.

depolarization of the atria takes place in an abnormal direction. The accompanying QRST complex is usually similar to that of previous beats of sinus origin because the pathway of ventricular depolarization is normal. Occasionally, the QRST complex is abnormally broad ('aberrant') because the impulse passes down only one of the bundle branches, the other still being refractory from the preceding beat. It then simulates the appearance of a ventricular ectopic beat (see p. 181) but is usually preceded by a P wave.

Atrial ectopic beats may presage the appearance of other atrial arrhythmias but they require no treatment.

Junctional (nodal) ectopic beats

Ectopic beats deriving from the junctional tissue are quite common and, like atrial ectopic beats, usually benign. They are responsible for an occasional irregularity in an otherwise regular pulse and cannot be diagnosed without an electrocardiogram, which shows the same features as with atrial ectopic beats except that the P wave is inverted in lead II and is either buried in the QRS complex, or precedes or follows it by a very short interval. No treatment is necessary.

Junctional (nodal) rhythm (Fig. 9.8)

In this condition the junctional tissue is acting as the pacemaker of the heart and the ECG appearance is that of a succession of junctional ectopic beats. It is usually a transient condition resulting from a depression of sinus node activity. It occurs in some normal individuals and may be provoked by digitalis or ischaemic heart disease. The heart rate is usually in the region of 50–60/min and no treatment is required. If the heart rate is undesirably slow, it can be accelerated by the use of atropine.

In patients with acute myocardial infarction treated with thrombolytic therapy, the occurrence of junctional rhythm is an indicator of successful reperfusion.

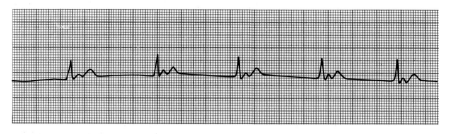

Fig. 9.8 Junctional rhythm. In this example retrograde conduction into the atria is relatively slow and a P wave can be distinguished after the QRS complex, interrupting the ST segment.

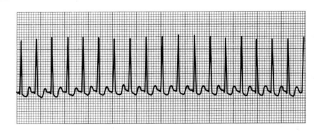

Fig. 9.9   Supraventricular tachycardia. Regular narrow QRS tachycardia at a rate of 220 beats/min.

Paroxysmal supraventricular tachycardias (Fig. 9.9)

In its broadest sense, the term paroxysmal supraventricular tachycardia might refer to any recurrent supraventricular arrhythmia. However. arrhythmias originating within the atrium (atrial tachycardia, atrial flutter and atrial fibrillation) are generally excluded. The term encompasses a number of different arrhythmias, which share certain characteristics — starting abruptly, usually being regular at a rate of 140–220/min, and being associated with narrow QRS complexes, closely resembling those seen in sinus rhythm. Aberrant conduction with broadening of the QRS may, however, occur as may rates above and below those quoted.

The majority of arrhythmias are due to re-entry. In the commonest form, re-entry involves dual pathways within the AV node which have different rates of conduction and refractoriness. In other cases re-entry is dependent on the presence of an additional connection (accessory pathway), linking atrium and ventricle. The best recognized form is Wolff–Parkinson–White syndrome, which is characterized in sinus rhythm by a short PR interval and delta wave (p. 190). During the common form of tachycardia, excitation passes from atrium to ventricle over the AV node and from ventricle to atrium via the accessory pathway. As the ventricles are excited over the normal route QRS complexes are narrow. The absence of a delta wave during sinus rhythm does not exclude the possibility of an accessory pathway, as some pathways only conduct retrogradely from ventricle to atrium. These pathways are hence 'concealed' during sinus rhythm, but can still conduct retrogradely giving rise to a re-entrant tachycardia.

The attacks may last only seconds, but they often persist for minutes or hours or, much less commonly, for days. They may recur at short intervals or be separated from one another by weeks, months or even years. It is sometimes possible to identify provoking factors such as tobacco, coffee, and alcohol. Paroxysms are most often encountered in otherwise normal people in whom they give rise to palpitation, but no serious haemodynamic effects. These tachycardias

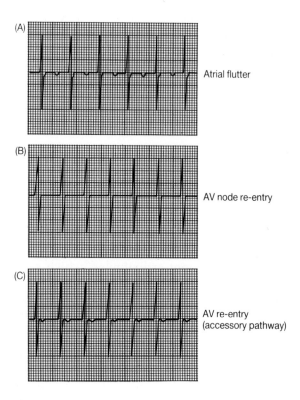

Atrial flutter

AV node re-entry

AV re-entry
(accessory pathway)

Fig. 9.10 Differential diagnosis of regular narrow QRS tachycardia. Schematic ECGs. (A) Atrial flutter with 2 : 1 AV block. Close examination of the trace reveals two flutter waves (arrowed) for every QRS complex. (See also Fig. 9.11). (B) Atrioventricular nodal re-entry tachycardia. Atrial depolarization is generally synchronous with ventricular depolarization. The P wave is either lost within the QRS complex or is in the terminal portion of the QRS complex. (C) Atrioventricular re-entry tachycardia due to the presence of an accessory pathway. A P wave is evident after the QRS complex, reflecting retrograde atrial activation over the accessory pathway. (See also Fig. 9.27.)

can, however, produce cardiac failure and hypotension in the presence of heart disease because of the increased workload of the heart and the inadequate filling time during diastole.

The patient usually complains of attacks of rapid regular palpitation of abrupt onset, sometimes accompanied by dizziness or even syncope. When the attack is prolonged or when it occurs in those with heart disease, there may be dyspnoea and ischaemic chest pain. There may also be polyuria.

The episodes are often so brief and infrequent that no doctor ever sees them; if the patient is observed at the time, the pulse is found to be regular at a rate between 140 and 220. Carotid sinus massage frequently terminates the attack, but if it fails to do so, it has no effect upon the pulse rate. The ECG usually reveals QRST complexes of normal or near normal configuration occurring rapidly and regularly. The presence and timing of a P wave is of diagnostic value (Fig. 9.10):

- a P wave which is 'absent' (hidden in the QRS or in the terminal portion of the QRS) suggests AV node re-entry as the underlying mechanism of tachycardia;
- a P wave following the QRS suggests the presence of an accessory pathway.
- Atrial flutter with a 2:1 AV block should also be considered in a differential diagnosis (Fig. 9.10).

It is difficult to obtain conventional ECG recordings of the attacks because of their unpredictability and brevity; the documentation of episodes is aided by dynamic electrocardiography (Holter monitoring), and by patient-activated ECG recorders.

The ECG between attacks is usually normal, but the appearances of the Wolff–Parkinson–White syndrome, the 'short PR syndrome' (with a normal QRS), or other abnormalities of conduction may be seen.

Termination of the acute attack. In the treatment of the individual attack, the patient may be taught to carry out the Valsalva manoeuvre and the doctor can use carotid sinus massage. If these procedures prove unsuccessful, drug treatment should be considered. As the majority of tachycardias arise by re-entry either within or involving the AV node, drugs slowing AV nodal conduction are indicated:

- intravenous verapamil is commonly chosen (5–10 mg i.v. over 30–60 s);
- verapamil should not be given if the patient is already receiving a beta-blocker;
- intravenous adenosine has recently been introduced as an alternative to verapamil. Adenosine causes a transient but profound inhibition of AV node conduction (p. 369).

In patients in whom the safety and efficacy of intravenous verapamil has been demonstrated, it is reasonable to provide the patient with a supply of oral verapamil to take a stat 120 mg dose in the event of an acute attack, hence avoiding the need for hospital attendance.

Prevention. Because of the repetitive paroxysmal nature of the tachycardia, prevention is often of greater importance than the treatment of the individual attack. When possible, a provoking factor such as strong coffee or tobacco should be identified and avoided. If episodes are infrequent and symptoms are not severe, drug treatment is not required and simple reassurance is all that is necessary. In other patients stat doses of verapamil as outlined above can obviate the need for continuous drug treatment. When drug therapy is required, a number of drugs can be considered. These include beta-adrenergic blockers and verapamil. Class I antiarrhythmic drugs such as flecainide are also effective for prophylaxis, but their long-term safety is in doubt and these drugs are best avoided if possible.

In some patients, antitachycardia pacing provides an alternative to drug treatment (see p. 195). Catheter ablation is a further alternative (see p. 197)

Atrial tachycardia with block

This is a relatively rare arrhythmia, which is commonly due to advanced digitalis intoxication. There is nearly always cellular potassium depletion, but the serum potassium is not necessarily low.

The ventricular rate depends upon the degree of AV block. Commonly, this is 2:1 and there are no adverse haemodynamic effects as the ventricular rate is about 80–100/min.

The clinical recognition of this rhythm disturbance is virtually impossible and the diagnosis must be made from the electrocardiogram, in which P waves are seen to occur at a rate of 140–220/min; there is either a prolongation of the PR interval or some of the P waves are not followed by QRS complexes. Carotid sinus pressure produces a transient increase in the atrioventricular block with a corresponding fall in the ventricular rate — a response quite unlike that of paroxysmal supraventricular tachycardia (see p. 178).

Atrial tachycardia with block is seldom dangerous in itself and generally does not require specific treatment. Digitalis should be stopped and potassium supplements given. Electrical shock should not be used unless it is certain that digitalis intoxication is not responsible, as it may induce more serious arrhythmias.

Atrial flutter (Fig. 9.11)

In this arrhythmia, the atria beat regularly at a rate of 250–350/min — usually close to 300/min. In most cases the arrhythmia arises due to micro re-entry circuits within the atria.

Some degree of AV block is almost invariable. In most instances the ventricles beat regularly because of a 2:1, 3:1 or 4:1 response to the regular atrial activity, but it is irregular if the degree of block varies from cycle to cycle. The commonest variety is that of 2:1 block which characteristically has a ventricular rate of 140–160. In cases with 2:1 block flutter waves are not always obvious. Any regular,

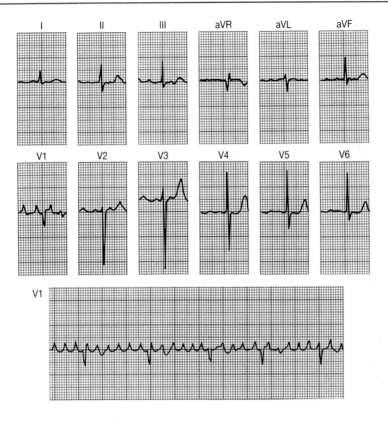

Fig. 9.11 Atrial flutter. Flutter waves are most readily apparent in the right-sided chest leads V1 and V2. They are also seen in inferior leads, III and aVF. A high degree of AV block is apparent with 5–6 flutter waves for every 1 QRS complex. Rhythm strip lead is V1.

narrow QRS complex arrhythmia in this rate band should be closely scrutinized for the presence of flutter waves (Fig. 9.10 and 9.11).

Atrial flutter is almost always a complication of underlying organic heart disease. Common associations include:

- rheumatic heart disease;
- ischaemic heart disease;
- myocarditis;
- hyperthyroidism.

It may be persistent or occur in paroxysms which are usually self-limited to hours or days, but it may progress to atrial fibrillation. The symptoms resemble those of atrial tachycardia, with palpitation, dizziness or syncope. The arrhythmia often provokes cardiac failure.

The pulse is usually regular at a rate of 140–160/min. It may be possible to see venous 'flutter' waves in the neck. Carotid sinus massage leads to a transient increase in the atrioventricular block, with a slowing of the ventricular rate only as long as the pressure is maintained.

The electrocardiogram is diagnostic with 'flutter' waves of a sawtooth appearance, best seen in leads VI and III occurring at approximately 300/min. The sawtooth nature of the complexes may be obscured by the QRS complexes when there is 2:1 block, but it is readily revealed when carotid sinus massage is applied.

Drug treatment is seldom effective in restoring sinus rhythm. Digitalis increases the AV block, brings the heart rate under control, and sometimes abolishes the arrhythmia. Intravenous amiodarone is more likely to restore sinus rhythm, but requires a central line for its administration. Shock (d.c.) is indicated if immediate correction is necessary and is almost invariably effective (see p. 194). In the patient liable to paroxysms of atrial flutter, beta-blockers, particularly sotalol, may be of some value. If this is ineffective, oral amiodarone is an alternative, but carries a risk of serious long-term side effects (see p.202).

Atrial fibrillation (Fig. 9.12)

In this arrhythmia, irregular atrial impulses occur at rates over 300/min. It may be due to multiple foci of ectopic activity or to wavelets of excitation following variable courses through the atrial myocardium depending upon the location of patches of excitable and refractory muscle. Some degree of AV block is invariable; the ventricular rhythm is slower than the atrial but it is also irregular.

The presence of atrial fibrillation suggests that there has been either a pathological process involving the atria, as in rheumatic heart disease, or that there has been a rise in pressure with atrial dilatation secondary to mitral valve or left ventricular disease. Common causes of atrial fibrillation include:

- rheumatic mitral valve disease;

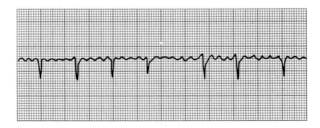

Fig. 9.12 Atrial fibrillation. The rhythm strip shows narrow QRS complexes which are irregularly irregular.

- ischaemic heart disease, particularly acute myocardial infarction;
- alcohol;
- thyrotoxicosis;
- hypertension;
- acute infections, particularly when these affect the lungs;
- cardiopulmonary surgery.

It is a rare complication of many other types of heart disease. In a substantial proportion of patients, no evidence of organic heart disease can be found — 'lone' atrial fibrillation. The incidence of lone atrial fibrillation is greater amongst younger patients.

Atrial fibrillation may be paroxysmal, with attacks lasting for a few minutes or hours. This is particularly likely in acute myocardial infarction, in chest infections, and in the early stages of thyrotoxicosis and mitral valve disease. In rheumatic cases, the arrhythmia usually becomes established eventually and persists for the rest of the patient's life.

Atrial fibrillation leads to untoward effects for three major reasons:

- the ventricular response may be so fast that there is inadequate time for diastolic filling and the cardiac output falls;
- the atrial contribution to ventricular filling is lost;
- stasis in the ineffectively contracting atrium encourages thrombosis. As a consequence, embolism is common, particularly in patients with mitral valve disease. Emboli from the right atrium produce pulmonary artery obstruction; those from the left atrium may lodge in cerebral, renal or other peripheral vessels.

The first symptom may be that of irregular palpitations, but in many patients atrial fibrillation leads to the sudden development of left ventricular failure and pulmonary oedema. The onset may also be insidious with gradually increasing dyspnoea.

The diagnosis is usually easy because the arterial pulse is totally irregular. The ventricular response to atrial fibrillation appears random. Because of the varying times available for filling of the ventricles, the output of the heart and the volume of the pulse alter from beat to beat. This chaotic pulse serves to differentiate atrial fibrillation from atrial or ventricular ectopic beats, which are the arrhythmias most likely to be confused with it. In these latter conditions some periods of regularity are usually observed, and often the irregularity will be noted to occur every second, third or fourth beat. The venous pulse in atrial fibrillation is also irregular. The heart rate at the apex ('the apex rate') is usually higher than the radial pulse rate because the heart expels so little blood in some beats that no pulsation can be appreciated in the peripheral arteries.

In the electrocardiogram, the P wave disappears but atrial activity produces an irregular undulation of the base line (Fig. 9.12). The QRS complexes are totally irregular in timing, except in the rare situation of atrial fibrillation complicated by complete heart block. In most cases of untreated atrial fibrillation, the ventricular rate lies between 100 and 160/min, but rates above or below this are not uncommon.

Although patients with the arrhythmia may survive for many years with few symptoms, atrial fibrillation is frequently a serious complication because of the risks of heart failure and embolism.

Treatment. There are four aspects to the treatment of atrial fibrillation:

- the control of ventricular rate;
- the restoration of sinus rhythm;
- the maintenance of sinus rhythm;
- prevention of embolism.

Control of the ventricular rate. Control of the ventricular rate is a priority because it is the fast ventricular rate that is most deleterious, rather than the atrial fibrillation *per se*, and also because the arrhythmia may terminate spontaneously. Depending upon the severity of the clinical situation, digoxin or one of the other cardiac glycosides may be given intravenously or orally. In most cases, oral administration is satisfactory, and brings the heart rate under control within 2–3 h. When full digitalization has been achieved, the ventricular rate at rest should be held at about 70–80/min. If the heart rate cannot be reduced to this level, a beta-adrenoceptor blocking drug or verapamil may be added. Amiodarone is useful in intractable cases.

Restoration of sinus rhythm. When atrial fibrillation has been present for many years, and there is associated and untreatable severe heart disease, there is little to be gained by trying to restore normal rhythm because this is not likely to be maintained. Even if it is, the atrial muscle has usually atrophied and is functionally ineffective. When the arrhythmia is of relatively recent onset, and particularly when the heart disease has been alleviated or some complicating condition such as thyrotoxicosis or pulmonary infection corrected, the patient is likely to benefit from its termination.

In some patients sinus rhythm can be restored by pharmacological means. Amiodarone is frequently used for this purpose. The class I antiarrhythmic drug, flecainide, has also been used successfully, but should be used with caution because of the risk of pro-arrhythmia.

Electric shock therapy is the most reliable means of restoring sinus rhythm and is effective in most instances, at least initially. However, there is a considerable relapse rate within the succeeding months.

The maintenance of sinus rhythm presents a difficult problem, particularly in patients with paroxysmal atrial fibrillation. Both amiodarone and class I antiarrhythmic agents are of proven value. However amiodarone may give rise to serious side-effects and there are serious concerns regarding the potential pro-arrhythmic effects associated with the long-term use of class I antiarrhythmic drugs. Other agents, such as the beta-blocker sotalol, have less troublesome side-effects, but are also less effective. Drug selection must therefore be tailored to the severity of the problem posed by recurrent episodes of atrial fibrillation. Digoxin is of no value in preventing recurrences of atrial fibrillation.

Anticoagulation. Patients with atrial fibrillation complicating rheumatic heart disease should be anticoagulated. Recent evidence has shown that patients with non-rheumatic atrial fibrillation, but with demonstrable underlying heart disease, also benefit from anticoagulation. The benefits of anticoagulation in patients with lone atrial fibrillation remain uncertain and aspirin should be considered as an alternative. Anticoagulation is also indicated for 1 month before and 1 month after elective cardioversion.

THE CAROTID SINUS AND ARRHYTHMIAS

The carotid sinus is situated at the bifurcation of the common carotid artery and is sensitive to changes in arterial pressure. Impulses arising from the stretch receptors in the carotid sinus pass to the medulla and reflexly slow the heart by stimulating the motor nucleus of the vagus nerve and by inhibiting cardiac sympathetic action. Usually, external pressure on the carotid sinus leads to a slight slowing of the heart rate by reducing the activity of the sinus node. In some individuals in whom the carotid sinus is hypersensitive, external pressure leads to extreme bradycardia and hypotension with resulting syncope.

Carotid sinus pressure plays an important part in the recognition and management of cardiac arrhythmias. It is best to locate the carotid artery on one side first and then to stroke it gently, but firmly. If this is ineffective, the manoeuvre should be repeated on the other side:

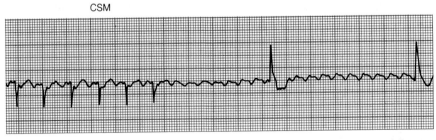

Fig. 9.13 Carotid sinus massage in atrial flutter. The initial tracing shows atrial flutter with 2:1 atrioventricular block. Carotid sinus massage causes a high degree of atrioventricular block, enabling the individual flutter waves to be clearly distinguished. The subsequent QRS complexes are ventricular escape beats.

- *sinus tachycardia*. Carotid sinus massage causes only slight slowing of the ventricular rate in patients with sinus tachycardia;
- *atrial fibrillation*. Carotid sinus massage causes slight slowing of the ventricular response;
- *paroxysmal supraventricular tachycardia*. Carotid sinus massage causes an abrupt termination of the arrhythmia, if it has any effect at all;
- *atrial flutter*. Carotid sinus massage produces an increase in atrioventricular block, temporarily decreasing the ventricular rate which rises again when the massage is discontinued (Fig. 9.13);
- *ventricular tachycardia*. Carotid sinus massage has no effect.

It is best to carry out carotid sinus massage with ECG control, as excessive bradycardia and even ventricular arrhythmias may result from this procedure. Other dangers include reflex hypotension and cerebrovascular insufficiency. The procedure carries additional hazard in the presence of a carotid bruit.

Ventricular ectopic rhythms

Ventricular ectopic beats (extrasystoles, premature beats)

An ectopic focus in the ventricles may arise because of ventricular escape, enhanced automatic activity, or re-entry. Ventricular ectopic beats are not uncommon in normal individuals but are encountered frequently in organic heart disease, especially in myocardial infarction. If they occur every second beat (bigeminy or 'coupling') they are frequently due to digitalis therapy.

Patients are seldom aware of ventricular ectopic beats, but may complain of the heart seeming to stop briefly, or of an occasional heavy beat. The diagnosis may be suspected from an irregularity of the pulse interrupting an otherwise regular rhythm, but cannot be made without an ECG, in which there are bizarre and broadened QRS

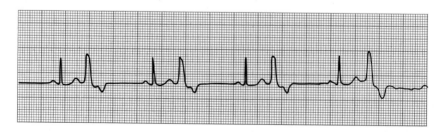

Fig. 9.14 Ventricular ectopic beats. Each sinus beat is followed by a broad complex ventricular ectopic beat. The constant coupling in this example is termed ventricular bigeminy.

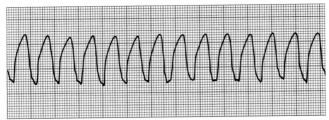

Fig. 9.15   Ventricular tachycardia. Regular wide QRS tachycardia at a rate of 170/min.

complexes followed by T waves pointing in the direction opposite to that of the main QRS component (Fig. 9.14). The QRST complexes are not preceded by a P wave and are usually succeeded by a long period (the compensatory pause) before the next sinus-activated beat appears.

The importance of ventricular ectopic beats depends upon their context. In normal individuals they are virtually of no consequence. Such individuals should undergo clinical examination, echocardiography and exercise testing to rule out structural heart disease or coronary disease. Ventricular ectopic beats are associated with an impaired prognosis in ischaemic heart disease. But there is no evidence that suppression of ventricular ectopics with antiarrhythmic drugs improves prognosis. On the contrary, the class I antiarrhythmic drugs flecainide and encainide have recently been shown to increase mortality in patients with ventricular ectopic beats following myocardial infarction, despite reducing the frequency of ectopic beats.

Ventricular tachycardia (Fig. 9.15)

In this condition a tachycardia arises in the ventricles at a rate of 120–220/min; the atria usually remain under the control of the sinus node. It may be a consequence of either re-entry or enhanced automaticity of ventricular pacemaker cells. It is nearly always a complication of serious heart disease, although occasionally seen in an otherwise normal individual. The attacks are liable to occur in paroxysms lasting for seconds or minutes, but may continue for several hours. Ventricular tachycardia frequently causes or aggravates heart failure and the shock syndrome.

As with supraventricular tachycardia, the first symptom may be that of rapid and regular palpitations, but because of the more serious effects on the circulation, acute breathlessness and ischaemic chest pain tend to be more severe. On examination there is a rapid, regular but small pulse. The independent atrial activity may be responsible for dissociated 'a' waves in the venous pulse and a variation in the intensity of the first heart sound, but these physical signs are difficult to elicit. The ECG shows rapidly occurring broad QRS complexes resembling those of bundle branch block (Fig. 9.17). P waves may be identified at a rate different from that of the ventricles. The RR intervals are usually equal, but may vary by up to 0.03 s from one another. The lack of response to carotid pressure assists in the differentiation from atrial tachycardia with bundle branch block (see also pp. 177 and 181).

Treatment. In the patient with good underlying heart function, urgent treatment may not be necessary. Most instances of ventricular tachycardia, however, call for immediate action, particularly in the context of acute myocardial infarction. Lignocaine, 100 mg, may be given intravenously and repeated if necessary. Alternative therapy includes flecainide and amiodarone. If these drugs fail to control the arrhythmia, electric shock may be used.

The drugs mentioned above may be used to prevent recurrences but should not be used empirically. The efficacy of drug therapy should be assessed by electrophysiological testing (see p. 34) to ensure that the arrhythmia is successfully controlled and to guard against the possibility of pro-arrhythmic effects.

In patients with ventricular tachycardia which fails to respond to drug therapy, alternative means of treatment should be considered. These include surgery to identify and remove or destroy the area of diseased muscle giving rise to the arrhythmia. An implantable cardioverter defibrillator (p. 197), to terminate automatically episodes of tachycardia represents another option. These devices detect the onset of tachycardia and pace or shock the heart back to its normal rhythm via implanted electrodes.

Torsades de pointes (Fig. 9.16)

This distinctive type of ventricular tachycardia is associated with a long QT interval, and may be idiopathic, due to hypokalaemia, or the result of the toxic action of such drugs as tricyclic antidepressants and type Ia antiarrhythmics. Its characteristic ECG feature is 'twisting of the points' of the QRS complexes. It usually occurs in repetitive bursts

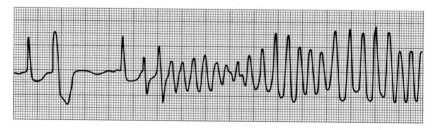

Fig. 9.16 Torsades de pointes. This is a form of polymorphic ventricular tachycardia in which the QRS axis undergoes progressive change. As a result the amplitude of the QRS complexes waxes and wanes.

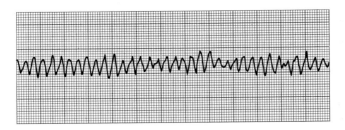

Fig. 9.17   Ventricular fibrillation.

lasting a few seconds; it may progress to ventricular fibrillation. The underlying cause should, if possible, be corrected. Treatment of the arrhythmia with antiarrhythmic drugs should be avoided. Episodes causing haemodynamic compromise should be terminated by d.c. shock. Recurrences can generally be prevented by atrial or ventricular pacing at 90–100/min. If pacing is not available, an infusion of isoprenaline to increase ventricular rate is an alternative.

Ventricular fibrillation (Fig. 9.17)

In this condition there is a chaotic electrical disturbance of the ventricles, with impulses occurring irregularly at a rate of 300–500/min. Ventricular contraction is uncoordinated and ventricular filling and emptying cease. The cardiac output falls precipitously to zero.

Ventricular fibrillation is the commonest cause of sudden death (see p. 137). It may occur as a primary arrhythmia or as a complication of acute myocardial infarction.

It may also result from drowning, electrocution and overdosage of drugs including digitalis, adrenaline and isoprenaline. Self-terminating episodes are rare but may complicate complete heart block.

Because of its catastrophic effects, ventricular fibrillation gives rise to the clinical features of cardiac arrest, with sudden disappearance of arterial pulses, cessation of respiration, loss of consciousness and dilatation of the pupils. Although it cannot be diagnosed clinically, it is to be suspected in any patient dying with apparent suddenness, particularly in the context of acute myocardial infarction. On the electrocardiogram, there is a chaotic rhythm with ventricular complexes of varying amplitude and rate (Fig. 9.17). Eventually asystole ensues.

Ventricular fibrillation is almost invariably fatal, and immediate treatment is necessary if death is to be prevented. As with other forms of cardiac arrest, an effective circulation and ventilation must be obtained within 4 min if irreversible brain damage is not to occur. Sinus rhythm can usually only be restored by electric shock, which should be administered as soon as possible. If an electrical defibrillator is not immediately available, the standard treatment of cardiac

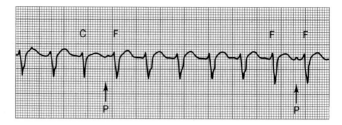

Fig. 9.18 Features of ventricular tachycardia. The ECG shows a slow ventricular tachycardia at a rate of 120/min. Several diagnostic features of ventricular tachycardia are evident: Dissociated P waves (P), narrow complex 'capture' beats, and intermediate morphology 'fusion' (F) beats.

arrest should be started with closed chest cardiac compression and artificial ventilation (see Chapter 20).

Recurrences of ventricular fibrillation should be prevented in the same way as ventricular tachycardia.

THE DIFFERENTIATION OF SUPRAVENTRICULAR FROM VENTRICULAR TACHYCARDIA

The rapid rate associated with some supraventricular tachycardias may result in bundle branch block, causing a broad QRS complex tachycardia which is difficult to distinguish from ventricular tachycardia. It is occasionally possible to distinguish between the two on clinical grounds. In ventricular tachycardia atrial activity is usually dissociated from that of the ventricles. There may be irregular cannon waves in the jugular veins (see p. 51) and variation in the intensity of the first heart sound. In junctional tachycardia, cannon waves may occur with every beat.

The response to carotid sinus massage is sometimes diagnostic (see p. 177), as this manoeuvre frequently abolishes supraventricular tachycardia but leaves ventricular tachycardia unaffected. However, one should delay applying this test if possible until a 12-lead ECG is available, as one may otherwise miss the opportunity of verifying the nature of the arrhythmia by obtaining a graphic record.

Commonly, a clinical diagnosis is not possible. A 12 lead ECG may provide additional formation. ECG evidence of atrial dissociation confirms a diagnosis of ventricular tachycardia (Fig. 9.18). The following findings are diagnostic:

- dissociated P waves;
- capture beats — the dissociated atrial activity 'captures' the ventricle over the normal conduction pathway, giving a single beat with narrow QRS morphology;
- fusion beats — the dissociated atrial activity is conducted into the ventricles fusing with the tachycardia beats and giving a QRS

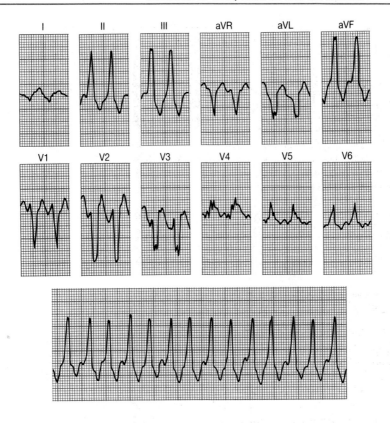

Fig. 9.19 Ventricular tachycardia. The QRS width (140 ms) suggests that the tachycardia is ventricular in origin. For further discussion see text.

morphology intermediate between a supraventricular morphology and the tachycardia morphology.

However, these classical diagnostic features are frequently absent and their absence should not be used to infer a supraventricular origin. There are a number of other ECG features which may be helpful in reaching a diagnosis (Fig. 9.19):

- *QRS width.* A tachycardia with a QRS width greater than 140 ms (3.5 small squares) is very likely to be ventricular;
- *QRS axis.* A tachycardia demonstrating left axis deviation is similarly likely to be ventricular.

If doubt remains it is important to remember that ventricular tachycardia is much more common than supraventricular tachycardia with bundle branch block. When in doubt a tachycardia is best treated

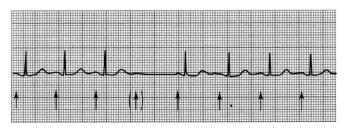

Fig. 9.20 Sinu-atrial exit block. The P waves are regular (arrowed). One P wave is absent (bracketed arrow), but the P wave rhythm is maintained without change in cycle length. The sinus discharge rate has therefore been maintained, although the impulse has failed to exit the sinus node.

as ventricular. Intravenous adenosine may also prove of value in distinguishing supraventricular tachycardia with aberration from ventricular tachycardia (see p. 369).

DISORDERS OF CONDUCTION

Sinu-atrial block and sinus arrest

In sinu-atrial block, an impulse from the sinus node fails to activate the atria. This results in a dropped beat; on the electrocardiogram a complete PQRST complex is absent, but the next sinus beat comes in at the predicted time (Fig. 9.20). It is of little clinical importance except that it may be a manifestation of intoxication by digoxin or other antiarrhythmic drugs. It may be a component of the sick sinus syndrome (see p. 166). If it is prolonged, syncope occurs. In sinus arrest, the sinus node fails to initiate an impulse; after a pause, junctional or ventricular escape occurs. Its significance is similar to that of sinu-atrial block.

Atrioventricular (heart) block

The term atrioventricular (AV) block implies that there is some defect in conduction of the impulse from the atria to the ventricles. In first-degree AV block, all the impulses reach the ventricles but they are delayed in their passage and the PR interval exceeds 0.20 s. In second-degree block, some impulses reach the ventricles while others fail to do so. In complete heart block, no impulses reach the ventricles from the atria, and the ventricles are under the control of a lower pacemaker situated in the junctional tissue, bundle of His, the bundle branches or Purkinje tissue. In bundle branch block, AV conduction is maintained through one branch, the other being blocked.

First-degree AV block (Fig. 9.21). First-degree AV block occurs

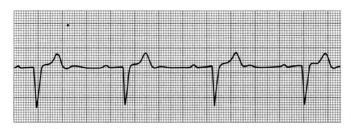

Fig. 9.21   First degree AV block. The PR interval is prolonged at 320 ms. In this example, bradycardia (rate 40) and QRS widening (130 ms) are also evident.

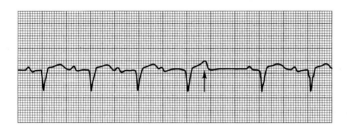

Fig. 9.22   Second degree AV block: Wenckebach. Progressive PR prolongation is evident, culminating in a P wave (arrowed) which fails to conduct to the ventricle.

occasionally in normal individuals, is a characteristic feature of the carditis of acute rheumatic fever, and digitalis overdosage. It cannot be diagnosed clinically and its recognition depends on observing a PR interval of greater than 0.20 s in the ECG. Its only importance is as an index of digitalis intoxication and as a precursor of the more advanced degrees of AV block.

Second-degree AV block.   There are two types of second degree heart block. In the first type (sometimes referred to as *Mobitz type 1* or *Wenckebach block*) the PR interval becomes progressively more prolonged from beat to beat until one P wave is not succeeded by a QRS complex (Fig. 9.22). The next atrial complex is followed at a normal or near normal interval by a QRS complex and the cycle of events recurs.

The pulse is correspondingly irregular. The Wenckebach phenomenon is frequently the result of digitalis intoxication, but both this and the other varieties of second-degree heart block are often due to ischaemic heart disease, particularly myocardial infarction, and to many other types of cardiac disease.

In the second type (*Mobitz type 2*), block occurs without progressive prolongation of the PR interval (Fig. 9.23). This is much rarer than Wenckebach block. Whereas Wenckebach block is indicative of diseased conduction in the AV node, sudden dropped beats, without progressive PR prolongation, suggest disease lower in the

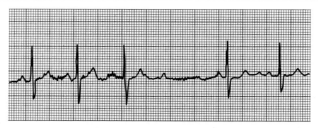

Fig. 9.23 Second degree AV block: Mobitz 2. A P wave fails to conduct to the ventricles, without any progressive PR prolongation beforehand. The tracing is taken from a Holter recording and high frequency artefact is apparent.

His–Purkinje system. In 2 : 1 block there is no opportunity to observe progressive PR prolongation and consequently it is difficult to categorise the site of conduction disturbance.

The main significance of second-degree heart block lies in the liability of the patient to develop complete heart block and the Adams–Stokes syndrome. However, if the ventricular rate in second-degree heart block is sufficiently slow, cardiac failure or hypotension may be precipitated. The more distal the site of block in the conduction system, the less reliable becomes the escape pacemaker if complete heart block develops. For this reason the two types of second degree AV block are of differing significance:

- *sudden dropped beats (Mobitz 2)* indicate disease low in the conduction system and a risk of a poor escape rhythm, should complete heart block develop. They are therefore an indication for pacing;
- *progressive PR prolongation (Mobitz 1)*, on the other hand, indicate AV node disease, is more likely to be succeeded by a satisfactory ventricular escape rhythm, should complete block occur. Pacing, therefore, generally is unnecessary.

Occasionally, the slow heart rate accompanying second-degree AV block is responsible for clinical deterioration and the heart must be accelerated. This may be achieved by administering atropine or by artificial pacing.

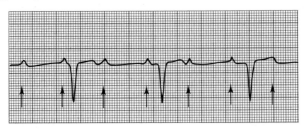

Fig. 9.24 Complete heart block. P waves (arrowed) are completely dissociated from the QRS complexes.

Complete AV (heart) block (Fig. 9.24)

The ventricular rate is slow (25–50/min). There are cannon waves in the venous pulse (see p. 51) and a varying first heart sound (see p. 56).

Acute complete heart block is most commonly a complication of myocardial infarction, but may also result from cardiac surgery and myocarditis. In myocardial infarction, it usually follows occlusion of the right coronary artery which is responsible for the blood supply of the junctional tissue and bundle of His (see also p. 118). The severely damaged heart may not be able to compensate adequately for the bradycardia by increasing its stroke volume; heart failure and hypotension may ensue. There is also a considerable risk of ventricular asystole. The bradycardia may be temporarily controlled by infusing isoprenaline in a dose of 2–5 mg in 500 ml of 5% dextrose, but insertion of an artificial pacemaker is preferable (see p. 375). If the patient survives, normal AV conduction is usually restored within a week.

In most cases of chronic complete heart block there is fibrosis of both bundle branches of unknown cause. This variety is most commonly seen in the elderly. A congenital form occurs either as an isolated finding or in association with other congenital heart defects. Heart block can also complicate rheumatic or ischaemic heart disease, or follow trauma to the conducting tissue at surgery. A proportion of patients with chronic complete heart block survive for years with no symptoms, but once heart failure or syncopal attacks of the Adams–Stokes variety develop, the expectation of life, if left untreated, is usually only a few months. For this reason, an artificial pacemaker is indicated when symptoms arise.

THE ADAMS–STOKES ATTACK

In an Adams–Stokes attack the patient loses consciousness for a period of some seconds because of transient cardiac arrest. It usually occurs in patients with second-degree or complete heart block who develop sudden loss of ventricular activity. It is particularly common during the progression from second-degree to complete heart block because the ventricular pacemaker necessary for survival may not have become firmly established. In some cases, the Adams–Stokes attack is due not to ventricular asystole but to a short burst of ventricular tachycardia or fibrillation.

The presenting symptom is syncope with or without a preceding period of dizziness. The attack usually lasts some 10–30 s and convulsions may occur. During the attack the patient is pulseless, pale or cyanosed. Consciousness returns rapidly with reappearance of the heart beat, the patient then flushing as blood courses through capillaries dilated by the hypoxia of the attack. Attacks of the

Adams–Stokes variety may be separated from one another by a number of months, but occasionally a series occurs over a period of minutes or hours. Sooner or later, the patient is likely to die of ventricular asystole or ventricular fibrillation.

The diagnosis should be considered in any patient presenting with syncope, but is unlikely to be the explanation in the absence of bundle branch block, second-degree block, or complete AV block between the episodes.

During an attack a blow over the cardiac apex may restore the heart action, but if it does not do so, the usual therapy for cardiac arrest should be undertaken (p. 344) with closed-chest cardiac compression and artificial ventilation. Adams–Stokes attacks can be prevented by an artificial pacemaker.

Bundle branch block

In this condition, either the right or the left branch of the bundle of His is not conducting impulses.

Right bundle branch block.   Block of the right bundle branch gives rise to a characteristic electrocardiographic appearance (Fig. 9.25). This is often an isolated congenital lesion of no importance but may be associated with other congenital heart defects, particularly atrial septal defect (p. 274); in middle or advanced age, it is usually due to ischaemic heart disease or idiopathic fibrosis. Right bundle branch block may be partial, with QRS width of less than 0.12 s, or complete,

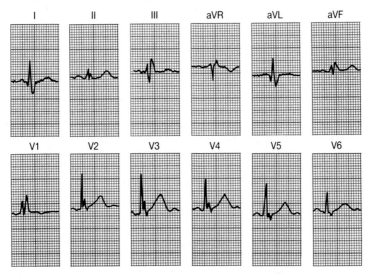

Fig. 9.25   Right bundle branch block and RsR' pattern is evident in lead V1. There is a late S wave in lead V6.

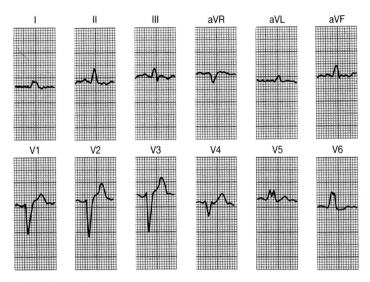

Fig. 9.26 Left bundle branch block.

in which case the QRS is of 0.12 s duration or more. It may be suspected clinically because the block leads to a delayed activation, and therefore contraction, of the right ventricle. This results in late closure of the pulmonary valve which can be recognized by a wide splitting of the second heart sound (p. 56). Right bundle branch block is of minor clinical significance, except as an indicator of possible heart disease and as a precursor of complete heart block (especially if associated with left or right axis deviation indicating block in one of the fascicles of the left bundle).

Left bundle branch block. Left bundle branch block is rare in the otherwise normal individual and is most commonly seen in ischaemic heart disease. It is difficult to recognize clinically, although there may be reversed splitting of the second heart sound (p. 57); it is readily identified on the ECG (Fig. 9.26). Because it is associated with severe ventricular disease (usually ischaemic) it carries a more serious prognosis than right bundle branch block, but patients with this lesion may survive for many years.

Neither form of bundle branch block requires treatment.

Pre-excitation (Wolff–Parkinson–White syndrome)

In this condition, an anomalous conduction pathway bypasses the AV node. This permits the abnormally early activation of part of one ventricle, the remaining ventricular muscle receiving its impulse normally. This leads to a short PR interval (less than 0.12 s) and a slurred upstroke and widening of the QRS (Fig. 9.27).

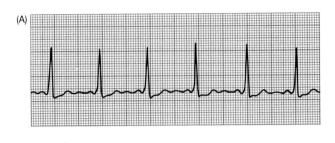

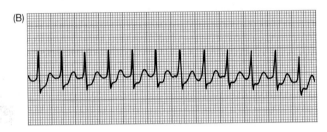

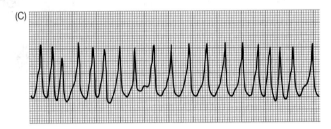

Fig. 9.27 (A) Sinus rhythm. A short PR interval and delta wave are evident. (B) Re-entrant tachycardia. This is the common form of reentrant tachycardia conducting from atrium to ventricle over the AV node and retrogradely from ventricle to atrium over the accessory pathway. It results in a narrow QRS tachycardia with loss of delta wave. (See also Fig. 9.2.) (C) Atrial fibrillation. The characteristic features of atrial fibrillation in Wolff–Parkinson–White syndrome are apparent. 1. Irregular QRS complexes. 2. Varying QRS morphology, reflecting differing degrees of activation over the AV node and accessory pathway. 3. Some very short RR intervals (less than 200 ms), reflecting rapid conduction over the accessory pathway.

The normal and abnormal conduction pathways are able to form part of a re-entry circuit (Fig. 9.2) (p. 164). This facilitates the occurrence of paroxysmal tachycardia. In the common form of re-entry tachycardia the ventricles are excited normally through the AV node and His–Purkinje system. Consequently there is no pre-excitation during tachycardia and the delta wave disappears. On presentation, this narrow QRS tachycardia may be indistinguishable from other causes of paroxysmal supraventricular tachycardia.

Sudden death occasionally occurs in patients with Wolff–

Parkinson–White syndrome. The danger lies not in re-entry tachycardia, but in atrial fibrillation. Normally in patients with atrial fibrillation, the ventricles are protected from the rapid rate of atrial depolarization by the gating effect of the AV node. In patients with an accessory pathway this protection is lost. If the refractory period of the pathway is short, impulses from the atrium can be conducted at very high rates to the ventricle and can result in ventricular fibrillation. Atrial fibrillation, complicating Wolff–Parkinson–White syndrome, should be treated with a drug acting selectively on the accessory pathway to abolish pre-excitation. Intravenous flecainide or intravenous amiodarone are the drugs of choice. Alternatively, the patient can be cardioverted to restore sinus rhythm.

Patients with Wolff–Parkinson–White syndrome and a history of atrial fibrillation or syncope should undergo electrophysiological testing to determine whether the pathway is dangerous and to assess the adequacy of drug treatment. Surgical division of the accessory pathway should be considered. Catheter ablation using radiofrequency currents has recently been introduced and is proving a highly successful alternative to surgery in destroying accessory pathways (p. 197).

MANAGEMENT OF ARRHYTHMIAS

Electrical therapy

CARDIAC PACING

Control over the electrical activity of the heart may be obtained by the use of an artificial pacemaker (Fig. 9.28). A pacemaking system consists of a pulse generator (containing batteries and electronic circuitry) and one or more electrodes. If pacing is to be maintained for only a short period of time, an external power source is used; if long-term pacing is necessary, the pulse generator is implanted.

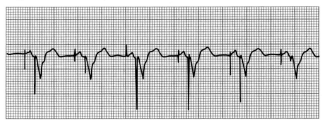

Fig. 9.28   Paced ECG. A dual chamber pacemaker is present, pacing both atrium and ventricle. The first pacing spike is followed by a P wave and the second by a QRS complex.

Electrical pacemaking is potentially hazardous. If the electrical impulse is of sufficient magnitude and falls during the period of ventricular repolarization, i.e. on the T wave of the ECG, ventricular fibrillation may be induced. This problem is overcome by the use of a 'demand' pacemaker which senses the patient's spontaneous beats and operates only when there is no ventricular complex generated by the patient's own heart. In the absence of a complex, the pacemaker discharges after a selected interval.

Temporary pacing

When pacing is employed in the treatment of heart block in acute myocardial infarction, it is customary to introduce the electrode through a peripheral vein and to position its tip in the apex of the right ventricle. The other end of the electrode is attached to a portable battery-operated demand pacemaker. The electrode is withdrawn when the risks of atrioventricular block have resolved. The procedure for insertion of a temporary pacemaker is described in Chapter 20.

Permanent pacing

In chronic heart block, an electrode is positioned with its tip in the right ventricle, and its proximal end attached to a pacemaker buried under the skin of the axillary region or the anterior chest. The pacing electrode may have a single pole, in which pacing is between this pole and the can of the pacemaker (unipolar pacing) or two poles in which case pacing is between the two poles (bipolar pacing). Occasionally electrodes may be placed directly on the surface of the myocardium at the time of a thoracotomy or laparotomy and the wires passed subcutaneously to a pacemaker positioned in the abdomen. However, epicardial pacing is less satisfactory than endocardial. Pacemakers should have a life of more than 10 years but regular checking for battery or other failure is necessary.

Numerous types of pacemaker are now available; most are 'programmable', that is the cardiologist can choose the particular type of pacing programme that is most suitable for an individual patient. Programmable functions include:

- *stimulus voltage and duration.* These factors are programmable to provide an adequate safety margin, exceeding the patient's threshold voltage. Excessive voltages should be avoided as these are an unnecessary drain on the generator and may lead to skeletal muscle twitching;
- *sensing threshold.* In patients with an underlying spontaneous rhythm, the threshold voltage for detection of sensed electrograms can be determined. The sensitivity of the pacemaker is then programmed to provide an adequate margin of safety for detection

of these electrograms. Problems may, however, arise if the pacemaker unit is made excessively sensitive — musculoskeletal potentials may be detected and misinterpreted as cardiac activity, inhibiting pacing. Most pacemakers have noise detection circuits which switch to fixed rate pacing when electrical noise is detected to guard against this possibility;

- *pacing rate*. This sets the rate at which the generator unit will discharge impulses. Many units feature, in addition, hysteresis, that is the heart rate must fall to a lower value than the generator's discharge rate, before pacing will be initiated. For example, a rate of 70/min with hysteresis of 20/min would mean that a pacemaker will only start pacing when the spontaneous heart rate falls below 50/min, at which time pacing will commence at 70/min.

Hazards of pacemaking include infection and failure of the components of the pacemaking unit, such as batteries, circuitry and electrodes.

Dual chamber pacing. Ventricular pacing successfully prevents bradycardias, but it fails to substitute for the heart's normal pacemaker function in two ways. Firstly, the rate of the pacemaker is fixed and cannot adapt to the differing needs of the body, as for example during exercise. Secondly, the normal sequence of atrial and ventricular contraction is lost, which leads to a fall in cardiac output.

In patients who continue to have a normal atrial rhythm, these problems can be prevented by insertion of a dual chamber pacemaker. Dual chamber pacing involves the use of two intra-cardiac leads, one in the atrium and one in the ventricle. This system ensures the maintenance of normal AV synchrony. The AV interval is a programmable function. The pacemaker may operate in a number of modes. In one it paces both atrium and ventricle. In another, the patient's underlying spontaneous atrial activity is sensed and this is followed, after the AV delay, by a ventricular impulse. This system has the advantage that the rate of discharge of ventricular impulses will be determined by the patient's own intrinsic atrial rate. Heart rate will, therefore, increase appropriately to meet the varying demands of the body.

Dual chamber pacing improves the exercise tolerance of patients with complete heart block in comparison with single chamber pacing. It also prevents the occurrence of pacemaker syndrome. *Pacemaker syndrome* is a problem which arises in occasional individuals with single chamber ventricular pacemakers. Patients experience transient hypotension and dizziness with the onset of pacing. This is due to loss of AV synchrony and is prevented by dual chamber pacing.

Dual chamber pacing is preferable to single chamber in patients with complete heart block and maintained atrial activity. It is also the preferred mode of pacing in patients with carotid sinus hypersensitivity, who are particularly prone to pacemaker syndrome. Finally, in patients with the bradycardia–tachycardia form of sick sinus syndrome, dual chamber pacing may help to prevent the occurrence of atrial fibrillation.

Rate-responsive pacing. In some patients, particularly those with atrial fibrillation, dual chamber pacing is not possible. A variety of rate-responsive pacing systems have been developed, to enable heart rate to rise with exercise in a single chamber ventricular pacing system. These pacemakers detect the onset of exercise and increase the ventricular pacing rate. Sensed parameters include the mechanical detection of vibrations, changes in QT interval of the ECG, changes in temperature of the blood returning to the right atrium and changes in respiratory rate. Rate-responsive systems have the advantage of increasing the patient's exercise capacity, in comparison with fixed-rate pacemakers.

Recently, dual chamber rate-responsive pacemakers have been introduced. These are indicated in patients requiring dual chamber pacing, in whom the response of the sinus node to exercise is reduced. These pacemakers enable the normal sequence of AV synchrony to be maintained, with an accompanying increase in heart rate with exercise.

ELECTRICAL THERAPY FOR TACHYARRHYTHMIAS

Direct current (d.c.) shock therapy

The d.c. shock must be timed to avoid the vulnerable period. It is customary to arrange for the defibrillator to discharge 0.02 s after the peak of the R wave. A synchronized discharge of this kind is not possible when there is ventricular fibrillation.

Because the procedure is a painful one, an anaesthetic is usually given, except when there is ventricular fibrillation (because the patient is unconscious). A short-acting barbiturate is often used, but an alternative is to supplement an analgesic such as morphine with diazepam 5–10 mg intravenously. One electrode, smeared with electrode jelly, is placed in the right parasternal region and the other either in the left axilla or posteriorly below the left scapula. The machine is charged to the chosen level and discharged by pressing a button on the electrode. The strength of shock needed varies with the arrhythmia being treated:

- *ventricular tachycardia and ventricular fibrillation.* An initial 200 J shock is appropriate, increased to 360 J for subsequent shocks if the initial shock is ineffective (see Fig. 20.1);
- *atrial fibrillation.* The initial amplitude should be 100 J and

subsequently increased to 200 and 360 J as necessary;

- 'organised' supraventricular arrhythmias (atrial flutter, paroxysmal supraventricular tachycardia), a low-amplitude shock is frequently successful; an initial amplitude of 25 J is appropriate.

Apart from slight skin burns, the procedure is usually free from undesirable effects. However, there is a danger of producing serious arrhythmias in the patient with digitalis intoxication, and it is wise to discontinue this drug for 1–2 days prior to electric shock administration if possible.

The indications for electric shock therapy are discussed under the individual arrhythmias, but in general it may be stated that electric shock therapy is almost invariably effective for all types of tachycardia including the supraventricular tachycardias, atrial flutter, atrial fibrillation, ventricular tachycardia and ventricular fibrillation. Some cases of chronic atrial fibrillation are resistant. Electric shock should not be given if it is thought that the arrhythmia is digitalis- or quinidine-induced.

Antitachycardia pacing

Some re-entrant supraventricular tachycardias, particularly AV node re-entry tachycardia, can be terminated by critically timed atrial extrastimuli. Antitachycardia pacemakers have been developed which have the ability to detect the onset of a tachyarrhythmia and deliver critically timed trains of extrastimuli to the right atrium, thereby restoring sinus rhythm (Fig. 9.29). These devices provide an alternative to drug therapy in the management of supra-ventricular tachycardias. They are particularly useful in patients who have failed multiple trials of drug therapy and in patients in whom drug therapy is contraindicated. For example, they are of value for women of child-bearing age who wish to become pregnant, in whom antiarrhythmic drug therapy would be contraindicated during pregnancy.

Antitachycardia pacemakers should only be implanted after very careful electrophysiological assessment and determination of an

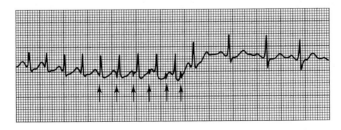

Fig. 9.29 Anti-tachycardia pacing. A supraventricular tachycardia is terminated by a train of six extra stimuli (arrowed), restoring sinus rhythm.

(A)

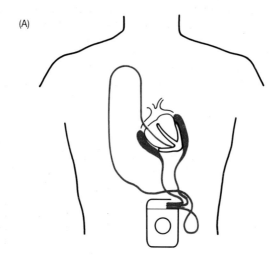

(B)

(C)

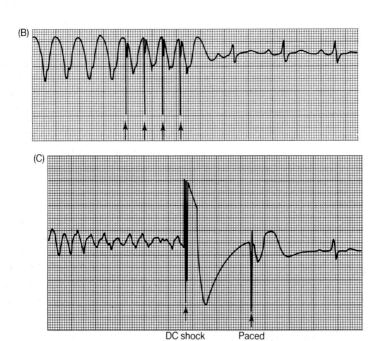

DC shock   Paced

Fig. 9.30 Implanted defibrillator. (A) Schematic representation of an implantable defibrillator. The defibrillator is sited in the abdomen. Epicardial patches and an endocardial pace-sense lead are also shown. (B) Ventricular tachycardia terminated by a train of four extrastimuli. (C) Ventricular fibrillation terminated by a DC shock delivered by the device (arrowed). The first beat after delivery of the shock is paced.

appropriate pace termination sequence for the arrhythmia. They are in general contraindicated in patients susceptible to atrial fibrillation, because of the possibility that a train of atrial extra-stimuli will cause atrial fibrillation rather than restoring sinus rhythm. Because of the special dangers of atrial fibrillation in patients with Wolff–Parkinson–White syndrome they are rarely indicated in this condition.

The implantable defibrillator

Implantable defibrillators have been developed which can deliver a d.c. shock to the heart to terminate episodes of ventricular tachycardia or ventricular fibrillation. These devices are implanted in the abdomen (Fig. 9.30). The onset of ventricular tachycardia or ventricular fibrillation is sensed via a conventional endocardial pacing lead in the right ventricle. Two patch electrodes are placed on the epicardial surface of the heart for delivery of the defibrillator charge. Because of the proximity of these electrodes to the myocardium, much lower energies are required than for external defibrillation. Shocks of 10–20 J are generally sufficient to defibrillate the heart and restore sinus rhythm.

Implantable defibrillators are particularly expensive. Their use should be restricted to patients resuscitated from sudden cardiac death and to patients with life-threatening ventricular tachyarrhythmias, which are not amenable to other forms of treatment. The technology is developing rapidly and in many cases it is now possible to substitute an endocardial lead and axillary patch for epicardial patches. This has the advantage of avoiding the need for major surgery for device implantation. Some devices offer the additional facility of antitachycardia pacing to terminate ventricular tachycardia (Fig. 9.30B).

Catheter ablation

A relatively new form of antiarrhythmic therapy is 'ablation'. With this technique, an electric current is delivered by an electrode positioned against the endocardium with the deliberate intention of damaging adjacent tissue. The method is particularly useful for supraventricular arrhythmias which have proved impossible to control with drug therapy. By ablating the bundle of His, heart block is produced. The ventricle is then protected from the fast rate, but a permanent pacemaker is needed.

The value of this technique has been greatly enhanced with the recent introduction of radio-frequency ablation. This is also proving of value in ablating accessory pathways in patients with Wolff–Parkinson–White syndrome (Fig. 9.31) and in modifying the AV node in patients with AV node tachycardia.

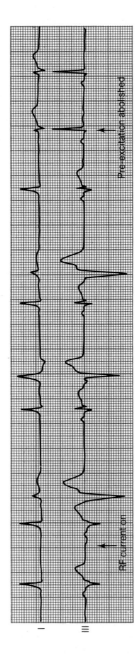

Fig. 9.31 Radiofrequency ablation of an accessory pathway in a patient with Wolff–Parkinson–White syndrome. Six seconds after commencing current application accessory pathway conduction is abolished, with loss of the delta wave and prolongation of the PR interval.

Antiarrhythmic drugs

Before commencing a patient on therapy with an antiarrhythmic drug, it is essential to consider the advantages and disadvantages of drug treatment. As a group, antiarrhythmic drugs have the potential to do harm as well as to do good. It is well established that under some circumstances antiarrhythmic drugs may exacerbate existing arrhythmias or even create new ones. In general, antiarrhythmic drug treatment should only be prescribed when clearly indicated either to treat symptoms or to prevent potentially life-threatening arrhythmias. They are not indicated simply to 'tidy up' the ECG. Although antiarrhythmic agents are highly successful in suppressing ventricular ectopic beats, they may have an adverse effect on more serious ventricular tachyarrhythmias.

Antiarrhythmic therapy is used to:

- Suppress or prevent arrhythmias;
- Slow the ventricular response rate in the case of supraventricular arrhythmias.

ANTIARRHYTHMIC DRUG CLASSIFICATION (Table 9.1)

There are four main classes of antiarrhythmic drug action:

Table 9.1   Classification of antiarrhythmic drugs

Class I Membrane-stabilizing drugs		
Subgroup	(A)	Quinidine
		Procainamide
		Disopyramide
	(B)	Lignocaine
		Mexiletine
	(C)	Flecainide
		Propafenone
Class II Anti-sympathetic drugs		
Beta-blockers		
Class III Drugs which prolong action potential duration		
Amiodarone		
Bretylium		
Sotalol		
Class IV. Calcium antagonists		
Verapamil		

- *class I* 'membrane-stabilizing' drugs, which also have a local anaesthetic action, block the inflow of sodium into the cell and, therefore, the rate of depolarization. This has the effect of

reducing the automaticity of ectopic pacemaker foci and of slowing conduction, which may abolish a re-entry circuit;
- *class II 'anti-sympathetic' drugs* — notably those which block beta-adrenoceptors;
- *class III drugs which prolong action potential duration.* Amiodarone is the main drug in this category, although sotalol and bretylium also have class III actions;
- *class IV drugs which block the inflow of calcium into the cell.* This affects the activity of certain cells, particularly those of the atrioventricular node, which are dependent more on the calcium inflow than on sodium. Verapamil belongs to this group.

Class I drugs

These are subdivided into three subclasses (Table 9.1).

Quinidine. This drug has been used for more than 50 years in the prevention and termination of atrial and ventricular ectopic rhythms. When given in adequate doses it is an effective antiarrhythmic agent, but frequently produces nausea, vomiting, headache, tinnitus and diarrhoea. More serious are its cardiotoxic effects, including heart block and asystole, and the provocation of ventricular tachycardia and ventricular fibrillation. Quinidine causes a clinically significant increase in digoxin plasma levels when they are given together; digoxin dosage should be halved in patients on this drug when quinidine is added. Other rarer toxic effects include respiratory depression, thrombocytopenia and skin rashes. Because of its toxicity, quinidine has been largely replaced by d.c. shock and by other antiarrhythmic drugs. The drug is of proven value in preventing recurrences of atrial fibrillation, but at a risk of provoking more serious arrhythmias.

Quinidine produces a variety of ECG effects including a prolonged QT interval, depression of the ST segment and T wave inversion. These do not necessarily indicate overdosage, but the appearance of conduction defects or ventricular arrhythmias (notably torsade de pointes) implies cardiac toxicity and the drug should be discontinued.

Procainamide. The actions of procainamide are similar to those of quinidine, but it is less effective in the treatment of atrial arrhythmias and is less toxic when used intravenously.

Procainamide may be administered intravenously, intramuscularly and orally. When given intravenously, it may produce a marked hypotensive effect due to peripheral vasodilatation, but this can be avoided with care. It should be given at a rate not exceeding 100 mg/min; an ECG should be recorded and the blood pressure taken every minute. Further procainamide should not be given if the systolic pressure falls below 90 mmHg, or if the QRS complex becomes more than 25% wider than it had been, or if the arrhythmia has been controlled.

By the oral route, nausea, vomiting and anorexia are common; nightmares, depression and convulsions are rare. Long-term oral procainamide therapy may lead to depression of the bone marrow, skin rashes and a syndrome simulating systemic lupus erythematosus.

Disopyramide. Disopyramide resembles quinidine in its antiarrhythmic effects but has atropine-like actions which cause a dry mouth and urinary retention and, rarely, glaucoma. It has a negative inotropic effect and should be avoided in cardiac failure. It may provoke arrhythmias including torsades de pointes. The oral dosage is 100–150 mg three to four times daily. Intravenously it may be given in a dosage of 2.0 mg/kg. Disopyramide should not be used in the management of atrial flutter. There is a danger that the drug will simultaneously slow the atrial rate through its class I effect and speed up AV conduction through its atropine-like effect, resulting in 1:1 conduction and an acceleration of the ventricular response rate.

Lignocaine. Lignocaine is the first choice drug in the acute management of ventricular tachycardia and ventricular fibrillation. It has virtually no myocardial depressant effect in therapeutic doses and is safer to give intravenously than other class I antiarrhythmic agents. It should not be given in the presence of AV block, which it may aggravate. The drug is used mainly intravenously, and by this route its duration of action is only 10–20 min. Initially, a dose of 50–100 mg (i.e. 5–10 ml of the 1% solution) can be given over a period of 1–2 min and repeated, if necessary, 2 min later. This may be followed by an intravenous infusion of 4 mg/min for 30 min, 3 mg/min for a further 30 min and thereafter 2 mg/min for 24–48 h, if necessary. Serious toxic effects from lignocaine are unusual, but include confusion, convulsions, respiratory depression and coma. The drug is not effective in controlling atrial arrhythmias.

Mexiletine. Mexiletine resembles lignocaine in its structure and actions but is well absorbed orally and is therefore useful in the chronic treatment of ventricular arrhythmias. Toxic effects include nausea, vomiting and tremor. The oral dosage is usually 200–250 mg thrice daily.

Flecainide. Flecainide is one of the most effective antiarrhythmic drugs, and usually abolishes all ventricular ectopic activity. It is a class Ic antiarrhythmic agent. However, like other drugs in this category it carries a particular risk of pro-arrhythmia. It has been found to be hazardous when given to patients after myocardial infarction, particularly if they have impaired left ventricular function, because it may cause cardiac failure and fatal arrhythmias. Its use in patients with ischaemic heart disease should be restricted to patients with life-threatening ventricular arrhythmias, in whom efficacy has been proven and pro-arrhythmic effects excluded by invasive electrophysiological investigations. The drug is also of value in the management of some supraventricular arrhythmias (particularly Wolff–Parkinson–White syndrome) in whom the risk of serious pro-arrhythmic effects is extremely low. Oral flecainide is given in a dosage of 100 mg twice daily.

Propafenone. Propafenone is a class Ic drug, which has been found particularly useful in the management of the Wolff–Parkinson–White syndrome. It is also effective in many cases of ventricular tachycardia but, like other drugs in its class, it is also prone to provoke ventricular arrhythmias. Oral propafenone is given in a dosage of 150–300 mg thrice daily.

Class II drugs — beta-adrenoceptor blocking agents

Beta-adrenoceptor blocking drugs oppose the effects of catecholamines on the beta-adrenoceptors.

Some block the receptors in the heart selectively (beta$_1$-receptor blocking agents). Others also block receptors in the bronchi and peripheral vessels. Consequently, they may induce bronchospasm in susceptible subjects and impair the circulation to the limbs.

Propranolol and similar drugs antagonize the ability of sympathetic substances to increase the rate and contractility of the heart. These drugs are sometimes effective in abolishing ventricular and atrial arrhythmias and are of value in slowing the ventricular response to atrial arrhythmias.

Individual beta-blockers are presented in the Appendix (p. 378).

Class III drugs

Amiodarone. This drug prolongs the action potential and the refractory period; it is therefore of value in blocking re-entrant pathways. It has proved particularly effective in the Wolff–Parkinson–White syndrome, but also in many resistant supraventricular and ventricular arrhythmias. Its toxic effects have precluded its widespread use. It causes corneal deposits, but these appear to be benign and reversible and seldom give rise to symptoms. Other side-effects include a bluish discoloration of the skin following exposure to the sun and thyroid disorders, especially thyrotoxicosis. More rarely, a pneumonitis may occur, which may be fatal. Oral amiodarone may not exert its antiarrhythmic action for up to a week and on stopping the drug may take several weeks for the effects to disappear. The usual dosage is 200 mg thrice daily for a week, gradually reducing thereafter to 200 mg daily. The incidence of side effects is dose related and patients should be reduced to the minimum drug dose compatible with arrhythmia control. In some cases of supraventricular arrhythmias, a 100 mg daily dose may be sufficient to provide arrhythmia control.

Bretylium.   Bretylium is an adrenergic blocking agent, which was at one time used in the management of hypertension, but was abandoned because of undesirable side-effects and tachyphylaxis in long-term use. It prolongs action potential without affecting the fast sodium current and is, therefore, categorized as a class III drug. It is relatively ineffective at suppressing ventricular ectopic activity but quite often prevents recurrences of ventricular tachycardia and ventricular fibrillation when other drugs have failed. It is given as 5 mg/kg intramuscularly every 6–8 h, or as a slowly administered intravenous infusion, at a dose of 1–2 mg/min.

Sotalol.   Sotalol differs from other beta-blockers in prolonging action potential duration. Its antiarrhythmic effects are weaker than those of amiodarone, but it may none the less prove useful, particularly in the management of supraventricular arrhythmias, when the risks of amiodarone are not thought to be justified. It is given orally in a dose of 80–160 mg twice daily.

Class IV drugs

Verapamil.   This calcium antagonist, when used intravenously in a dosage of 5–10 mg is usually effective in abolishing supraventricular tachycardia. It is administered over 30–60 s and should be avoided in those receiving beta-blocking drugs, and given cautiously to patients with compromised ventricular function. Oral verapamil (40–120 mg three times a day) is useful in slowing the ventricular rate in atrial fibrillation.

Digoxin and adenosine

Neither digoxin nor adenosine are included in the traditional classification of antiarrhythmic drug actions. Both act to slow conduction through the AV node and are of use in supraventricular arrhythmias. Digoxin is considered further in Chapter 8 (p. 151).

Adenosine is a selective inhibitor of AV node conduction. The drug is administered intravenously (see Appendix, p. 393) and causes a transient AV block lasting a few seconds. It can hence be used to terminate re-entry tachycardias which include the AV node in the re-entry circuit. The drug is also of value in distinguishing broad complex tachycardias, when the diagnosis is in doubt (see p. 369).

General principles of antiarrhythmic drug selection

The above classification of antiarrhythmic drugs is of value in comparing the similarities and differences between the actions of

Sites of action of anti-arrhythmic drugs

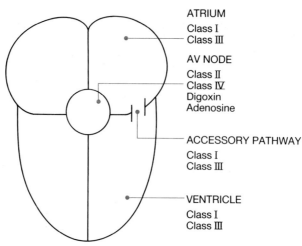

ATRIUM
Class I
Class III

AV NODE
Class II
Class IV
Digoxin
Adenosine

ACCESSORY PATHWAY
Class I
Class III

VENTRICLE
Class I
Class III

Fig. 9.32 Sites of action of antiarrhythmic drugs. Antiarrhythmic drugs can be considered to act at four sites within the heart: the atrium, AV node, accessory pathway and ventricle. For further discussion see text.

different drugs. However, it is of limited value clinically, when selecting which drug to treat a particular arrhythmia. That is best considered from the anatomical and functional viewpoint of which parts of the conduction system are involved in an arrhythmia. There are four functionally distinct regions, the atrium, the AV node, accessory pathways and the ventricle (Fig. 9.32).

Atrium

The two common examples of intra-atrial arrhythmias are atrial flutter and fibrillation. Either class I or class III drugs may be effective in restoring sinus rhythm. Alternatively, treatment may be selected to limit ventricular response, with drugs limiting AV nodal conduction.

AV node

Digoxin remains the mainstay of treatment to slow AV conduction, and is widely used in the management of atrial fibrillation. Beta-blockers are similarly of value and can be used in combination with digoxin, when digoxin slows the heart rate inadequately. Verapamil is also of value in this context, but should not be given with beta-blockers.

Several re-entrant arrhythmias arise within the AV node or involve the AV node. These commonly present as paroxysmal supraventricular tachycardia. Verapamil is frequently an effective treatment. Class I agents, particularly flecainide, may also be of value.

Accessory pathways

Accessory pathway conduction is slowed by class I agents and once again flecainide is particularly effective. Amiodarone is also of value, increasing the refractory period of the pathway. These drugs are specifically indicated in cases of atrial fibrillation complicating Wolff–Parkinson–White syndrome. They are also of value for re-entrant arrhythmias which involve conduction over an accessory pathway.

Ventricle

Class I drugs are the first line of treatment of ventricular tachyarrhythmias. Amiodarone is particularly effective, but is generally restricted in its use because of potential side-effects. However, if left ventricular function is severely impaired, amiodarone is the treatment of choice. Beta-blockers are of value in patients with exercise or ischaemic-induced arrhythmias.

Although class I drugs are the mainstay of treatment, there is little to guide selection of drugs from within the class. It is not possible to predict from the characteristics of an arrhythmia whether a Ia, Ib or Ic agent is likely to be successful. Choice of treatment is initially empirical, perhaps based on which drug is least likely to cause side-effects. However, treatment should then be validated by electro-physiological testing to prove drug efficacy and exclude the possibility of pro-arrhythmic effects.

Further reading

Bennett, D.H. (1985) *Cardiac Arrhythmias*, 2nd edn. Bristol: Wright.

Bloomfield, P. & Miller, H.C. (1987) Permanent pacing. *British Medical Journal* **295**: 741.

Camm, A.J. (1986) Asystole and electromechanical dissociation. *British Medical Journal* **292**: 1123.

Fisher, J.M. (1986) Recognising a cardiac arrest and providing basic life support. *British Medical Journal* **292**: 1002.

Kuck, K.H. & Schluter, M. (1993) Functional tachycardia and the role of catheter ablation. *Lancet* **341**: 1386.

Kulbertus, H.E. (1986) *Medical Management of Cardiac Arrhythmias*. Edinburgh: Churchill Livingstone.

Marsden, A.K. (1989) Basic life support. *British Medical Journal* **299**: 442.

Mason, J.W. (1987) Amiodarone. *New England Journal of Medicine* **314**: 455.

Opie, L. (1984) *The Heart*. London: Grune & Stratton.

Parsonnet, V. & Bernstein, A.D. (1986) Pacing in perspective: concepts and controversies. *Circulation* **73**: 1087.

Shenasa, M. et al. (1993) Arrhythmia Octet. Ventricular tachycardia. *Lancet* **341**: 1512.

Diseases of the Pericardium, Myocardium and Endocardium

THE PERICARDIUM

The pericardium has several functions: it helps to fix the heart and prevent excessive movement, it acts as a barrier against the spread of infection and malignancy from adjacent organs, and it reduces friction between the heart and its neighbouring tissues. It also limits acute cardiac dilatation and plays a part in the distribution and equalization of hydrostatic forces on the heart, being responsible for 'diastolic coupling', such that the diastolic pressures in the two ventricles are closely correlated when the pericardium is intact, but not when it is absent.

Pericardial disease, which may be acute or chronic, is usually associated either with a generalized disorder or with pulmonary disease.

Pathology

Pericarditis may be fibrinous, purulent or constrictive. In acute fibrinous pericarditis, the serous pericardium is inflamed and covered with an adherent layer of fibrin. There may be an accompanying effusion. In purulent pericarditis, there is usually a thick fibrinous exudate, containing polymorphonuclear cells and organisms. In pericardial constriction, the pericardium is a dense mass of fibrous tissue which is often heavily calcified. Sometimes a mixed picture of effusion and constriction is seen ('effusive-constrictive pericarditis').

Acute pericarditis

Aetiology

The causes of acute pericarditis are diverse (Table 10.1). Frequently no cause is identified. It seems probable that most idiopathic cases are due either to an unrecognized viral infection or to allergy or autoimmunity. The viruses most frequently identified have been of the Coxsackie B group, but influenza, measles, mumps, chickenpox and human immunodeficiency virus (HIV) may also be responsible. Purulent pericarditis usually results from the spread of infection from adjacent lung. Tuberculous pericarditis is preceded by infection in contiguous mediastinal lymph nodes.

Table 10.1   Causes of pericarditis

Infective
    Viral —Coxsackie B, influenza, measles, mumps, chicken-pox,
             human immunodeficiency virus
    Pyogenic
    Fungal
    Tuberculous

Connective tissue disorder
    Rheumatic fever (p. 231)
    Rheumatoid arthritis (p. 339)
    Systemic lupus erythematosus (p. 339)
    Polyarteritis (p. 339)
    Scleroderma (p. 339)
    Sarcoid (p. 340)

Myocardial infarction

Autoimmune
    Post-myocardial infarction syndrome — Dressler's syndrome (p. 135)
    Post-cardiotomy syndrome (p. 251)

Neoplastic invasion

Metabolic and endocrine
    Uraemia
    Gout

Trauma

Cardiac surgery

Clinical features and diagnosis

Chest pain is the commonest symptom but is not invariable. Its distribution simulates that of acute myocardial infarction, being central and sometimes radiating to the shoulder and upper arm. The pain may be most severe in the xiphisternal or epigastric regions. It is often sharp and severe, but may be aching or oppressive. Unlike ischaemic cardiac pain, it is accentuated by inspiration, by movement and by lying flat.

The most definitive sign of pericarditis is a pericardial rub,

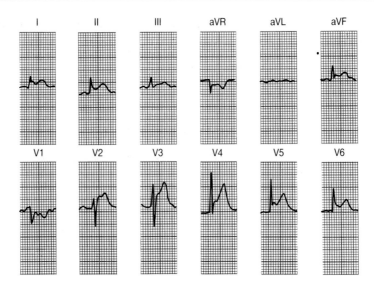

Fig. 10.1   Acute pericarditis. There is widespread ST elevation, with characteristic upward concavity of the ST segments.

although this is not always present. A to-and-fro scratchy or grating noise may be heard in systole, mid-diastole and presystole, or in only one of these phases. It is often localized to a small area but varies in position from time to time. It is usually accentuated if the patient leans forward, with the breath held in expiration, but is sometimes heard better towards the end of inspiration. Although the rub may disappear with the development of the pericardial effusion, it does not necessarily do so. Other signs may include those of pericardial effusion and, occasionally, of pericardial tamponade.

Investigations.   In the early stages, the ECG usually shows widespread ST elevation with the ST segment concave upwards (Fig. 10.1). After a few days the ST segment returns to the iso-electric line and the T wave becomes inverted. The ECG may simulate that of myocardial infarction, but Q waves are not seen and the ST segment elevation is of a different configuration (see Fig. 2.12).

The chest radiograph is not helpful unless there is a large pericardial effusion or there is concomitant pulmonary or pleural disease. Echocardiography is of value in the detection of pericardial effusion.

Differential diagnosis.   Acute pericarditis is most likely to be confused with acute myocardial infarction, spontaneous pneumothorax and pleurisy. In differentiating it from acute myocardial infarction, the following points are of importance:

- *history*. The character of the pain, the absence of pre-existing angina, and the history of an upper respiratory infection or of pyrexia preceding the onset of chest pain;
- *the absence of Q waves* and of the characteristic infarction type of ST elevation on the ECG;
- *the absence of serum enzyme changes.*

In spontaneous pneumothorax, the diagnosis can usually be made without difficulty by the detection of hyper-resonance and absent breath sounds over the affected lung or by the radiological demonstration of air in the pleural space. There is sometimes a coexistent pneumo-mediastinum which can cause a crunching or crackling sound with each heart beat. Pleurisy can be distinguished by the location and character of the pain, the presence of a pleural rub and, sometimes, by the clinical and radiological evidence of pleural effusion. Pleurisy and pericarditis commonly coexist.

Aetiological diagnosis

Viral pericarditis should be suspected if there is a history of an upper respiratory infection and fever preceding the chest pain, and can be confirmed by the demonstration of changing titres of viral antibodies in the blood, or the culture of viruses from the stools.

Tuberculous pericarditis may be difficult to diagnose, because there is often no evidence of either pulmonary or miliary infection. Usually, however, there is a history of malaise and weight loss for some weeks prior to the pericarditis. Tuberculosis is unlikely if tuberculin skin tests are negative. If necessary the diagnosis may be confirmed by pericardial aspiration or biopsy.

In pericarditis due to staphylococci, streptococci or pneumococci, there is usually infection in the lungs or elsewhere in the body. In rheumatic fever, there is accompanying evidence of the rheumatic process as well of myocarditis and endocarditis. In pericarditis due to hypersensitivity or autoimmunity, there is no preceding respiratory infection but there is often a history of similar episodes in the past.

Acute pericarditis may also occur in patients with acquired immunodeficiency syndrome (AIDS). Some cases are idiopathic, while others are related to specific viral pathogens, particularly cytomegalovirus. Tuberculous pericarditis may also occur in patients with AIDS.

Treatment

This consists of the symptomatic relief of pain by salicylates (600 mg orally every 3–4 h) or indomethacin (25–75 mg orally four times daily), the removal of fluid when this is causing pericardial tamponade (see p. 374), and the treatment of the underlying cause when this is possible. No specific therapy is usually necessary for viral or allergic pericarditis, although corticosteroids may be used to abbreviate their course if this is protracted. Tuberculous pericarditis requires prolonged treatment with antituberculous drugs and corticosteroids. Pericardial resection may be necessary even during the acute phase if pericardial constriction develops. Bacterial pericarditis should be treated with the appropriate antibiotics; surgical removal of pericardial pus may be necessary.

Pericardial effusion

Pericardial effusion may result from:

- transudation (in cardiac failure);
- exudation of serous fluid or pus (in pericarditis);
- blood (from trauma or malignant disease).

It is also a feature of myxoedema. The hydropericardium of cardiac failure causes few, if any, symptoms, although it may cause compression of the lungs and reduce the vital capacity. Pericardial effusion due to other causes may produce pain and pericardial tamponade.

Large effusions may be detected by percussion. With the patient lying flat, increased dullness may be noted in the second left interspace, as well as in the fourth and fifth right interspaces, and to the left of the apex beat.

Auscultation may reveal pericardial friction and heart sounds which are often, but not always, soft.

Investigations. The chest radiograph is valuable in diagnosis, particularly if several films are taken over a period of days — a sudden increase in the cardiothoracic ratio being very suggestive of pericardial effusion. When there is a considerable effusion, the cardiac silhouette is enlarged and the normal demarcation between the chambers is obliterated (Fig. 10.2). Similar abnormalities may be seen in some cases of cardiac failure, but the presence of a very large heart shadow in the absence of pulmonary vascular congestion makes the diagnosis of pericardial effusion likely.

Pericardial effusion produces low-voltage ECG complexes which may vary considerably in amplitude from cycle to cycle, ('electrical alternans'), reflecting changes in the position of the heart within the pericardial effusion.

Echocardiography is the most useful diagnostic method. When fluid separates the contracting and relaxing posterior wall of the heart from the stationary posterior pericardium, an echo-free space is produced (Fig. 10.3). Similarly, the anterior wall of the heart is

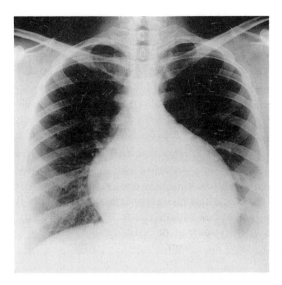

Fig. 10.2 Chest X-ray of pericardial effusion. The cardiac contour is markedly enlarged with a rounded appearance.

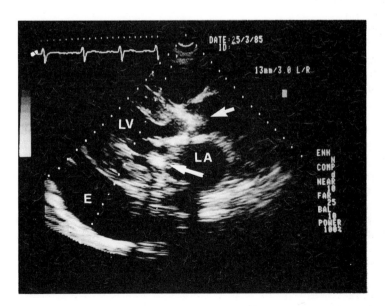

Fig. 10.3 Cross-sectional echocardiogram in the long axis parasternal view of a patient with a large pericardial effusion. An echo-free space is seen behind the posterior left ventricular wall. No anterior effusion is seen. LV = left ventricle. E = pericardial effusion. The arrows point to a thickened aortic valve and a calcified mitral valve.

separated from the chest wall.

Paracentesis may occasionally be required for diagnostic purposes, e.g. to identify a causative organism. No specific treatment is required for a pericardial effusion unless there is tamponade.

Pericardial tamponade

The pericardium does not normally impede ventricular distension during diastole. An accumulation of pericardial fluid, or pericardial fibrosis or calcification may prevent adequate filling. This may develop acutely, as when the pericardium fills with fluid, or slowly, as in chronic pericardial constriction. Probably the commonest causes are neoplasm and idiopathic or viral pericarditis, but it may develop in such conditions as uraemia, myocardial infarction, and after a traumatic cardiac catheterization, perforation by a pacing wire, cardiac surgery and chest injury.

The inability of the ventricles to fill during diastole leads to raised diastolic pressures in right and left ventricles, an increase in systemic and pulmonary venous pressures, and a fall in cardiac output.

Clinical features

Clinical features include:

- sinus tachycardia;
- elevation of jugular venous pulse. A further rise may occur during inspiration — Kussmaul's sign;
- fall in systemic blood pressure and shock in severe cases;
- variation in systemic blood pressure in relation to the respiratory cycle — pulsus paradoxus.

Investigations. Echocardiography shows the presence of a pericardial effusion with right ventricular diastolic collapse.

Treatment

The management of cardiac tamponade depends on the extent of haemodynamic compromise. Severe cases may be rapidly fatal, and relief by emergency paracentis may be required (see p. 374). In less critical cases, particularly if the underlying cause of tamponade is likely to recur, formal surgical drainage is preferable.

Pericardial constriction ('constrictive pericarditis')

Constriction of the heart by a fibrosed or calcified pericardium is relatively uncommon. In most patients, no identifiable cause can be found, although in some communities a tuberculous infection is responsible for the majority of cases. Constriction can also be a late complication of other types of infection, neoplastic invasion and intrapericardial haemorrhage.

Adequate filling of the ventricles during diastole is prevented by thick, fibrous and, often, calcified pericardium. Although extension of the disease process may affect the superficial areas of the myocardium, the rest of the heart is usually normal.

Clinical features and diagnosis

The inability of the ventricles to distend during diastole leads to an increase in diastolic pressure and to a consequent rise in pressure in the left and right atria and in both pulmonary and systemic veins. The stroke volume is low and there is a compensatory tachycardia.

The onset may be subacute or chronic. Symptoms resemble those of right-sided cardiac failure. The presenting complaint is often that of abdominal swelling due to ascites, but dyspnoea and ankle swelling are also common.

- *The pulse* is of small volume and may exhibit paradox. Sinus tachycardia is usually present, but atrial fibrillation develops in the advanced case.
- *The neck veins* are grossly engorged and show two characteristic features: a rapid 'y' descent (Fig. 4.4, p. 50) and an increase in pressure on inspiration.
- *The first and second heart* sounds are soft, and there is nearly always an early diastolic sound heard best at the lower end of the sternum. This is an unusually early third heart sound associated with rapid but abbreviated ventricular filling.
- *The liver* is enlarged and often tender, although it may be difficult to feel because of gross ascites. In contrast with the severity of the ascites, peripheral oedema is comparatively slight.

Investigations.   One of the most characteristic features of pericardial constriction is a shell-like rim of calcified pericardium, which is particularly well seen in lateral radiographs of the heart (Fig. 10.4). However, calcification is not invariable, nor does its presence necessarily imply constriction. The heart is usually small or of normal size, but is occasionally large. CT scan is of value, as this demonstrates thickening of the pericardium in almost all cases.

The ECG is not diagnostic, but usually shows low voltage QRS complexes associated with flattened or slightly inverted T waves. If

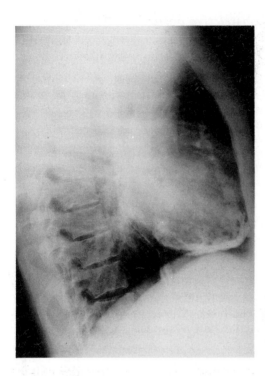

Fig. 10.4 Lateral chest X-ray showing a rim of calcification over the inferior aspect of the ventricles.

atrial fibrillation is not present, the P waves are often broad and bifid. Cardiac catheterization reveals:

- raised left ventricular diastolic, left atrial, pulmonary arterial, right ventricular diastolic and right atrial pressures. Characteristically, the diastolic pressures are identical in all four cardiac chambers;
- the right ventricular pressure pulse shows an early diastolic dip followed by a plateau (Fig. 10.5). This appearance is not specific to pericardial constriction and may be seen in restrictive cardiomyopathy.

Differential diagnosis. Pericardial constriction is suggested by a small and paradoxical pulse, a high venous pressure, a quiet heart with an early third heart sound and pericardial calcification, although not all these features are necessarily present. An important clue to the diagnosis is the combination of advanced right-sided failure with a normal-sized heart.

Pericardial constriction is most likely to be confused with cirrhosis of the liver, but the characteristic arterial and venous pulses in pericardial constriction should permit differentiation. In other forms of right-sided heart failure, cardiac valve lesions or pulmonary

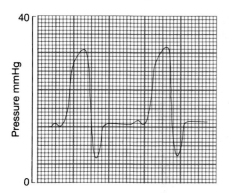

Fig. 10.5 Characteristic right ventricular pressure pulse in pericardial constriction. Note early diastolic dip, followed by a plateau.

disease are usually evident.

Differentiation of pericardial constriction from restrictive cardiomyopathy may be difficult. In restrictive cardiomyopathy:

- the heart is generally enlarged;
- the left ventricular end diastolic pressure generally exceeds the right ventricular end diastolic pressure;
- there is no pericardial thickening.

Treatment

The medical treatment of the failure associated with pericardial constriction is seldom successful, although some improvement may follow the use of diuretics. Digoxin is of value only if atrial fibrillation supervenes.

The only effective treatment is surgical removal of the thickened pericardium. However, pericardial constriction sometimes occurs during the acute or subacute phase of tuberculous pericarditis, and preliminary treatment should then be undertaken with antituberculous drugs and corticosteroids. In some patients the pericardium may be densely calcified and adherent to the underlying heart muscle. In such cases, ultrasonic debridement can provide a useful surgical adjunct.

Progress following pericardiectomy is usually satisfactory but may not be so if there has been extensive myocardial involvement or severe liver damage. In such patients, a low output syndrome may ensue.

MYOCARDIAL DISEASE

The myocardium is involved in most types of heart disease. The terms *myocarditis* and *cardiomyopathy* are reserved for those relatively uncommon types of myocardial disease which cannot be attributed to coronary atherosclerosis, congenital or valvar heart disease or hypertension.

Myocarditis is used to describe inflammatory disorders of the myocardium due to infection and toxins. *Cardiomyopathy* is used for chronic disorders of heart muscle; the term may be restricted to those disorders whose cause is unknown, and the term 'specific heart muscle disease' for those of identified aetiology.

Myocarditis

Myocarditis usually forms part of a generalized infection (particularly viral) but can also be due to physical and chemical agents (see Table 10.2). It is often associated with pericarditis. Occasionally, septicaemia may lead to focal suppurative lesions. Myocarditis is an important component of acute rheumatic fever (see Chapter 11).

Table 10.2   Causes of myocarditis

Infective
      Viruses — Coxsackie B, cytomegalovirus, infectious mononucleosis,
                    human immunodeficiency virus
      Mycoplasma
      Bacteria
      Spirochaetes
      Rickettsiae
      Fungi
      Parasites and protozoa

Radiation

Drugs — Sulphonamides, doxorubicin, lithium, emetine, cyclophosphamide

Heavy metals

Hypersensitivity states

Insect stings

Mild forms of myocarditis occur in a large number of infectious diseases but often cause only sinus tachycardia and non-specific ECG changes. They may, however, give rise to arrhythmias such as atrial fibrillation or supraventricular tachycardia without producing other overt cardiac effects.

Clinical features

There are three basic ways by which an infectious agent can lead to myocardial damage:

- direct invasion of the myocardium;
- toxin production e.g. diphtheria;
- immunologically mediated damage.

In the case of viral myocarditis, immune mechanisms are predominantly responsible for myocardial damage, rather than direct damage caused by the virus itself.

In severe cases, tachycardia may be marked, or, particularly in diphtheria, there may be a bradycardia due to heart block. The symptoms and signs of left and right cardiac failure may develop, with dyspnoea, gallop rhythm, cardiac enlargement and murmurs due to dilatation of the ventricles. Chest pain is common, but usually attributable to associated pericarditis. There is a risk of acute circulatory failure (shock) and of sudden death. Minor ECG abnormalities are common, but such changes may occur in infections even in the absence of myocarditis. Occasionally, there is ST elevation (due to pericarditis) or depression, or inversion of T waves, or disturbances of conduction and rhythm. There may be enzyme evidence of myocardial necrosis. Echocardiography and radionuclide imaging may be useful in demonstrating ventricular dysfunction.

Viral myocarditis

The diagnosis may be supported by the isolation of a virus from tissue or fluid specimens, or by increases in the titre of virus-neutralizing, complement-fixing, or haemagglutination-inhibiting antibodies. Endomyocardial biopsy is of some limited value in confirming the diagnosis. In Europe and North America most cases of myocarditis are thought to be viral in origin. In South America, Chagas' disease (caused by *Trypanosoma cruzi*) is the commonest cause of myocarditis.

There is a spectrum of clinical expression of myocarditis, ranging from mild local inflammation which may only be inferred from ST-segment changes in the ECG, to fulminant congestive cardiac failure. The outcome after viral myocarditis is similarly variable. In most cases, the myocarditis is self-limiting and recovery is complete. However, in a small minority of patients, myocarditis may culminate in dilated cardiomyopathy as a consequence of viral-mediated immunological damage.

There is no specific treatment. Therapy is primarily supportive, treating the complications of heart failure and arrhythmias if they occur. The role of corticosteroids remains controversial. Corticosteroids are frequently administered to patients with progressive disease who have evidence of an inflammatory cell infiltrate on endomyocardial biopsy, although the benefits of such treatment are not proven.

A large number of viruses may cause viral myocarditis. Coxsackie B is a particularly common cause, but other possibilities include cytomegalovirus, infectious mononucleosis, influenza and human immunodeficiency virus (HIV).

Human immunodeficiency virus (HIV). Clinically apparent cardiac involvement occurs in about 10% of patients with the acquired immunodeficiency syndrome (AIDS). Manifestations include, myocarditis, pericarditis, endocarditis, dilated cardiomyopathy and metastatic involvement from Kaposi's sarcoma. Most cases of myocarditis are thought to be related to the HIV virus itself, although myocarditis secondary to opportunistic pathogens may also occur.

Congestive heart failure is the commonest clinical manifestation. Conventional drug treatment with diuretics and ACE inhibitors provides effective short term treatment of the failure, but is unlikely to alter the course of the underlying myocarditis.

Cardiomyopathy related to specific heart muscle diseases

Aetiologically, cardiomyopathies fall into two groups: those in which the heart disease is the major or only abnormal feature, and those in which the myocardial disease is a complication of a generalized disorder. Systemic diseases associated with cardiomyopathy are listed in Table 10.3.

Table 10.3   Systemic disorders causing cardiomyopathy

Connective tissue disorders (systemic lupus erythematosus, scleroderma and polyarteritis)
Amyloidosis
Sarcoidosis
Neuromuscular diseases (Friedreich's ataxia, progressive muscular dystrophy and myotonic dystrophy)
Haemochromatosis
Glycogen storage diseases

There are three distinctive clinical patterns of cardiomyopathy:

- dilated;
- hypertrophic;
- restrictive.

DILATED CARDIOMYOPATHY

Dilated (congestive) cardiomyopathy is the commonest type of heart muscle disease. In many patients no aetiological agent can be identified, but it is likely that a substantial proportion follow a viral myocarditis. Alcohol abuse is an important factor in many cases. Other causes of dilated cardiomyopathy are listed in Table 10.4.

Table 10.4 Some causes of dilated cardiomyopathy

Infection

    Viral myocarditis

    Human immunodeficiency virus

Toxins and drugs

    Ethanol

    Anthracyclines (e.g. doxorubicin, daunorubicin)

    5-Fluorouracil

Nutritional and related deficiencies

    Thiamine deficiency

    Hypocalcaemia

    Hypophosphataemia

Pregnancy

The major physiological defect is the decreased contractile force of the left ventricle, with slow and inadequate systolic emptying. The ventricle dilates and the pressure rises in the left atrium. Subsequently, pulmonary hypertension and right ventricular failure occur.

Clinical features

Patients usually present with dyspnoea and oedema whose onset may be abrupt or insidious. Tachycardia is common as are ventricular ectopic beats and atrial fibrillation. The venous pressure is raised and there may be systolic venous pulsation from tricuspid regurgitation. Cardiac enlargement affects both left and right ventricles. Third and fourth heart sounds are common. There may be the pansystolic murmurs of mitral or tricuspid regurgitation.

Investigation.   The ECG frequently demonstrates arrhythmias, as well as abnormalities of the ST segment and T waves. The absence of Q waves (suggesting previous myocardial infarction) is an important negative finding. The chest radiograph confirms cardiac enlargement affecting all chambers. Echocardiography and radionuclide imaging reveal dilated, poorly contracting ventricles. Contractile impairment is global, in contrast to the regional impairment which occurs following myocardial infarction. Cardiac catheterization and angiocardiography are of little value in diagnosis as they merely demonstrate evidence of ventricular failure and, occasionally, tricuspid and mitral regurgitation.

Differential diagnosis.   The diagnosis requires the exclusion of coronary artery disease, thyrotoxicosis, hypertension, rheumatic heart disease and congenital heart disease as aetiological factors: it is supported by evidence of one of those generalized disorders which is associated with cardiomyopathy. Endomyocardial biopsy is occasionally of value in confirming an underlying aetiology, but most often simply shows an end stage fibrotic process, without providing clues as to the pathogenesis.

Treatment

The prognosis is poor, 50% dying within 2 years of diagnosis and nearly all within 5 years. Treatment depends on the stage of disease. Alcohol should be forbidden. Bed rest may be necessary in severe cases; diuretics are first-line drug treatment. Digitalis is valuable in controlling atrial fibrillation; vasodilators, especially the angiotensin converting enzyme (ACE) inhibitors, are usually effective in helping to combat the features of congestive failure, at least temporarily. Cardiac transplantation is indicated if disability is severe and life expectancy short (p. 159).

Alcoholic cardiomyopathy

Excessive alcohol consumption is one of the commonest causes of dilated cardiomyopathy in the Western world. Myocardial damage may arise by three basic mechanisms:

- direct toxic effects of alcohol;
- nutritional deficiencies, particularly thiamine deficiency;
- toxic effects of additives (e.g. cobalt) in alcoholic beverages.

Identification of the aetiological role of alcohol is of particular importance because, in contrast to other causes of dilated cardiomyopathy, ceasing alcohol consumption can halt the progression of the disease and may lead to an improvement in ventricular function. In patients with associated thiamine deficiency, thiamine administration may improve ventricular function.

HYPERTROPHIC CARDIOMYOPATHY

In this condition there is massive hypertrophy of the ventricles. The rigid non-compliant chambers impede diastolic filling. The ventricular septum is often the site of the most conspicuous hypertrophy, which may obstruct the left ventricular outflow tract (obstructive cardiomyopathy). The obstruction increases as systole progresses, and the more vigorously the ventricle contracts the more severe is the obstruction.

Hypertrophic cardiomyopathy is frequently familial and one may obtain a history of heart disease or sudden death in relatives. In approximately half the affected individuals the disease is transmitted as a single gene autosomal dominant trait.

Clinical features

The symptoms are often those which occur in aortic stenosis, including dyspnoea, angina and syncope. Arrhythmias are common and there is a high risk of sudden death.

Physical signs include:

- steep pulse upstroke due to the rapid ejection of blood by the hypertrophied ventricle during early systole;
- the venous pulse may show a large 'a' wave, and there may be evidence of both left and right ventricular hypertrophy;
- left ventricular outflow obstruction causes the systolic murmur and thrill of subaortic stenosis, maximal at the lower left sternal edge or apex;
- the pansystolic murmur of mitral regurgitation is frequent; less often there may be the signs of tricuspid regurgitation or of pulmonary stenosis;
- a fourth heart sound.

Both the 'a' wave and fourth heart sound are due to forceful atrial contraction against the non-compliant hypertrophied ventricle.

Investigations. The ECG shows left ventricular hypertrophy and, sometimes, conduction defects.

The echocardiogram is of great value. Characteristic features are:

- asymmetrical hypertrophy of the septum (ASH);
- systolic anterior movement of the mitral valve (SAM) (Fig. 10.6);
- midsystolic closure of the aortic valve;
- cross-sectional echocardiography demonstrates the asymmetric hypertrophy and the obliteration of the ventricular cavity during systole.

The chest radiograph may show left ventricular hypertrophy.

On cardiac catheterization, a systolic pressure difference can be demonstrated between the body and the outflow tract of the left ventricle if there is obstruction. This difference is increased by drugs such as isoprenaline, which increase myocardial contractility, and may be abolished by drugs such as propranolol, which decrease myocardial contractility. Angiocardiography demonstrates a small left ventricular cavity with narrowing of the outflow tract and, often, mitral regurgitation.

Differential diagnosis. Obstructive cardiomyopathy has usually to be differentiated from other types of aortic stenosis. In valvar aortic stenosis, the pulse is usually small and flat and there is either an early systolic click or calcification of the aortic valve. In congenital

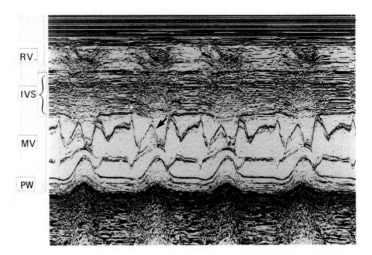

Fig. 10.6 M-mode echocardiogram in hypertrophic cardiomyopathy. The arrow indicates a systolic anterior movement of the mitral valve (SAM). The interventricular septum is grossly thickened.

subaortic stenosis, the pulse is small and flat and there is frequently aortic regurgitation, which is not a feature of obstructive cardiomyopathy.

Treatment

The prognosis is very variable. Minor forms of the disease are quite common and patients with severe hypertrophy may remain alive and well for many years. The main concern is sudden death; often this is preceded by ventricular arrhythmias.

Beta-blockers and calcium antagonists are both helpful in relieving chest pain (especially the combination of beta-blocker and nifedipine). In patients with frequent ventricular arrhythmias, on 24-h ECG recording, amiodarone is indicated, as there is some evidence that amiodarone treatment can prevent sudden death. Resection of part of the intraventricular septum is occasionally indicated for relief of severe symptoms which fail to improve with medical management. Recently, dual chamber pacing with a short AV delay has been introduced and appears to provide symptomatic benefit.

RESTRICTIVE AND INFILTRATIVE CARDIOMYOPATHIES

Restrictive cardiomyopathy is the least common of the three major functional categories of cardiomyopathy (dilated, hypertrophic and restrictive). In restrictive cardiomyopathy the ventricles are abnormally stiff and impede ventricular filling, with the result that there is abnormal diastolic function. Systolic function, by contrast, may remain normal.

Restrictive cardiomyopathy may arise due to a variety of pathological processes (Table 10.5). These may involve infiltration of the myocardium or endomyocardial scarring.

Table 10.5 Causes of restrictive cardiomyopathy

Infiltrative
    Amyloid
    Sarcoid

Storage diseases
    Haemochromatosis
    Glycogen storage diseases

Endomyocardial
    Endomyocardial fibrosis
    Hypereosinophilic syndrome
    Carcinoid

The haemodynamic presentation and clinical features closely resemble constrictive pericarditis (p. 213). Differentiation from cases of constrictive pericarditis may be extremely difficult. There is frequently cardiac enlargement in patients with restrictive cardio-myopathy, whereas it is unusual for the heart to be enlarged in constrictive pericarditis. Conversely, CT scan generally shows pericardial thickening in constrictive pericarditis and a normal pericardium in restrictive cardiomyopathy.

Clinical features

Shortness of breath is the commonest presenting symptom. Other patients may present with signs of right heart failure. Features on clinical examination include:

- tachycardia. Because of compromised ventricular filling, heart rate increases to maintain cardiac output;
- elevated jugular venous pulse, with a further increase on inspiration (Kussmaul's sign);
- enlarged liver, ascites and peripheral oedema;
- S_3, S_4 or both.

Conduction disturbances and arrhythmias may occur if the disease process involves the conduction system. Sudden death is common.

Management

There is no specific therapy. Treatment is seldom effective and disease is commonly progressive. Use of low doses of diuretics and vasodilators may provide symptomatic benefit. Caution is necessary as decreased ventricular filling pressures may reduce cardiac output and cause excessive hypotension. In patients with eosinophilia, steroids and cytotoxic drugs may be helpful.

ENDOCARDIAL DISEASE

Endocarditis is an inflammation of the inner lining of the heart, affecting predominantly the valve structures. It may be infective or non-infective. The non-infective processes, which include rheumatic fever and systemic lupus erythematosus, are considered in more detail elsewhere.

Infective endocarditis

Infective endocarditis may be due to bacteria, fungi, *Coxiella* or *Chlamydia*. Endocarditis has classically been described as subacute or acute, based on the clinical course observed before the advent of antibiotic therapy. Acute endocarditis denoted aggressive organisms which rapidly destroyed the heart valve and caused death within 6 weeks. Subacute referred to less aggressive organisms which resulted in a much more protracted course of many months and even years.

The commonest variety is bacterial in origin and subacute in its course. Infective subacute endocarditis seldom affects a previously normal heart. The process is most frequently superimposed upon pre-existing disease. Prosthetic valves may also become infected and an increasing number of cases are being seen in intravenous drug abusers. Acute endocarditis (most frequently *Staphylococcus aureus*) may occur on previously normal hearts.

Native valve endocarditis. The majority of patients have a predisposing cardiac lesion. The pattern of underlying cardiac disease has been changing, reflecting the decline in the incidence of rheumatic heart disease. Currently the commonest underlying lesions in decreasing frequency are mitral valve prolapse, degenerative aortic and mitral lesions and rheumatic heart disease. The most common congenital lesions predisposing to endocarditis in the adult are bicuspid aortic valve, ventricular septal defect, coarction of the aorta and pulmonary stenosis.

Endocarditis in intravenous drug abusers. Endocarditis in the absence of underlying cardiac disease is common amongst intravenous drug abusers. The tricuspid valve is the focus of infection in about 50% of cases, with the mitral and aortic valves each accounting for about 20% of cases. Pulmonary valve endocarditis also occurs but is quite rare.

The presentation of right-sided endocarditis differs from left-sided. Typically, patients may present with pneumonia or multiple septic pulmonary emboli.

Prosthetic valve endocarditis. Prosthetic valve endocarditis is divided into categories of early and late. By definition endocarditis is early when symptoms occur within 60 days of valve implantation and late if they occur after this time. Early infection is generally due to contamination in the perioperative period, from sources such as i.v. cannulae, central lines, or urinary catheters. The majority of cases are due to staphylococcal infection. The bacteriology of late prosthetic valve endocarditis more closely resembles native valve endocarditis.

Pathology

A large number of different organisms may cause bacterial endocarditis. Common organisms include:

- *Streptococcus viridans.* An oral commensal of several varieties, this is the organism most frequently responsible for endocarditis, accounting for some 50–70% of cases. Most are highly sensitive to penicillin;
- *Streptococcus faecalis.* These organisms normally inhabit the gastrointestinal tract. The organisms are generally resistant to penicillin. High doses must be used and an aminoglycoside added to achieve a bactericidal effect;
- *Streptococcus bovis.* This organism is frequently associated with the presence of colonic polyps or colonic malignancy. It is generally penicillin sensitive;
- *Staphylococcus aureus.* This skin organism accounts for about 25% of cases of native valve endocarditis. It is the commonest cause of endocarditis amongst intravenous drug abusers, in whom it is responsible for some 60% of cases. The majority of organisms are highly resistant to penicillin. Multiple metastatic abscesses are common;
- *Staphylococcus epidermis.* This organism is a relatively rare cause of native valve endocarditis, but a common cause of prosthetic valve endocarditis. Different strains vary in their sensitivity to penicillin.

Other rare causes of endocarditis include *Neisseria gonorrhoeae,*

Coxiella burnetii (Q fever) and Chlamydia psittaci (psittacosis).

The infection leads to the formation of friable vegetations which have necrotic tissue, platelets, fibrin, white cells and red cells in their base, with superficial layers of fibrin and micro-organisms. Ulceration may lead to erosion or perforation of the valve cusps or of a sinus of Valsalva. The location of the endocarditis depends upon the underlying lesion. In aortic regurgitation, endocarditis affects the ventricular surface of the valve; in mitral regurgitation it involves the atrial surface of the mitral valve. In a ventricular septal defect, the vegetations may form around the defect itself but are often located either on the tricuspid valve or where the jet impinges on the right ventricular wall. Invasion of the adjacent myocardium is common and may proceed to abscess formation, and to pericardial involvement.

Embolization from the vegetations is frequent and is responsible for many of the clinical features of the disease. Large emboli may cause occlusion of the cerebral, renal or splenic arteries. Micro-emboli affect nearly all parts of the body and, in particular, lead to skin lesions and a glomerulonephritis. Pulmonary emboli develop when the right side of the heart is involved, as it is when there is a ventricular septal defect or persistent ductus arteriosus.

Several of the manifestations of the disease, including arthritis and glomerulitis, are thought to be due to immune complex deposition.

Clinical features

A history of dental treatment or infection is present in some patients, and in a small proportion there has been preceding urethral, pelvic or cardiac surgery.

The onset is often insidious with malaise and feverishness being the earliest complaints. The symptoms often mimic those of influenza. If left untreated, a characteristic clinical picture develops which was common in the days before antibiotic therapy. The complete syndrome of fever, anaemia, petechiae in the skin, clubbing, splenomegaly, a cardiac murmur and microscopic haematuria is seldom seen nowadays.

Abnormal physical signs in patients with endocarditis include:

- *heart murmurs*. The appearance of a new murmur or change in character of an existing murmur are particularly suggestive of endocarditis. A murmur may also disappear because of worsening valvar regurgitation;
- *petechiae*. These may develop on any part of the body. They may be embolic or vasculitic. They should be sought particularly in the conjunctivae, in the mouth and in the ocular fundi (Roth's spots are small oval, retinal haemorrhages with a pale centre). Haemorrhagic lesions on the palms and soles are termed Janeway lesions;

- *splinter haemorrhages.* These are small linear streaks in the nailbed of fingers and toes;
- *Osler's' nodes.* These are small tender nodules in the tips of the fingers and toes;
- *clubbing.* This only arises if the disease is present for several months;
- *splenomegaly.* This too takes several months to develop and is a feature of longstanding disease.

Most patients with infective endocarditis are anaemic, but the anaemia is not of a specific type. The spleen is often enlarged and occasionally tender. Proteinuria and microscopic haematuria are usual.

Neurological complications are common and are due to embolic occlusion of cerebral vessels or to mycotic aneurysms. Coma, convulsions and hemiplegia may occur and meningitis, encephalitis and subarachnoid haemorrhage may be mimicked.

Investigations.   The chest X-ray and ECG are of little value except in the diagnosis and assessment of the underlying cardiac abnormality. Echocardiography is the most important investigation in this disorder, both because of its ability to demonstrate vegetations, and because it can help in the assessment of the severity of valvar involvement. Vegetations can be seen in about 60% of cases by the cross-sectional technique. Trans-oesophageal echo is achieving even higher success rates, and can identify the presence of vegetations in some 90% of patients with endocarditis (Fig. 10.7).

Confirmation of the diagnosis depends on obtaining a positive blood culture, which is possible in some 90% of cases. At least six specimens of blood should be obtained over a period of 1–2 days. The

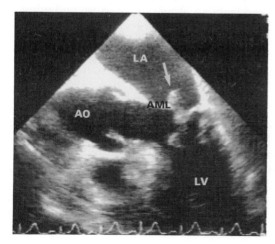

Fig. 10.7 Transoesophageal echocardiogram. A large vegetation (arrowed) is present, attached to the anterior mitral leaflet. LA, left atrium; LV, left ventricle; AML, anterior mitral leaflet; AO, aorta.

blood should be incubated aerobically and anaerobically, and special cultures should be set up for fungi. If the patient has received penicillin previously, penicillinase should be incorporated in the culture medium. Complement fixation tests must be undertaken for the diagnosis of *Coxiella* and *Chlamydia* infection.

Prognosis. Recovery from infective endocarditis is rare unless effective and prolonged antibiotic therapy is given. Death, which may be due to heart failure, emboli or renal failure, often does not occur until several months after the onset. Even if the infection is cured, damage to the valves may be so serious as to lead to intractable heart failure. Even with modern antibiotic treatment, mortality is still in the region of 30%.

Complications. Complications are a common occurrence in patients with endocarditis:

- *congestive heart failure* may occur due to progressive valve destruction;
- *systemic emboli* are a particular concern, and may result in stroke or myocardial infarction;
- *mycotic aneurysm formation* may lead to occlusion of vessels or to haemorrhage. Neurological complications may be due either to emboli or to the presence of a mycotic aneurysm;
- *renal failure.* This may arise due to immune complex deposition causing glomerulonephritis. Aminoglycoside antibiotics may also impair renal function;
- *intracardiac abscess formation.* Aortic root abscess formation is a serious complication and an indication for surgical intervention. It should be suspected in patients with persistent or recurrent pyrexia. Septal extension from an abscess may cause widening of the PR interval and heart block.

Treatment

It is important that the responsible organism should be identified without delay, so that the appropriate antibiotics can be given. However, the start of therapy should not be postponed beyond 2–3 days in spite of negative blood cultures. Bactericidal agents should be employed, because bacteriostatic drugs produce only temporary suppression of the infection. Following isolation and identification of an organism, careful discussion with the microbiology department is advisable to guide antibiotic selection. The microbiology department can also undertake back titrations to ensure that adequate antibiotic levels are achieved to kill the organism.

Antibiotic selection

- When the organism is penicillin-sensitive, a penicillin (penicillin G or ampicillin) is given. Administration is usually intravenous, at least for the first 2 weeks and adequate dosage (e.g. penicillin G, 8 million units/day), preferably confirmed by laboratory testing, is essential. Change to oral therapy may be possible later, given a good response.
- In penicillin-resistant infection (e.g. *Streptococcus faecalis*) a combination of a penicillin (penicillin G or ampicillin) and an aminoglycoside (e.g. gentamicin, vancomycin) will be necessary.
- Penicillin-sensitive staphylococci will respond to penicillin, but the more common penicillin-resistant strains demand large doses of penicillinase-resistant drugs (e.g. flucloxacillin 2 g intravenously every 4 h). Vancomycin can be used as an alternative. Oral rifampicin is also of value in the management of penicillin-resistant staphylococci.
- Blood–culture negative endocarditis should be treated as for *Streptococcus faecalis* infections, infection with *Coxiella* and *Chlamydia* having first been excluded.

A minimum of 4 weeks therapy is thought necessary in all cases. Antibiotic therapy is constantly changing as new drugs become available and as organisms become resistant to those in current use.

The temperature usually falls to normal within 3 days of the start of effective antibiotic therapy. If pyrexia recurs, there are several possible explanations:

- emergence of resistant organisms;
- superinfection with another organism;
- development of a reaction to the antibiotic;
- development of an abscess.

Surgery

In most cases it is appropriate to undertake medical management and first to attempt to control and cure the infection. Surgery is indicated in patients with:

- refractory heart failure due to valvar regurgitation;
- a paravalvar abscess;
- ineffective therapy or repeated relapses;
- multiple embolic episodes.

In patients with prosthetic endocarditis, achieving a cure with antibiotics alone is particularly difficult. For this reason the threshold for surgical intervention should be correspondingly lower.

Anticoagulation. The use of anticoagulants in the management of endocarditis is problematic. On the one hand embolic phenomena are common. On the other, anticoagulation will not necessarily reduce the incidence of emboli and increases the potential risk of bleeding from a mycotic aneurysm. In general, if a patient is already on anticoagulant therapy (e.g. for a mechanical valve prosthesis), this should be continued, but anticoagulants should not be commenced *de novo* unless very clear-cut indications exist.

Prophylaxis

Although endocarditis may occur in the absence of any obvious cause and in patients without known heart disease, many cases are probably preventable. All patients known to be at risk should pay great attention to oral hygiene, and should be aware of the need to have antibiotic cover for dental extractions, genito-urinary surgery and other procedures in which infection is likely. For dental extractions, it is recommended that oral amoxycillin 3 g is given prior to the procedure. Prophylaxis for genital or urinary operations, and for patients with prosthetic valves should also include an aminogly-coside, e.g. gentamicin.

Further reading

Abelmann, W.H. & Lovell, B.H. (1989) The challenge of cardiomyopathy. *Journal of the American College of Cardiology* **13**: 1219.

Goodwin, J.F. (Ed.) (1985) *Heart Muscle Disease.* Lancaster: MTP Press.

Maron, B.J. et al. (1987) Hypertrophic cardiomyopathy. *New England Journal of Medicine* **316**: 780, 844.

Rahimtoola, S.H. (1978) *Infective Endocarditis.* New York: Grune & Stratton.

Shabetai, R. (1978) The pericardium: an essay on some recent developments. *American Journal of Cardiology* **42**: 1036.

Shulman, S.T. et al. (1984) Prevention of bacterial endocarditis. *Circulation* **70**: 1123A.

Working Party of the British Society for Antimicrobial Chemotherapy (1982) The antibiotic prophylaxis of infective endocarditis. *Lancet* **i**: 1323.

Rheumatic Fever and its Sequelae

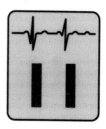

Acute rheumatic fever is a disease which follows infection by group A haemolytic streptococci and produces manifestations in many tissues and organs. Arthritis is often the most conspicuous feature, but cardiac involvement is of much greater importance. The duration of rheumatic activity is very variable; it may cease in 2 weeks or persist for many months. Recurrences are common. Death is rare in the acute phase but chronic rheumatic heart disease is responsible for a considerable morbidity and mortality.

Aetiology

Rheumatic fever seems to occur only after a group A streptococcal infection. It is complication of less than 1% of episodes of streptococcal pharyngitis, developing some 10–20 days after the onset of the sore throat. No history of sore throat, however, can be obtained in some 30–50% of cases; none the less virtually all patients with acute rheumatic fever have a streptococcal antibody response.

It is still far from clear how the infection leads to rheumatic fever. It seems probable that rheumatic fever is a result of a hyperimmune reaction either to bacterial allergy or to autoimmunity.

Over the last 50 years, rheumatic fever has been becoming progressively less frequent and is now rare in many countries, including the UK, the United States and Scandinavia. However, in the rapidly expanding cities of Asia, Africa and South America, rheumatic heart disease is the commonest cause of cardiac death. The decline of rheumatic fever in Western countries is not solely the result of the use of antibiotics for it preceded their discovery. It may be attributed both to a change in the virulence of streptococci and to improving social conditions, for poverty and, especially, overcrowding are associated with a relatively high risk of the disease. Rheumatic fever most commonly occurs between the ages of 5 and 15, with the peak about the age of 8. It is rare under the age of 4 and becomes progressively less common after the age of 15, although occasional cases are seen even after the age of 30. Rheumatic fever affects males and females equally often, but females are more susceptible to chorea. Rheumatic fever or its sequelae are often seen in more than one member of the same family. Although this may in part be due to the sharing of unfavourable social circumstances, there is good evidence of a genetic predisposition to the disease.

Microscopic evidence of acute rheumatic fever is widespread, but particularly affects tissues lined by endothelium such as blood vessels, the endocardium, the pericardium and synovial membranes. The earliest lesion is one of swelling in and around collagen fibres, accompanied by oedema and lymphocytic infiltration. Later, and more specifically, granulomatous Aschoff nodules appear. These are formed by collections of round cells, fibroblasts and multinucleated giant cells, and are usually surrounded by an area of polymorphonuclear cells, lymphocytes and plasma cells. The Aschoff nodules occur throughout the heart and are common in the interstitial tissue close to small blood vessels situated beneath the endocardium of the left ventricle.

Macroscopically, the lesions of rheumatic fever are most obvious in relation to the heart valves and the pericardium. The valve cusps become thickened by oedema and by the infiltration of capillaries. Grey or yellow warty vegetations ('verrucae') form along the lines of closure. These are common on the mitral and aortic valve cusps, and seldom affect the tricuspid or pulmonary valves. When the pericardium is involved, it becomes thickened and may contain a fibrinous straw-coloured effusion.

Chronic rheumatic heart disease is a sequel to acute rheumatic carditis, and many of its features are the result of fibrosis occurring during the healing of the acute lesion. Its pathology will be discussed in more detail later in this chapter.

Clinical features

In most cases, some 2–3 weeks after the onset of acute pharyngitis, the child begins to feel unwell, loses his appetite and complains of pains in the limbs. Fever is present, but it is not usually high. The major clinical features are carditis, polyarthritis, subcutaneous nodules, erythema marginatum and chorea.

Carditis.   The heart is involved in about half of the first attacks of rheumatic fever.

Endocarditis, with valvar involvement, is suggested by the appearance of cardiac murmurs; of all patients who develop carditis, three-quarters have murmurs in the first week. An apical pansystolic murmur indicates either mitral valve damage or functional mitral regurgitation associated with myocarditis. Rheumatic involvement of the mitral valve is also strongly suggested by the appearance of a low-pitched and short mid-diastolic apical murmur (Carey Coombs). This murmur is usually transient, but may persist for months or years until the characteristic features of mitral stenosis develop. However, the presence of a short mid-diastolic murmur at the apex in rheumatic fever cannot be taken as evidence of mitral stenosis or of its subsequent development. Midsystolic murmurs in the aortic or pulmonary area are less certain evidence of cardiac involvement, as they are common in febrile children without heart disease and usually disappear as recovery takes place. The diastolic murmur of aortic regurgitation is not uncommon, and usually persists after the acute rheumatic process has subsided.

Myocarditis is an important and common feature of acute rheumatic fever, but is difficult to diagnose with confidence. It is suggested by a tachycardia which is greater than would be expected from the height of the fever or which persists after the temperature falls, and by cardiac enlargement. More diagnostic is the appearance of left-sided or right-sided heart failure when this cannot be attributed to valve damage. The symptoms include dyspnoea, orthopnoea and oedema. Gallop rhythm is common but does not necessarily imply myocarditis, as it may occur in any child with fever and tachycardia.

When clinical evidence of *pericarditis* is present, the carditis is usually severe and involves the myocardium and endocardium as well (pancarditis). Retrosternal pain and pericardial friction occur and there may be a pericardial effusion.

When rheumatic activity has subsided, there are often residual signs of valve damage. Because of this, abnormal cardiac signs cannot be taken as evidence of continuing activity.

Polyarthritis.   Arthritis is common but its severity is variable. Characteristically, the joints become swollen, painful and hot, but in the younger child there may be only vague aches. The arthritis usually affects one joint after another, giving the impression of 'flitting', but it may involve several joints simultaneously. The knees, ankles, shoulders, wrists and elbows are most commonly involved, but the smaller joints of the hand and feet may be affected, particularly in the older patient. The inflammation in each joint usually develops within a few hours and may take up to a week to subside. Salicylates and corticosteroids produce relief of symptoms and signs promptly and are of some diagnostic value in this respect. Even in the absence of treatment, the polyarthritis usually disappears within 3 weeks and leaves no residual abnormality.

Subcutaneous nodules. These seldom give rise to symptoms but are of diagnostic importance. They are firm painless structures which are attached to tendon sheaths, joint capsules and fascia, and the skin is movable over them. They occur mainly over the extensor surfaces of the wrists, elbows, knuckles, knees and Achilles tendons and also over the scalp. They usually last about a week.

Erythema marginatum. This consists of lesions which develop rapidly from small macules or papules into large circles with pink, slightly raised, sharply circumscribed edges and pale centres. As these circles intersect, a pattern of segments develops. These appear and disappear within a period of hours. Erythema marginatum affects the trunk and limbs, but never involves the face. It is neither painful nor itchy; recurrences may ensue after all other features of rheumatic fever have disappeared.

Chorea (St Vitus' dance). This is a neurological manifestation of the acute rheumatic process. It often occurs without the other features, but cardiac involvement is common. It can affect children of either gender, but after puberty, it is confined to females. The onset is usually insidious with the development of an apparent clumsiness in an otherwise healthy child. Jerky and non-repetitive movements occur and muscle tone is reduced. When the arms are extended the wrist is flexed and the fingers hyperextended, giving rise to a 'dinner fork' configuration. Chorea must be differentiated from tics, which are also jerky but are repetitive, and from athetosis, in which the movements may not be repetitive but are of a more writhing character.

Laboratory investigations

In most cases there is a moderate leucocytosis of 12 000–15 000 white blood cells/mm^3 and an increased erythrocyte sedimentation rate (ESR). These features suggest rheumatic activity, but they are not reliable indices when steroids are given as the leucocytosis may persist or rise, and the ESR fall as a result of the therapy itself. However, a persistently raised ESR suggests, but does not prove, continuing activity.

In only about one-quarter of patients can a group A streptococcus be grown from the throat. The presence of a high antistreptolysin 'O' (ASO) titre provides good evidence of recent infection, particularly if it rises and falls. Other antibody tests, such as those for anti-DNase B and anti-streptozyme (ASTZ) are also of value.

A number of electrocardiographic abnormalities occur in acute rheumatic fever. Amongst these are a prolonged PR interval and, more rarely, more advanced degrees of atrioventricular block. Non-specific T wave changes are common and the ST and T wave changes characteristic of pericarditis may be seen.

The diagnosis of rheumatic fever

There is no certain way of establishing the presence of rheumatic fever, but the combination of certain clinical features and laboratory findings is highly suggestive. It may be diagnosed with some confidence if evidence of a recent streptococcal infection is present together with two or more of the following:

- carditis;
- polyarthritis;
- chorea;
- erythema marginatum;
- subcutaneous nodules.

The diagnosis is also probable if evidence of streptococcal infection is combined with *one* of the clinical features mentioned together with two or more of the following:

- previous evidence of rheumatic fever or rheumatic heart disease;
- arthralgia;
- fever;
- raised ESR or white cell count;
- prolonged PR interval.

(Revised Jones Criteria, American Heart Association, 1984.)

Differential diagnosis

The diagnosis of rheumatic fever is often difficult because the complete picture is seldom present. Furthermore, although the criteria described are valuable, they depend upon accurate observation and the correct timing and performance of laboratory tests. A history of sore throat may be misleading, as this is often due to organisms other than streptococci. Likewise, polyarthritis may be wrongly diagnosed when only the vague limb pains so common in childhood have occurred. Cardiac signs can also be deceptive, as functional systolic murmurs often come and go in the child with pyrexia from any cause. Another problem is posed by the patient with chronic rheumatic heart disease who develops a sore throat. Nevertheless, if the above-mentioned criteria are adhered to, the correct diagnosis will usually be made.

Diseases which are particularly important to differentiate from rheumatic fever are bacterial arthritis, rheumatoid arthritis and subacute infective endocarditis. In most cases of acute septic arthritis, the disease process is confined to a single joint and the inflammation is liable to extend into adjacent soft tissue. The diagnosis can be confirmed by bacteriological examination of fluid from the joint. Staphylococcal and meningococcal septicaemias can be diagnosed from blood cultures. Rheumatoid arthritis tends to involve smaller joints than rheumatic fever, but observation over a long period may be necessary in order to be certain of the diagnosis. Subacute infective endocarditis may be difficult to differentiate from rheumatic fever if blood cultures are negative, but a polyarthritis is rare, and some of the characteristic features such as microscopic haematuria and anaemia, which are seldom found in rheumatic fever, are usually present.

Course and prognosis

The course of rheumatic fever is variable and unpredictable. In some apparently severely ill patients, complete recovery takes place within a few days, whereas in others the disease drags on for months. In either case, the liability to recurrences of rheumatic activity following further streptococcal infection remains and it is common for the victim of one attack to experience one or more further episodes over the succeeding years.

The first attack is seldom fatal, but recurrences may lead to increasing cardiac damage and heart failure. By contrast, if the patient has escaped cardiac damage in the first attack, it is unlikely to develop subsequently. It has been estimated that more than two-thirds of patients who have experienced rheumatic fever eventually develop chronic rheumatic valve disease.

It is rare for the young child with rheumatic fever to escape cardiac damage. The risk of developing valve disease after an acute episode diminishes with age and it is not unusual for those first affected in adult life to have no sequelae. There can be no doubt that many cases of rheumatic fever escape diagnosis because about half of the patients with proven chronic rheumatic disease give no history of an acute episode.

Treatment

During the acute phase of the disease the subject wants and needs bed rest. When the temperature, pulse rate and ESR have returned to normal and the evidence of acute arthritis and carditis has disappeared, the patient may be gradually mobilized and rehabilitated. Active carditis requires complete rest, and this may have to be continued for several weeks. Subsequent increases in activity must depend upon the individual response, and a full resumption of normal physical activity usually has to be delayed to 6 months from the time when the last signs of active carditis have resolved.

Both salicylates and corticosteroids have a dramatic effect on the fever and polyarthritis of rheumatic fever. Although controversy continues as to the relative merits of the two forms of drug therapy, it is now common practice to use salicylates for rheumatic fever without carditis, and to add or substitute corticosteroids if there is undoubted evidence of cardiac involvement. However, it does not seem that any drug prevents the development of chronic valve damage. It is important not to give large doses of salicylate which can lead to salicylate intoxication; it is particularly undesirable to administer large doses of sodium salicylate as the sodium may precipitate cardiac failure. For children, 50 mg of acetylsalicylic acid per kilogram body weight may be given daily, and the dose subsequently adjusted to control symptoms. For adults, 4–8 g a day may be appropriate, in divided doses, given every 4 h. Salicylates should be continued until signs of rheumatic activity have ceased. There is great variation in the dosage of corticosteroids necessary to control activity. An initial dose of 40 mg of prednisone daily may be given and subsequently reduced to 20 mg daily, continued for 6 weeks and gradually withdrawn. Some patients have a rebound of rheumatic activity subsequently, and it is best to try to control this with salicylates.

The manifestations of cardiac failure are often suppressed by corticosteroids but diuretics and digitalis should be administered if necessary.

Prevention of rheumatic fever

Rheumatic fever may be prevented by the prophylaxis and treatment of acute streptococcal infections.

Acute streptococcal infections are probably most effectively treated by a single injection of 0.6–1.2 mega-units of benzathine penicillin, but this is painful. Alternatively, phenoxymethylpenicillin may be given for 10 days.

All patients who have experienced acute rheumatic fever should receive long-term prophylactic therapy. For this purpose, benzathine penicillin may be injected monthly in a dosage of 0.6–1.2 mega-units, or oral therapy given as 125 mg phenoxymethylpenicillin twice daily or sulphadiazine 0.5 g twice daily. It is not known how long prophylaxis should be continued, but it is common practice to recommend this up to the age of 25.

The healing of rheumatic carditis and the development of chronic rheumatic heart disease

Chronic rheumatic heart disease is the result of damage produced by recurrent attacks of acute rheumatic carditis and the subsequent healing process. These changes are largely confined to the valve structures, although in some instances myocardial damage may also be severe. Rheumatic pericarditis heals without residual effects. It is difficult to know to what extent the chronic lesions are the result of continuing and smouldering rheumatic activity. It is unusual for adult patients with chronic rheumatic heart disease to exhibit clinical evidence of acute rheumatic infection, but laboratory investigations may reveal evidence of repeated sub-clinical streptococcal infections, and biopsy of myocardial muscle in the adult frequently shows Aschoff bodies.

Because valve damage predominates in patients with chronic rheumatic heart disease, this condition will be considered in detail under the individual valve lesions. Nevertheless it is important to recognize that myocardial damage coexists and that correction of a valve abnormality will not necessarily restore normal cardiac funcion.

The pathological processes that cause valve deformity include thickening and distortion of the cusps at the time of rheumatic fever, contracture of the valve structures, fusion of the commissures, shortening of the chordae tendineae and, finally, calcification during the phase of healing. The nature of the valve lesion depends upon the relative importance of these factors in the individual case. Stenosis occurs if fusion of the cusps predominates; regurgitation is produced by shortening of the chordae tendineae and contracture of the valve leaflets.

The valve deformities may take many years to develop and, in particular, narrowing is not critical until the affected orifice is reduced to less than a quarter of its normal size. Regurgitation may be important from the time of the attack of acute rheumatic fever but its appearance as a symptomatic disorder, also, is likely to be delayed. Therefore, although the signs of mitral and aortic regurgitation may be present in childhood or early adult life, symptoms due to these lesions seldom develop until the third or fourth decade. The same is true for mitral stenosis; in aortic stenosis symptoms are often postponed even longer.

Further reading

Ad Hoc Committee to Revise the Jones Criteria (modified) of the Council on Rheumatic Fever and Congenital Heart Disease of the American Heart Association (1984) Jones Criteria (revised) for guidance in the diagnosis of rheumatic fever. *Circulation* **69:** 203A.

Committee on Rheumatic Fever and Infective Endocarditis of the Council on Cardiovascular Disease in the Young (1984) Prevention of rheumatic fever. *Circulation* **70,** 1118A.

Disciasco, G. & Taranta, A. (1980) Rheumatic fever in children. *American Heart Journal* **99:** 63.

Disorders of the Cardiac Valves

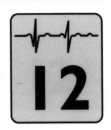

MITRAL VALVE DISEASE

The normal mitral valve (Fig. 12.1) consists of the valve ring, two unequal cusps (leaflets), chordae tendineae and papillary muscles. The larger antero-medial (or aortic) cusp is interposed between the mitral and aortic orifices, and forms part of the outflow tract of the left ventricle (Fig. 12.2). The papillary muscles arise from the ventricular wall opposite the commissures and are attached to the cusps on either side of the commissures by the chordae tendineae (Fig. 12.3). The chordae are collagenous strands, which, when tensed by the contracting papillary muscles, prevent the cusps from prolapsing into the left atrium during ventricular systole.

Chronic mitral valve disease may take the form of mitral stenosis with or without some degree of regurgitation, in which case it is virtually always the consequence of rheumatic endocarditis. Pure

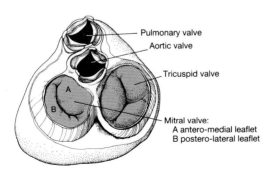

Fig. 12.1 Appearances of the heart valves during systole, with the atria and great vessels removed. The heart is viewed from behind, with the left ventricle and mitral valve on the left.

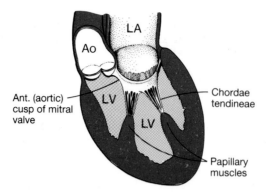

Fig. 12.2. Diagrammatic representation of relationships of left atrium (LA), left ventricle (LV) and aorta (Ao). Note that the aortic cusp of the mitral valve separates the mitral valve orifice from the outflow tract of the left ventricle.

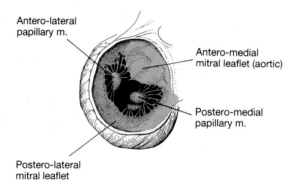

Fig. 12.3 Open mitral valve viewed from the left atrium. Note that the papillary muscles arise opposite the commissures and are attached to the cusps on either side of the commissures by the chordae tendineae.

mitral regurgitation in Western Countries is seldom rheumatic in origin; mitral valve prolapse is the common abnormality. Regurgitation may also be due to ruptured or defective chordae tendineae, papillary muscles or valve cusps, or to dilatation of the valve ring following left ventricular enlargement from a variety of causes.

Mitral stenosis

Pathology

Mitral stenosis is usually the result of recurrent rheumatic inflammation followed by healing. The leaflets adhere at their commissures, leaving a central orifice. In some instances the valve cusps remain pliant and mobile; in others fibrosis and calcification make them rigid. In about 10% of cases severe shortening of the chordae tendineae produces a funnel-shaped orifice.

Pathophysiology

Serious haemodynamic consequences develop only when the mitral valve orifice is reduced from the normal size of approximately 5 cm^2 to about 1 cm^2. In severe mitral stenosis, the orifice is a slit less than 1 cm long and 0.5 cm across.

In the normal heart there is little pressure difference across the mitral valve between its opening in early ventricular diastole and its closure. In mitral stenosis, a pressure difference develops which depends upon the area of the mitral valve orifice and the volume of blood flowing through it (Fig. 12.4).

When the stenosis is relatively mild, the mean pressure in the left atrium may be normal at rest (i.e. less than 12 mmHg) but increases on exercise as the cardiac output rises. In more severe stenosis, the pressure is raised even at rest, and in the most severe grades is persistently elevated to 25 mmHg or more. The left ventricular pressure is normal, provided there is no disease affecting this chamber.

When the stenosis is slight, the cardiac output may be normal, but as the narrowing increases, the cardiac output diminishes to about half the normal value, and may not rise in response to exercise.

The pressure in the pulmonary veins and capillaries parallels that in the left atrium. If the pulmonary capillary pressure rises rapidly to 30 mmHg, pulmonary oedema develops as the hydrostatic pressure exceeds plasma osmotic pressure. If the process takes place slowly, fluid exudes into the alveolar wall and a physical barrier eventually develops between capillaries and alveoli consisting of a thickened capillary basement membrane, increased collagen and oedema. These changes increase the tissue tension of the alveolar wall and limit the exudation of fluid. As a consequence, patients with mitral stenosis can sometimes tolerate high pulmonary capillary pressures without developing severe pulmonary oedema. Because of the increased fluid in the interstitial tissues, the lymphatics become engorged.

As the pulmonary capillary pressure increases, there is a concomitant rise in pulmonary arterial pressure. However, in many cases of tight mitral stenosis, pulmonary arterial hypertension is much more severe than can be accounted for by this passive rise. The disproportionate elevation of pulmonary arterial pressure is largely due to an increase in tone in the small pulmonary arteries. Severe pulmonary arterial hypertension is disadvantageous in that it leads to right ventricular hypertrophy and failure. However, the increased resistance of the pulmonary arterial vessels prevents an abrupt rise in

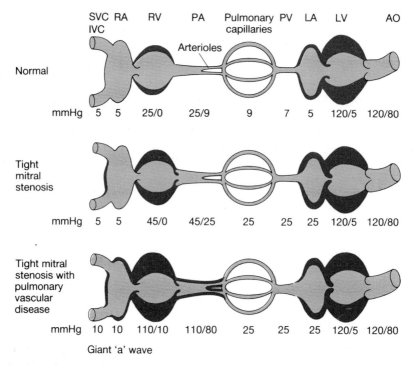

	SVC RA IVC	RV	PA	Pulmonary capillaries	PV	LA	LV	AO
Normal mmHg	5 5	25/0	25/9	9	7	5	120/5	120/80
Tight mitral stenosis mmHg	5 5	45/0	45/25	25	25	25	120/5	120/80
Tight mitral stenosis with pulmonary vascular disease mmHg	10 10	110/10	110/80	25	25	25	120/5	120/80

Giant 'a' wave

Fig. 12.4 The haemodynamic effects of mitral stenosis. In the normal heart, the pressure in the left atrium is similar to that of the left ventricle during ventricular diastole. With the development of mitral stenosis, the pressure in the left atrium rises, and this rise is transmitted to the pulmonary veins, capillaries and arteries. When pulmonary vascular disease develops, there is a narrowing of the pulmonary arterioles which leads to a disproportionate rise in the pulmonary arterial and right ventricular systolic pressures. With right ventricular failure, both the right ventricular end-diastolic pressure and the mean right atrial pressure may rise to 10 mmHg.

right ventricular output on exercise and therefore protects the lungs from a sudden increase in pulmonary capillary pressure.

The pulmonary vascular congestion typical of mitral stenosis leads to increased rigidity (decreased compliance) in the lungs. As a consequence, patients with severe mitral stenosis may have to double or treble the work of breathing.

Complications

- Atrial fibrillation develops sooner or later in most cases of mitral stenosis. At first this may be paroxysmal, but it is usual for it to become permanent. At its onset the ventricular rate is often more than 140/min and the patient may be rapidly precipitated into acute pulmonary oedema. It is an important complication, both because it contributes to the development of cardiac failure and because it is responsible for atrial stasis and the consequent risk of thrombosis and embolism.

- Pulmonary embolism and infarction frequently occur, especially when the disease is far advanced, as thrombosis is encouraged by atrial fibrillation, cardiac failure and bed rest.
- Systemic embolism is common and often follows the onset of atrial fibrillation. The embolism is cerebral in a high proportion of cases but may involve the mesenteric, renal or other arteries.
- The congested respiratory tract makes the patient liable to attacks of acute bronchitis and to the development of chronic bronchitis.
- Infective endocarditis is rare in pure mitral stenosis but is commoner as a complication of mixed mitral stenosis and regurgitation.

Symptoms

The patient with mitral stenosis, who is often symptom-free for many years, eventually develops features of left-sided cardiac failure and, later, those of right-sided failure. Various factors, such as pregnancy and the onset of atrial fibrillation, may suddenly precipitate the patient from one of these stages into the next.

The major symptom of mitral stenosis is shortness of breath. This occurs at first only on strenuous exercise, but as time passes less and less exertion is required to evoke it. Eventually, orthopnoea develops and the patient is liable to attacks of paroxysmal dyspnoea and acute pulmonary oedema. Acute pulmonary oedema is less likely when severe pulmonary arterial hypertension has developed.

Haemoptysis occurs in some 10–20% of patients with mitral stenosis but is seldom severe. In some cases, the sputum is frothy and pink due to acute pulmonary oedema, but frankly bloody sputum may be expectorated by a patient who is almost free of breathlessness. This is probably due to the rupture of dilated pulmonary or bronchial veins. Another important cause of haemoptysis is pulmonary infarction.

Patients may also complain of palpitation, cough and angina pectoris. Severe breathlessness and orthopnoea have usually been present for years before right-sided heart failure develops. The earliest symptom of this is oedema of the legs, but abdominal discomfort due to engorgement of the liver or to ascites also occurs.

Physical signs

Patients with long-standing mitral stenosis often have a characteristic facies — a dusky malar discoloration. This may be attributed to peripheral cyanosis associated with a low cardiac output and vasoconstriction.

The arterial pulse is usually normal in volume but may be small, and is often irregular due to atrial fibrillation. In the earlier stages, the venous pressure is normal, but rises with the onset of right-sided heart failure. When there is severe pulmonary hypertension, there may be a large venous 'a' wave due to forceful right atrial contraction against the hypertrophied non-compliant right ventricle.

The apex beat is usually in the normal place but may be deviated to the left by right ventricular hypertrophy. It often has a tapping quality, which is associated with the characteristic loud first heart sound. In more advanced cases, right ventricular hypertrophy produces a heaving impulse to the left of the lower sternum. Mid-diastolic and presystolic thrills may be present at, or internal to, the apex beat.

There are four cardinal auscultatory features of mitral stenosis (Fig 12.5):

- a loud first sound;
- an opening snap;
- a mid-diastolic murmur;
- a presystolic murmur.

The first sound is accentuated and the opening snap loud when the cusps are mobile; these signs may disappear with the development of rigidity and calcification of the valves (see p. 56). A mid-diastolic murmur is usually present, and its length, but not its intensity, gives an indication of the severity of the lesion. The presystolic murmur is often an early sign but may not be heard unless the patient is exercised and then turned into the left lateral position. A mitral systolic murmur signifies concomitant mitral regurgitation.

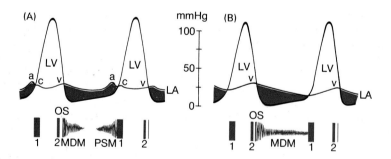

Fig. 12.5 (A) The pressure pulses in left ventricle and left atrium and the phonocardiographic appearances in mitral stenosis. A pressure difference is present throughout diastole (shaded area), and is accentuated by atrial contraction ('a' wave). Mid-diastolic and presystolic murmurs result. (B) Atrial fibrillation has developed with loss of the 'a' wave and of the presystolic accentuation of the murmur.

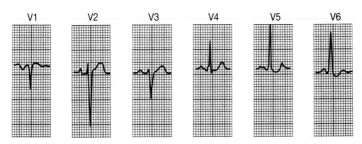

Fig. 12.6 P mitrale. There is a biphasic P wave in lead V1, with deep inversion of the terminal segment. In the left-sided leads the P wave is bifid, most clearly seen in leads V4 and V5 in this example.

The second sound splits normally, but the pulmonary component is often accentuated because of pulmonary hypertension. An apical third heart sound is impossible in significant mitral stenosis because the rapid filling of the left ventricle necessary for its production cannot occur.

The ECG

If sinus rhythm is present, there is usually P mitrale (Fig. 12.6). Atrial fibrillation is common; other atrial and ventricular arrhythmias occur occasionally. Evidence of right ventricular hypertrophy develops in cases with severe pulmonary hypertension.

Radiological appearances

The most characteristic radiological feature of mitral stenosis is the selective enlargement of the left atrium, which, in the posteroanterior view, produces a bulge below the pulmonary artery on the left border of the heart, and a rounded dense shadow within or outside the middle part of the right border of the heart (see Fig. 5.4). Left atrial enlargement can be confirmed by observing the displacement of the barium-filled oesophagus in the lateral view. Other radiological features may include calcification of the mitral valve, a normal or small left ventricle, and a normal or small aorta. The upper pulmonary veins are usually prominent. When the pulmonary capillary pressure is high, horizontal septal lines (Kerley's B lines) appear in the costophrenic angles, and the radiological features of pulmonary oedema may be seen. Haemosiderosis may produce mottling of the lungs. Pulmonary artery, right ventricular and, occasionally, right atrial enlargement may also be present when there is pulmonary arterial hypertension (Fig. 12.7).

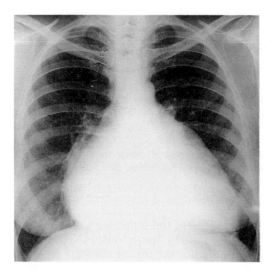

Fig. 12.7 Mixed mitral valve disease. Gross cardiac enlargement in a severe case of mixed mitral valve disease.

Echocardiography

In mitral stenosis, the M shape normally seen in diastole is lost, and the diastolic (EF) slope is reduced (Fig. 12.8A). Echoes from the valve are increased if it is fibrotic or calcified, and make the leaflets appear thickened. Separation of the leaflets is diminished, and the two leaflets may move in the same direction. Crosssectional echocardiography allows visualization of the stenotic mitral valve orifice (Fig. 12.8B), and estimation of the rate of filling of the left ventricle. Doppler ultrasound permits quantification of the rate of flow through the valve.

Cardiac catheterization

Cardiac catheterization reveals the haemodynamic changes previously described. This investigation is seldom required for diagnostic purposes, but may be helpful in assessing the severity of the lesion. This is most accurately done by simultaneously measuring the pressure on either side of the mitral valve and estimating the cardiac output. Angiocardiography is mainly of value in assessing the severity of any associated mitral or aortic regurgitation.

Combined valve disease

Mitral stenosis is frequently complicated by disease of the other cardiac valves. The combination of rheumatic aortic regurgitation with mitral stenosis is a common one; in most cases the aortic regurgitation is the less important defect. The severity of the aortic regurgitation can be judged with reasonable assurance by the pulse volume, and by the diastolic pressure, which in severe cases is usually less than 60 mmHg. The combination of severe mitral stenosis and aortic stenosis is unusual but important, because one may mask the presence of the other.

Severe tricuspid stenosis complicates about 3% of cases of mitral stenosis and often obscures its signs.

Tricuspid regurgitation is common in advanced mitral stenosis because the tricuspid valve ring dilates with right ventricular enlargement. The associated pansystolic murmur may be heard not only at the left sternal edge but as far out as the apex. This may lead to the erroneous diagnosis of mitral regurgitation. Systolic venous pulsation in the neck, the increase in the murmur on inspiration, and the lack of transmission of the murmur to the axilla serve to identify its tricuspid origin.

Diagnosis

The presence of mitral stenosis can often be suspected from a history of rheumatic fever combined with progressive dyspnoea, a small and irregular pulse, and a mitral facies. In the milder case, these features may be absent, and palpation and auscultation first reveal the diagnosis. A high proportion of patients have a tapping apex beat, right ventricular heave, loud first sound, opening snap, and mid-diastolic and presystolic murmurs. The experienced auscultator is usually first struck by the loud first sound and the opening snap rather than by the diastolic murmurs, which may be audible only if they are specifically sought with the patient lying in the left lateral position. The diagnosis is supported by P mitrale in the ECG, by the demonstration of left atrial enlargement in the radiograph and by the characteristic echocardiographic and catheterization features.

Probably the commonest cause for the mistaken diagnosis of mitral stenosis is the misinterpretation of normal splitting of the first sound for a presystolic murmur (a presystolic murmur is seldom the only auscultatory abnormality in mitral stenosis). A third heart sound may be wrongly interpreted as being an opening snap or a mid-diastolic murmur, and differentiation may be impossible without a phonocardiogram. One should hesitate to diagnose mitral stenosis on the basis of either a presystolic murmur or a short 'mid-diastolic murmur' alone without collateral evidence.

When an apical pansystolic murmur complicates the physical signs in mitral stenosis, it may be difficult to establish whether there is a significant degree of mitral regurgitation. This is unlikely if there is a loud first sound and an opening snap, or if there is evidence of advanced pulmonary hypertension. Important mitral regurgitation is probable if the systolic murmur is loud and radiates to the axilla, or if there is left ventricular hypertrophy, a soft first heart sound or a third

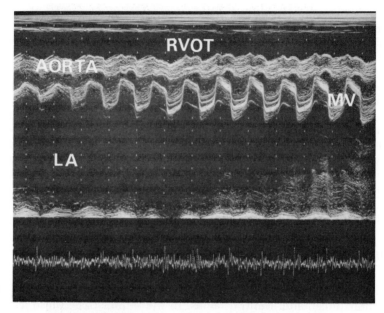

(A)

Fig. 12.8 (A) Severe mitral stenosis — an M-mode parasternal echocardiogram. The left atrium is hugely enlarged and the mitral valve shows the characteristic slow diastolic closure rate. RVOT = right ventricular outflow tract. MV = mitral valve. LA = left atrium. (B) Cross-sectional echocardiogram in mitral stenosis. The upper panel shows a short axis parasternal view. The mitral valve orifice is small and there is considerable thickening particularly on the left hand side of the orifice. The lower panel shows the long axis parasternal view with the hammocking appearance of the anterior cusp as it comes to the end of its opening movement.

sound rather than an opening snap. Doppler ultrasound and angiography are valuable in the diagnosis and assessment of regurgitation.

Mitral stenosis may be simulated by the mid-diastolic murmurs encountered in conditions leading to high flow through the mitral valve, such as ventricular septal defect and persistent ductus arteriosus, and by the Austin Flint murmur associated with severe aortic regurgitation as well as by the mid-diastolic murmur of left atrial myxoma. The possibility that a mid-diastolic murmur is not due to mitral stenosis should be considered particularly if there is neither a loud first sound nor an opening snap. In left atrial myxoma, the signs may entirely mimic those of mitral stenosis, but tend to vary from time to time (see also p. 341). Echocardiography is particularly valuable in differentiating the mid-diastolic murmur of mitral stenosis from that due to other causes.

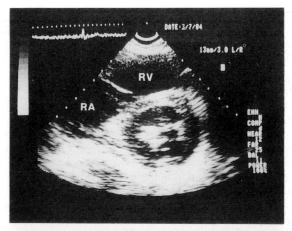

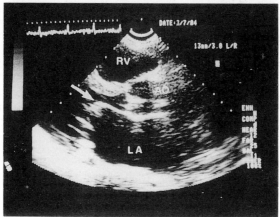

(B)

Fig. 12.8 continued.

Course and prognosis

The characteristic physical signs of mitral stenosis, which can be present within a year of acute rheumatic fever, may precede the development of symptoms by 10–20 years. Breathlessness, usually the first complaint, is most likely to start between the ages of 20 and 30 but may be delayed much longer. In those in whom complications do not develop, the course is slowly but steadily downhill over a number of years. However, in Western countries, patients with signs of rheumatic mitral valve disease are now mainly seen in middle or old age, whereas in parts of Asia and Africa, it is predominantly found in adolescents and young adults.

Sooner or later, some complication usually arises which leads to temporary or permanent deterioration. In young women, pregnancy is often responsible for the onset or aggravation of breathlessness; in the patient with severe stenosis, parturition may lead to pulmonary oedema and death. Once right-sided heart failure has developed, the prognosis without direct intervention on the valve is poor.

Medical treatment

Surgery or balloon valvotomy are eventually required in most cases, but it is usually necessary to prepare the patient for these procedures by appropriate medical therapy. Even after relief of the stenosis, treatment is often needed for the control of arrhythmias and the prevention of emboli.

Patients with mitral stenosis should be encouraged to live reasonably normal lives, but to avoid excessive exertion. They should be advised against being overweight, and discouraged from smoking. Infections must be promptly treated with appropriate antibiotics; anticoagulants should be used if there is evidence of venous thrombosis or of pulmonary or systemic embolism and considered in all patients with atrial fibrillation. Careful supervision is required during pregnancy (see p. 344).

Digitalis is required for atrial fibrillation, but is of no value in pure stenosis in sinus rhythm. Cardiac failure is otherwise treated by the usual means (see Chapter 8). An attempt to restore sinus rhythm should be made after mitral valve surgery in patients with atrial fibrillation, if this is known to be of fairly recent onset.

Surgical treatment and balloon valvotomy

Pure mitral stenosis can be treated by balloon valvotomy or by surgery. In the past, patients with pliant valves could be treated by a closed valvotomy (i.e. without direct vision of the valve and without cardiopulmonary bypass), but this procedure is being largely replaced by balloon valvotomy in which one or more balloons are passed through the atrial septum into the left atrium using the trans-septal technique, and the balloon(s) dilated within the valve. If the valve is rigid or there is much regurgitation, mitral valvotomy or replacement are performed with cardio-pulmonary bypass.

When the valve cusps are pliant and mobile, valvotomy leads to relief of the stenosis for many years, but restenosis of the valve frequently takes place after 5–10 years. When the valve is rigid or calcified, valvotomy is seldom successful for more than a few years, if at all. The mortality of mitral valve surgery depends upon the severity of the disease and the presence of complications. If the patient is in reasonably good health prior to the operation, and free of severe pulmonary hypertension and mitral regurgitation, the mortality should be less than 5% and, in the most favourable cases, less than 1%. Where there is advanced pulmonary hypertension or right-sided failure, the mortality may rise to 10% or more. In reaching a decision as to whether valvotomy should be undertaken, one must take into account the mortality even in relatively mild cases, the possibility of producing mitral regurgitation, the relatively high incidence of restenosis and the risk of causing cerebral embolism. Operation should be avoided in the presence of rheumatic activity. Surgery should also be deferred until cardiac failure has been brought under control or if there has been recent pulmonary or systemic embolism.

Mitral valvotomy is indicated when there are symptoms attributable to pure or almost pure mitral stenosis. It should be considered when there are signs indicating severe stenosis, particularly if there is advanced pulmonary arterial hypertension, even in the absence of symptoms. 'Prophylactic' valvotomy should be undertaken in young women with moderate or severe stenosis to avoid operating during pregnancy.

Atrial fibrillation develops shortly after the operation in about one-quarter of cases but often resolves spontaneously within 3 weeks. If it fails to do so, correction with d.c. shock should be undertaken.

The postcardiotomy syndrome, which is characterized by pericarditis, pleurisy, pyrexia and malaise, may arise 1–8 weeks after surgery. It has been attributed to an autoimmune reaction to heart muscle, or to the presence of blood in the pericardium. Corticosteroids relieve the symptoms but are usually unnecessary.

Successful valvotomy is effective in reducing symptoms, but signs of residual stenosis usually persist. The loud first heart sound and opening snap remain, but the diastolic murmurs are shortened or abolished.

Mitral regurgitation

Mitral regurgitation can be caused by a number of different disease processes:

- rheumatic endocarditis is the major cause in areas where rheumatic fever is prevalent, and is often accompanied by mitral stenosis. The valve cusps are usually rigid and deformed and the chordae tendineae fused and shortened. Calcification is common. In a small proportion of cases, however, the valve cusps are preserved, but the orifice enlarges as a consequence of scarring and dilatation of the mitral valve ring. Regurgitation may develop at the time of rheumatic fever, especially if this is severe, but does not usually produce major haemodynamic effects for several years because the progression of valve damage is slow;
- mitral valve prolapse (see p. 252);
- infective endocarditis may produce destruction or perforation of the cusps, or rupture of chordae tendineae;
- congenital mitral regurgitation occurs with or without other

congenital abnormalities (see 'atrial septal defect', p. 274);
- *papillary muscle malfunction* or rupture may result from myocardial infarction;
- *mitral valvotomy* may produce tearing of cusps;
- *left ventricular dilatation* from any cause, such as hypertension, coronary artery disease and aortic valve disease may lead to dilatation of the valve ring. The mitral regurgitation so produced leads to further enlargement of the left ventricle, and therefore further dilatation of the valve ring, with the development of a vicious circle;
- *spontaneous rupture of chordae tendineae* of unknown aetiology may occur.

Mitral valve prolapse

Prolapse of the mitral valve (billowing or ballooning of the posterior mitral valve leaflet) is a common condition which may be associated with rheumatic and ischaemic heart disease and with the Marfan syndrome. Usually, however, there is no other disease process; in such cases, there is a myxomatous change of the valve leaflets, which are voluminous and redundant. The usual auscultatory finding is a midsystolic click and/or a late apical systolic murmur, but the click and murmur may occur at other times during systole. In any individual, the auscultatory features may vary considerably from time to time, and can be made to do so by standing, sitting, and straining in the Valsalva manoeuvre. Most patients are asymptomatic, but some complain of left-sided chest pain or palpitation. The ECG may show minor ST abnormalities. Echocardiography (Fig. 5.20), which has demonstrated this abnormality in some 5% of normal young people, characteristically reveals a midsystolic 'buckling' of one or both leaflets into the left atrium. Some cases have a posterior 'hammocking' of the leaflets throughout systole. Although there is a slight risk of infective endocarditis and of serious arrhythmias, the prognosis is usually excellent. Patients with definitive evidence of mitral regurgitation should receive prophylaxis against infective endocarditis. Reassurance is an essential part of management; an anxiety state is the commonest complication of this lesion.

Pathophysiology

The severity of mitral regurgitation depends on a number of factors:

- the size of the mitral valve orifice during ventricular systole. Although this can be of fixed size, as it is when the valve is calcified, it may be variable, depending on the degree of left ventricular dilatation;
- the pressure relationships between the left ventricle, aorta and

left atrium;
- the left ventricular output.

Any factor which augments left ventricular output or raises aortic impedance increases mitral regurgitation. The degree of mitral regurgitation is limited by the distensibility of the left atrium and pulmonary veins. However, the pressure in the left atrium is much lower than that in the aorta, so that with a large valve orifice, as much blood may regurgitate into the left atrium during systole as is ejected into the aorta. A feature of chronic severe mitral regurgitation is that the left atrium is much larger than is usual in mitral stenosis.

During systole, the pressure in the left atrium may rise to a high 'v' peak, but will not do so if the regurgitated blood is readily accommodated in a voluminous left atrium. When mitral regurgitation develops abruptly, as with the rupture of papillary muscles or chordae tendineae, the left atrium is often small and the 'v' wave tall (Fig. 5.13).

In diastole, there is a large flow from left atrium to left ventricle, consisting of the blood received from the pulmonary circulation combined with that which regurgitated during the preceding systole. At this time the pressure in the left atrium falls rapidly to the ventricular level. Therefore, although there may be a high 'v' wave the mean left atrial pressure is often not greatly raised, and the pulmonary capillary pressure is seldom as high as that encountered in mitral stenosis. Eventually, however, with the development of left ventricular failure, the pulmonary capillary pressure rises and, with it, the pulmonary arterial pressure. Severe pulmonary hypertension and right-sided cardiac failure are unusual unless there is also an appreciable degree of mitral stenosis.

Complications

The complications are similar to those of mitral stenosis. Atrial fibrillation is frequent when mitral regurgitation is of rheumatic origin but less so when other disease processes are responsible. Infective endocarditis is not uncommon when the regurgitation is rheumatic or due to prolapse.

Symptoms

In cases of rheumatic origin, the physical signs precede symptoms by many years. When symptoms do occur, they usually increase slowly. Fatigue, perhaps attributable to the low cardiac output, may be the first complaint, but eventually dyspnoea on exertion, orthopnoea and, rarely, paroxysmal nocturnal dyspnoea develop.

When mitral regurgitation is due to perforation of a cusp, or to rupture of chordae tendineae or papillary muscles, the onset of symptoms is abrupt; the patient may present with acute pulmonary oedema.

Physical signs

The pulse is usually of normal volume; irregularity due to atrial fibrillation is common. The venous pressure is normal except when there is right-sided cardiac failure. The apex beat, which may be displaced downwards and outwards, often has the vigorous thrusting character of left ventricular hypertrophy and dilatation, and there is sometimes a systolic thrill.

The first sound is usually soft and introduces an apical pansystolic murmur which radiates to the axilla. The murmur may be of the same intensity throughout systole, but often increases towards the end of this period. When the regurgitation is due to papillary muscle malfunction or ballooning of a mitral cusp, the murmur may be exclusively in late systole. Rarely, it may radiate to the left sternal edge rather than to the axilla and may be mistaken for aortic stenosis. The intensity of the murmur bears some relation to the severity of the regurgitation, but is not a reliable guide. In most severe cases there is a third heart sound, followed by a short mid-diastolic murmur due to rapid filling of the left ventricle.

The ECG

The ECG may be normal but P mitrale is often present if atrial fibrillation has not supervened. Left ventricular hypertrophy occurs in severe mitral regurgitation, but if there is significant stenosis there may be evidence of biventricular hypertrophy or no abnormality.

Radiography and echocardiography

Radiologically, the most conspicuous feature is the marked enlargement of the left atrium, but there may also be left ventricular enlargement. Calcification of the mitral valve is often visible in rheumatic cases. Evidence of pulmonary dilatation and pulmonary oedema develops when there is left ventricular failure.

When mitral regurgitation is of acute onset due to malfunction or rupture of valve cusps, papillary muscles or chordae tendineae, there may be little left atrial or left ventricular enlargement in spite of high left atrial pressure and pulmonary oedema.

Echocardiography may not reveal any abnormality in mitral regurgitation, but if the reflux is large, there is dilatation of the left atrium and left ventricle. Calcification or thickening of the cusps may be seen. Other possible findings include mitral valve prolapse or a flail valve due to ruptured chordae or papillary muscles. Doppler ultrasound is a good technique for demonstrating mitral regurgitation, but does not allow accurate estimation of its severity.

Cardiac catheterization and angiocardiography

These procedures are seldom used for diagnosis, but quantitation can be obtained by injecting radio-opaque contrast medium into the left ventricle. Left ventriculography is of particular value in assessing the severity of mitral regurgitation complicating mitral stenosis. The presence of left ventricular failure may be confirmed by finding a high left ventricular end-diastolic pressure. A tall 'v' wave in the left atrial or pulmonary arterial wedge pressure tracing is suggestive of, but not diagnostic of, mitral regurgitation (see Fig. 5.13).

Diagnosis

The diagnosis is usually based on the finding of an apical pansystolic murmur radiating to the axilla. The pansystolic murmur of tricuspid regurgitation may reach the apex, but does not radiate further and is usually increased on inspiration. The systolic murmur of aortic stenosis may be heard best at the apex, but is midsystolic and does not radiate to the axilla. The murmur of ventricular septal defect is heard best at the lower left sternal edge.

It may be difficult to differentiate mitral regurgitation from a benign systolic murmur, but benign murmurs are never pansystolic, are seldom of grade 3 or greater intensity and tend to vary with posture and respiration.

Suggestive evidence of mitral regurgitation is provided by left atrial and left ventricular enlargement on the chest radiograph, and by P mitrale and left ventricular hypertrophy on the ECG. Echocardiography is valuable in prolapse of the mitral cusps and in ruptured chordae and papillary muscles. The definitive diagnosis is made by Doppler ultrasound or left ventriculography.

In mitral regurgitation of non-rheumatic origin, the diagnosis may be suggested by the sudden appearance of a loud apical systolic murmur accompanied by left ventricular failure.

Course and prognosis

The course of patients with mitral regurgitation is very variable. Those with mild regurgitation and without cardiomegaly may live a normal life span, although exposed to the risk of infective endocarditis. In rheumatic mitral regurgitation of moderate severity, the course is one of slow deterioration over 10–20 years with gradually increasing heart size until left ventricular failure develops. Unless this has been precipitated by a complication that can be corrected, the prognosis is then poor and death is likely to occur within a few years. When mitral regurgitation has been due to ruptured chordae tendineae, papillary muscles or cusps, the prognosis is generally poor, although the regurgitation is occasionally slight and well tolerated.

Medical treatment

Medical treatment does not differ from that for mitral stenosis, except that inotropic drugs, such as digitalis, may be of value even in sinus rhythm. Reduction in afterload, by vasodilator therapy, is helpful, particularly in acute mitral regurgitation.

Surgical treatment

Mitral regurgitation can be successfully treated surgically only under direct vision, with cardiopulmonary bypass. In some instances, it is possible to restore valve function by plicating the ring or ruptured chordae. In many cases, however, it is necessary to insert a mitral valve prosthesis. The problems associated with this are discussed on p. 359.

Because of the risks of open-heart surgery and of prosthetic valves, patients with mitral regurgitation should be considered for surgery only if they are becoming increasingly disabled and it is likely that they will succumb to their disease within a few years.

AORTIC VALVE DISEASE

The normal aortic valve consists of three semi-lunar cusps attached to a fibrous valve ring. Immediately above the insertion of the valve cusps are the sinuses of Valsalva, from two of which the coronary arteries arise. In about 1% of individuals the aortic valve has only two cusps.

The aortic valve and adjacent structures may be involved in congenital, rheumatic, bacterial, syphilitic and atherosclerotic changes. Both stenosis and regurgitation may occur as isolated lesions but are often combined. Calcification of the cusps is an important factor in the development of aortic valve disease and is often responsible for the stenosis that occurs in those with congenitally bicuspid valves.

Aortic stenosis

Aortic stenosis is most commonly the result of disease of the aortic valve cusps, but may also be due to narrowing in the outflow tract of the left ventricle below the cusps (subvalvar) and, very rarely, a constriction in the first part of the aorta (supravalvar stenosis).

Aetiology and pathology

Aortic valve stenosis may be congenital, rheumatic or sclerotic. Most instances of aortic stenosis occur in middle-aged or elderly patients, in whom there is no evidence of involvement of other valves. Calcification of the valve is usually severe and largely responsible for the stenosis. Even at necropsy it is seldom possible to determine the aetiology, but many have congenitally bicuspid valves. Rheumatic aortic stenosis results from adherence of adjacent cusps with thickening, fibrosis and subsequent calcification.

Subvalvar aortic stenosis may result from a congenital membrane or from fibrous tissue situated in the outflow tract of the left ventricle. This may be combined with valve stenosis, and thus form a tunnel in the outflow tract. A distinctive form of subvalvar stenosis is caused by hypertrophy of the muscle of the outflow tract of the left ventricle, particularly affecting the interventricular septum. This disorder has received a large variety of names including 'idiopathic hypertrophic subvalvular aortic stenosis' and 'hypertrophic obstructive cardio-myopathy' (see also p. 220).

Supravalvar aortic stenosis is congenital and may be associated with a distinctive facial appearance and mental deficiency.

Aortic stenosis is commonly associated with regurgitation. This is especially so in rheumatic and congenital valve stenosis and in congenital subvalvar stenosis. It is seldom severe in the calcific stenosis of the elderly and almost unknown in hypertrophic subaortic stenosis. Mitral valve disease usually predominates over aortic stenosis in rheumatic valve disease.

The left ventricle hypertrophies in response to the pressure load imposed upon it. The weight of the heart is often doubled in severe cases. There is usually little ventricular dilatation unless there is associated aortic regurgitation. Coronary artery disease may coexist with aortic stenosis, but commonly the coronary arteries are larger than normal. In aortic valve stenosis, there is a dilatation of the ascending aorta (an effect of the jet of blood which is propelled through the valve).

Pathophysiology

A minor degree of stenosis has little or no effect upon the function of the heart; only when the area of the valve orifice is reduced to a quarter of the normal are there serious consequences. The left ventricle responds to the pressure load by contracting more forcibly, and the left ventricular systolic pressure increases (see Fig. 12.9). A systolic pressure difference develops between the left ventricle and aorta (Fig. 12.10). The magnitude of this difference in pressure depends on the size of the orifice and the flow of blood through it. The obstruction delays emptying of the left ventricle, so that the phase of ejection becomes prolonged. The cardiac output is usually maintained within the normal range but at the expense of a considerable increase in left ventricular work. In consequence, left ventricular hypertrophy

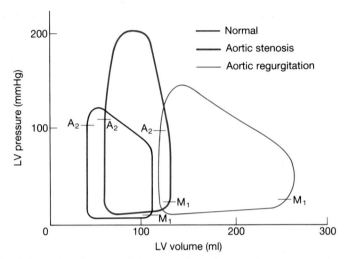

Fig. 12.9 Relationships between left ventricular volume and pressure in the normal heart, in aortic stenosis and in aortic regurgitation. M_1 = mitral valve closure. A_2 = aortic valve closure. Note high pressure generated in aortic stenosis and large end-diastolic volume (at M_1), with increased stroke volume in aortic regurgitation.

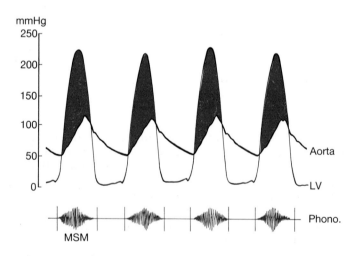

Fig. 12.10 Simultaneous pressure recordings and phonocardiographic appearances in aortic stenosis. Note the systolic pressure difference ('gradient') between the left ventricle and aorta, and the corresponding midsystolic murmur (MSM).

increases progressively as the valve orifice narrows. Although the hypertrophy is a compensatory phenomenon, it eventually contributes to the burden on the heart. The thickened ventricle is less compliant and is therefore less easily filled during diastole; atrial contraction contributes more and more to the filling process. The hypertrophied muscle increasingly outstrips the ability of the coronary arteries to supply it with blood.

Symptoms

There is a characteristic triad of symptoms:

- breathlessness;
- syncope on exertion;
- angina pectoris.

To these may be added the liability to sudden death.

Breathlessness is the earliest symptom in most cases. Later orthopnoea and paroxysmal nocturnal dyspnoea may occur. Eventually, right-sided heart failure with peripheral oedema may develop.

Syncope is much commoner in aortic stenosis than in other types of valvar heart disease and its relationship to exertion is of diagnostic value. Its mechanism is uncertain, but it may be due to the inability of the heart to increase its output sufficiently, or to reflex vasodilatation, or to arrhythmias.

Like syncope, anginal pain is much commoner in aortic stenosis than in other valve lesions. It does not differ in character from that seen in coronary artery disease.

Death is often sudden and may not be preceded by any symptoms. However, it is particularly likely to occur in those who have experienced syncope or angina pectoris. It is believed that ventricular fibrillation is usually responsible.

Physical signs

An aortic systolic murmur is the first abnormality to appear and may be present for decades before evidence of severe stenosis develops.

The pulse is abnormal in most severe cases (Fig. 12.11). Characteristically it is small in volume, rises slowly to its peak, and takes an unusually long time to pass the finger. The pulse pressure is correspondingly small. When there is an appreciable degree of aortic regurgitation as well, the pulse pressure may be normal or large, and the pulse may take on a 'bisferiens' quality in which a double pulse is felt.

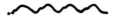

Fig. 12.11   Small, flat pulse in aortic stenosis.

The apex beat may be in the normal position or displaced downwards and to the left. It has a slow heaving quality. A systolic thrill can often be felt in the second right intercostal space, and also in the carotid arteries and along the left edge of the sternum.

There is a midsystolic murmur, which is usually loud and harsh. This may be best heard in the second right interspace, along the left sternal edge, or even at the apex. It is often audible over the carotid arteries. It is accompanied by an early systolic ('ejection') click in those cases in which there is aortic valve stenosis without heavy calcification. This sign is probably due to sudden tension of the valve cusps at the time of opening. Other signs may include a fourth (atrial) heart sound over the left ventricle and reversed splitting of the second heart sound. This latter sign is due to delay in left ventricular emptying and aortic valve closure. The aortic component of the second heart sound may not be audible if there is calcification.

ECG, chest radiography, echocardiography and Doppler ultrasound

The ECG usually shows left ventricular hypertrophy, the extent of which roughly parallels the severity of the stenosis. Other abnormalities which sometimes occur include asymmetrical inversion of T waves and left bundle branch block. The chest radiograph may be normal, but the ascending aorta is usually dilated in aortic valve stenosis. Left ventricular enlargement may be evident (Fig. 12.12). Calcification of the valve when present is best visualized by fluoroscopy. Apex cardiography is of value in demonstrating large 'a' waves which provide an index of severity.

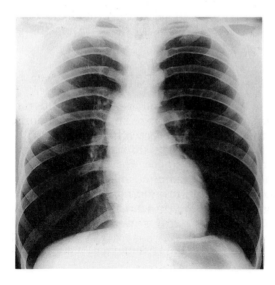

Fig. 12.12 Aortic stenosis. The rounded configuration of the left ventricular outline suggests left ventricular hypertrophy. The ascending aorta shows post-stenotic dilatation.

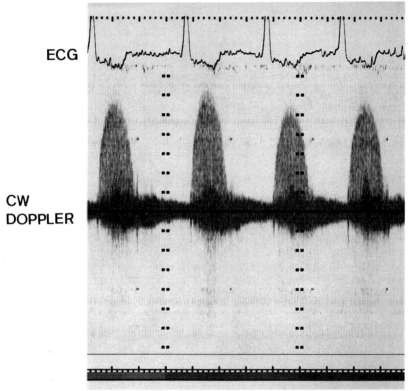

Fig. 12.13 Continuous wave Doppler recording in a patient with aortic stenosis and atrial fibrillation. The height of the signal varies with the velocity of the jet and in this case varies from cycle to cycle depending on the preceding cycle length. The maximum velocity is 6 metres per second which calculates out at a gradient of 144 mmHg.

Echocardiography may reveal thickening and calcification of the cusps; bicuspid valves are seen to open eccentrically. The supravalvar or subvalvar location of the obstruction may be apparent. Doppler ultrasound (Fig. 12.13) can be used to estimate the severity of aortic stenosis, and may obviate the need for cardiac catheterization.

Cardiac catheterization

The systolic pressure difference across the stenosis is measured with catheters in left ventricle and aorta or by the withdrawal of a catheter from left ventricle to aorta (Fig. 12.14). If the stenosis is severe, the left ventricular systolic pressure exceeds that in the aorta by more than 50 mmHg. In advanced cases the cardiac output falls, and the gradient may be less than this in spite of extreme narrowing.

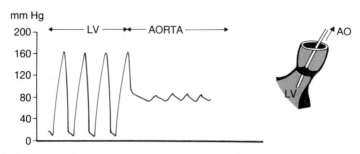

Fig. 12.14 Pressure tracing recorded as catheter is withdrawn from left ventricle to aorta in aortic valve stenosis. Note sudden fall in systolic pressure as the catheter tip enters the aorta.

Complications

The most frequent cause of death is cardiac failure, but there is considerable risk of sudden death. Infective endocarditis may occur and, by eroding the cusps, cause severe aortic regurgitation.

Diagnosis and differential diagnosis

The diagnosis is often suggested by the triad of symptoms (dyspnoea, angina, syncope on exertion), or by the finding of the typical murmur associated with a thrill and a small pulse. Calcification of the valve seen on fluoroscopy provides confirmatory evidence. Hypertrophic subaortic stenosis can be differentiated from other varieties by the pulse, which rises rapidly rather than slowly, and by the absence of an ejection click, valve calcification and aortic regurgitation; the diagnosis is established by echocardiography.

Systolic murmurs in the aortic area occur not only in aortic stenosis, but also when the aortic valve is sclerosed, and when the aorta is dilated by hypertension, atherosclerosis or syphilis. These conditions are not associated with the small pulse and massive left ventricular hypertrophy characteristic of aortic stenosis.

Prognosis

Cases of mild aortic stenosis have a good prognosis; if there is no appreciable degree of left ventricular hypertrophy, the patient is likely to survive for many years. Once the symptoms of breathlessness, angina or syncope have developed, death is likely to occur suddenly at any time, or within 5 years from heart failure.

Treatment

Little or no benefit can be expected from medical treatment. When symptoms have developed, strenuous activity should be avoided and the conventional treatment of heart failure and angina pectoris employed. Surgery is indicated for nearly all patients; this necessitates open-heart techniques. In some cases of non-calcific aortic valve stenosis and in sub-valvar stenosis, corrective operations to widen the stenosed orifice may be successful. When there is calcification of the aortic valve, it must be replaced. For this purpose, either prosthetic valves, homograft or heterograft valves can be inserted (see p. 357). The mortality of aortic valve replacement varies greatly from centre to centre, but averages about 5%. This risk must be weighed against the grave prognosis in those with advanced symptoms. Balloon valvotomy is an alternative to surgery in some patients, but it is by no means as satisfactory a means of producing an adequate orifice. It is indicated for patients with severe stenosis for whom surgery would be unduly risky, such as the very elderly or those suffering from other disabling diseases.

Aortic regurgitation (synonyms: aortic incompetence, insufficiency)

Aetiology

Aortic regurgitation is commonly due to rheumatic heart disease. It can also be of congenital origin, in which case it is usually of less importance than the lesions which accompany it, such as aortic and sub-aortic stenosis and ventricular septal defect. Other causes include bicuspid valves, hypertension, infective endocarditis, the Marfan syndrome, dissecting aneurysm, syphilitic aortitis, ankylosing spondylitis and Reiter's disease. In a substantial proportion of cases no cause can be found, i.e. they are 'idiopathic'.

Pathology

Aortic regurgitation can result either from damage to the cusps or from dilatation of the aorta and the valve ring. In rheumatic heart disease, the cusps are thickened and shortened and there may be some fusion of commissures. Varying degrees of stenosis and regurgitation occur. Calcification of the valve, which is usually severe in aortic stenosis, is seldom of importance in pure aortic regurgitation.

Syphilitic aortitis leads to aortic regurgitation as a result of dilatation of the aorta and the valve ring; stenosis is not a feature.

Infective endocarditis can cause erosion or perforation of the cusps, which have usually had some pre-existing abnormality.

Pathophysiology

In aortic regurgitation, a large volume of blood is regurgitated into the left ventricle in each diastole. The left ventricular output may be more than doubled. The increased stroke volume necessary to achieve this is associated with dilatation of the left ventricle (see Fig. 12.10). The regurgitant flow is greatest in early diastole when the difference in pressure between the aorta and left ventricle is maximal. The amount of blood that regurgitates is largely determined by the severity of the aortic valve disease but is also influenced by the compliance of the left ventricle and the systemic vascular resistance.

The dilated left ventricle contracts more powerfully in accordance with Starling's law, but there is an increased tension in the myocardium and increased oxygen consumption. The initial dilatation thus leads eventually to hypertrophy.

The diastolic pressure in the aorta is abnormally low, partly due to the leak and partly to peripheral vasodilatation. The left ventricular end-diastolic pressure is normal in the milder case but rises when cardiac failure supervenes.

Clinical features

Rheumatic aortic regurgitation usually develops at the time of acute rheumatic carditis and persists subsequently. Many years elapse between the appearance of the murmur and the onset of symptoms.

Almost invariably the first complaint is that of dyspnoea on exertion, although fatigue is also frequent. Other minor symptoms include dizziness and an awareness of the vigorous heart action.

The dyspnoea progresses slowly; eventually orthopnoea and paroxysmal dyspnoea may develop. Typical angina pectoris is infrequent except when the regurgitation is severe. In the advanced case, signs of right-sided failure complicate those of left-sided failure.

The arterial pulse in aortic regurgitation, often called 'collapsing' or 'water-hammer', rises rapidly and falls abruptly. This is most easily appreciated by placing the palm of one's hand on the anterior aspect of the patient's forearm (the arm being held vertically upright) because by this means one may accentuate the backflow of blood during diastole. Sometimes the pulse is of bisferiens type, i.e. is felt to have two equally prominent waves, particularly if the regurgitation is accompanied by stenosis. The cardiac rhythm is usually normal unless there is associated mitral valve disease. The systolic pressure is often abnormally high and the diastolic low. In a severe case the systolic pressure may be 250–300 mmHg and the diastolic 30–50 mmHg. Vigorous arterial pulsation is often visible in the neck.

If the regurgitation is substantial, the apex beat is displaced outwards and downwards and is overactive and heaving. The essential feature on auscultation is an early diastolic murmur, usually best heard over the midsternal region or at the lower left sternal edge. In some cases, particularly in syphilitic aortitis, it is loudest in the second right intercostal space. There is often an accompanying systolic murmur; this does not necessarily indicate coexistent aortic stenosis but may be due to the increased stroke volume. The early (or 'immediate') diastolic murmur is often difficult to hear, and is frequently overlooked by the inexperienced. It must be specifically sought, with the stethoscope diaphragm placed at the lower left sternal edge, with the patient sitting up, his breath held in expiration.

In some patients with advanced aortic regurgitation, a mid-diastolic murmur may be heard even in the absence of mitral stenosis. This murmur (known as the Austin Flint murmur) has been attributed to the effect of the regurgitant jet on the aortic leaflet of the mitral valve which is interposed between the mitral and aortic valve orifices (see Fig. 12.2). One should hesitate to diagnose an Austin Flint murmur in rheumatic heart disease because concomitant mitral stenosis is likely, particularly if there is a loud first sound or opening snap.

ECG, chest radiography, echocardiography and Doppler ultrasound

The ECG shows increasing evidence of left ventricular hypertrophy as the disease process advances. On the chest radiograph, there is usually left ventricular enlargement, with an elongated heart shadow and dilatation of the ascending aorta. Echocardiography often shows a vibration of the anterior leaflet of the mitral valve, and, if the regurgitation is severe, the mitral valve is seen to close abnormally early. Doppler ultrasound is a sensitive technique for demonstrating the presence, but not the severity, of aortic regurgitation.

Cardiac catheterization

Gross aortic regurgitation is so readily recognized clinically and by non-invasive methods that cardiac catheterization is seldom required for diagnostic purposes. This investigation is, however, necessary when the degree of severity is in doubt; it is of particular value in evaluating the significance of an aortic diastolic murmur in a patient needing surgery for concomitant mitral valve disease. The cine-angiographic demonstration of the regurgitation of contrast medium injected into the aorta provides a good estimate of severity.

Differential diagnosis

The clinical diagnosis of aortic regurgitation is usually not difficult if it is moderate or severe. A large pulse pressure is also observed in other conditions, such as persistent ductus arteriosus, arteriovenous fistulae, pregnancy, anaemia and thyrotoxicosis. The early diastolic murmur may be confused with that of pulmonary regurgitation, but this rare lesion is seldom found in the absence of severe pulmonary hypertension. Doppler ultrasound is useful in differentiating the two conditions, and echocardiographic demonstration of fluttering of the mitral valve is very suggestive of the aortic origin of the regurgitation.

In determining the aetiology of aortic regurgitation, it is important to look for other valve lesions and for evidence of disease in other systems. The signs of mitral stenosis or regurgitation suggest a rheumatic origin. Syphilis should be suspected particularly when there is aneurysmal dilatation of the aorta or calcification of the ascending aorta. Congenital aortic regurgitation is usually over-shadowed by aortic or subaortic stenosis.

Clinical course and prognosis

Minor degrees of aortic regurgitation are compatible with freedom from symptoms and a normal life span although the risk of infective endocarditis is ever present. In the moderate to severe case, symptoms and signs develop slowly, and it is usually not until the fourth or fifth decade that disability sets in. The severity of aortic regurgitation can be judged, to a large extent, by the pulse pressure and the size of the left ventricle. Increasing dyspnoea and an enlarging heart are signs that the patient is unlikely to survive for more than a few years. Sudden death is unusual in asymptomatic patients but may occur when an advanced stage has been reached.

Treatment

In less severe cases, considerable symptomatic improvement can be obtained by conventional treatment of cardiac failure such as the restriction of activity, and the use of digitalis and diuretics. When symptoms or heart size are increasing in spite of medical measures, surgery should be considered. In good hands the results of aortic valve replacement, either by artificial valves or bioprostheses are reasonably satisfactory, but there is an operative mortality of about 5%. Artificial prostheses necessitate anticoagulant therapy; bioprostheses do not. Successful surgery is accompanied by a diminution in heart size, although not necessarily to normal. Symptoms are relieved, but medical measures may still be required.

Combined aortic stenosis and regurgitation

Aortic stenosis and regurgitation are often combined. When the lesion is congenital, atherosclerotic or calcific, the stenosis is usually the more important. In rheumatic heart disease, all gradations between the two can occur. In deciding which is dominant, the character of the pulse and the pulse pressure are of great value. A collapsing pulse is incompatible with severe stenosis; a small pulse makes major regurgitation unlikely. The murmurs can be deceptive as loud aortic systolic murmurs are not uncommon in aortic regurgitation even when stenosis is slight or absent. Likewise, the intensity of an aortic diastolic murmur is an unreliable guide to the severity of regurgitation. Echocardiography and Doppler ultrasound supplemented, if necessary, by cardiac catheterization and angiocardiography permit adequate assessment of the relative contribution of each lesion.

TRICUSPID VALVE DISEASE

The structure of the tricuspid valve is similar to that of the mitral valve, except for the presence of three cusps. It may be affected by either stenosis or regurgitation. Tricuspid stenosis is nearly always rheumatic in origin and is rarely the dominant cardiac lesion. Some degree of tricuspid stenosis occurs in about 10% of cases of rheumatic heart disease, but is of significance in only about 3%. Organic tricuspid regurgitation, which is uncommon, is usually due to rheumatic heart disease. Functional tricuspid regurgitation is a frequent complication of right ventricular failure whatever the cause.

When tricuspid valve lesions are due to rheumatic heart disease, the pathological appearances are similar to those seen in the mitral valve. The valve cusps are thickened and the chordae may be adherent and shortened. Dilatation of the tricuspid valve ring is a major factor in regurgitation and occurs as a result of either dilatation of the right ventricle or the rheumatic process.

Tricuspid stenosis

The narrowed valve obstructs flow from the right atrium to the right ventricle during ventricular diastole. As a consequence, right atrial pressure rises, cardiac output falls, and the right atrium and venae cavae dilate. Atrial contraction becomes increasingly forceful and produces large 'a' waves in the venous pulse if sinus rhythm is preserved as it usually is. Hepatic engorgement follows and ascites and peripheral oedema eventually develop.

In most cases of tricuspid stenosis, mitral stenosis is also present and dominates the clinical picture. For this reason, breathlessness is the commonest symptom, but because tricuspid stenosis restricts right ventricular throughput, pulmonary congestion is often less severe than it is in isolated mitral stenosis. The patient with mitral stenosis may become less breathless as tricuspid stenosis progresses, but at the expense of right-sided cardiac failure.

Large flicking venous 'a' waves may be seen even in early cases. When the lesion is more advanced the venous pressure as a whole is elevated. The 'a' wave disappears when atrial fibrillation develops.

The flow of blood from the atrium into the ventricle during diastole is slow and the 'y' descent of the venous pulse is therefore prolonged. The liver is enlarged and may exhibit presystolic pulsation corresponding with the large 'a' waves. On auscultation, mid-diastolic and presystolic murmurs may be heard at the lower left sternal edge which are similar in timing to those of mitral stenosis but of a rather more scratchy quality. The murmurs are accentuated by inspiration, because of increased venous return to the right atrium at this time. The signs of mitral stenosis may be masked.

On the ECG the only characteristic feature is the presence of the tall P waves of right atrial enlargement. The chest radiograph shows enlargement of the right atrium and superior vena cava; the features of mitral stenosis are also usually present. The lung fields are often relatively clear. Echocardiography may reveal reduced movement or thickening of the cusps.

On cardiac catheterization, a diastolic pressure difference can be demonstrated between right atrium and right ventricle, and there is usually a large 'a' wave in the right atrial pulse.

The prognosis of patients with tricuspid stenosis is often relatively good. However, if the lesion is severe, progressive signs of right-sided cardiac failure develop; ascites, jaundice and cachexia are characteristic.

In the majority of patients with tricuspid stenosis, the lesion is insufficiently severe to warrant surgery, which should be undertaken only if the stenosis is responsible for major symptoms. Valvotomy seldom restores normal valve function; replacement by a prosthesis is usually necessary.

Tricuspid regurgitation

As mentioned, functional tricuspid regurgitation is a common complication of right ventricular failure and pulmonary hypertension. Since most patients with this condition have evidence of rheumatic heart disease, it is often difficult to be sure whether or not there is organic tricuspid disease as well. One can, however, deduce that the regurgitation is functional if the signs disappear with the use of digitalis and diuretics or the successful treatment of mitral valve disease.

The features of tricuspid regurgitation are the consequence of a large volume of blood being regurgitated through the valve from the right ventricle. As a result, the forward flow into the pulmonary circuit is reduced and the right ventricle has to cope with a large volume load. When regurgitation is severe, large systolic ('cv') waves develop in the right atrium, which are transmitted to the peripheral veins and liver. There is a high flow of blood through the tricuspid valve during diastole, as both the regurgitated and the forward flow must be transported at this time. Both diastolic and systolic flow through the valve is increased on inspiration as an increased volume of blood is drawn into the heart.

Coexistent mitral valve disease usually dominates the clinical picture and dyspnoea is the major symptom. Tricuspid regurgitation may reduce the effects of the mitral valve disease on the lungs at the expense of producing right-sided heart failure. As the disease progresses, there is an increase in venous pressure, hepatic enlargement, ascites and peripheral oedema. Large systolic waves are present in the jugular veins; systolic pulsation of the liver may be felt. A systolic murmur is heard at the lower left sternal edge; this is usually increased on inspiration. There may also be a tricuspid diastolic murmur due either to concomitant tricuspid stenosis or to high flow through the orifice during this phase.

There are no specific ECG features of tricuspid regurgitation; the chest radiograph usually shows right atrial enlargement. If the tricuspid regurgitation is secondary to mitral valve disease and pulmonary hypertension, the characteristic radiological features of these lesions will be present.

On cardiac catheterization, the chief feature is the large systolic venous wave of the right atrial pulse. The finding of severe pulmonary hypertension suggests the regurgitation is functional. A near normal pulmonary artery pressure is an indication that the tricuspid disease is organic.

It is often difficult to differentiate mitral regurgitation from tricuspid regurgitation, or to determine whether there is a combination of the two. Mitral regurgitation is suggested by radiation of the murmur to the axilla and by left ventricular enlargement, tricuspid regurgitation by systolic venous pulsation and by inspiratory accentuation of the murmur. Doppler ultrasound is a sensitive technique for detecting tricuspid regurgitation and gives some impression of its severity.

Tricuspid regurgitation is often tolerated for a long time, but sooner or later the features of advanced right-sided cardiac failure become disabling, often with jaundice and cachexia. Severe oedema and ascites develop and are progressively less responsive to treatment.

If the tricuspid regurgitation is functional, there may be striking improvement with digitalis and diuretic therapy. Usually, surgery for associated mitral valve disease is required, and, if successful, leads to the disappearance of the tricuspid leak. When severe tricuspid regurgitation does not diminish in response to these measures, repair or replacement of the valve by a prosthesis becomes necessary.

PULMONARY VALVE DISEASE

Pulmonary valve disease is relatively uncommon. Pulmonary stenosis is usually of congenital origin and is discussed in Chapter 13. Other causes of pulmonary stenosis include rheumatic heart disease, and malignant carcinoid. Obstruction of the outflow tract of the right ventricle may occur in hypertrophic cardiomyopathy and mediastinal tumours.

Pulmonary regurgitation is usually secondary to pulmonary hypertension, but occasionally occurs as a consequence of infective endocarditis, as a complication of the surgical relief of pulmonary stenosis, and as a congenital anomaly. It is nearly always overshadowed by the heart disease to which it is secondary. In most cases, there are signs of pulmonary hypertension, and the only feature which suggests the diagnosis is an early diastolic murmur (the Graham Steell murmur) in the second or third left intercostal spaces which becomes louder on inspiration. It is often difficult to decide whether a murmur in this position is due to pulmonary or aortic regurgitation. Pulmonary regurgitation is unlikely in the absence of signs of pulmonary hypertension and right ventricular hypertrophy. Aortic regurgitation is suggested by a collapsing pulse and the signs of left ventricular hypertrophy, although these signs may be absent if the regurgitation is slight. The diagnosis may be confirmed by Doppler ultrasound. Pulmonary regurgitation seldom produces serious haemodynamic effects and its prognosis and treatment are those of the associated pulmonary hypertension.

Further reading

Greenberg, B.H. & Murphy, E. (Eds) (1987) *Valvular Heart Disease*. Littleton: PSG.

Hall, R.J.C. & Julian, D.G. (1989) *Diseases of the Cardiac Valves*. Edinburgh: Churchill Livingstone.

Hall, R.J.C. & Kirk, R. (1992) Balloon dilatation of heart valves. *British Medical Journal* **305**: 487.

Congenital Heart Disease

A congenital abnormality of the heart is present in nearly one in every hundred babies born. About half of the affected babies die either from their heart disease or from some associated congenital anomaly during the first year of life if untreated. The prognosis of those who survive this period is reasonably good; from 5 years of age until early adult life, the prevalence of congenital heart disease remains at about three per thousand. The less severe types of lesion then begin to take their toll and it is unusual for patients with uncorrected congenital heart disease to survive much beyond the age of 40. Most forms of congenital heart disease are amenable to surgery; in some cases this leads to cure, but in others some residual abnormality is left that may require continuing attention.

Embryology

At an early stage, the heart consists of a simple tube of endocardium surrounded by myocardium and epicardium. As it grows, the tube twists into an S shape and by the fourth week of pregnancy it is divided by constrictions into five segments:

- the sinus venosus, which receives the systemic veins;
- the common atrium;
- the common ventricle;
- the bulbus cordis;
- the truncus arteriosus (Fig. 13.1).

Between the fifth and eighth week, changes of the greatest importance occur; it is at this time that congenital abnormalities are most likely to arise through arrested or faulty development. Septa develop in the atria and in the ventricles to sub-divide each of these chambers into two. Simultaneously, the atria are divided from the ventricles by endocardial cushions from which the mitral and tricuspid valves are formed (Fig. 13.2A). A spiral septum divides the bulbus cordis into

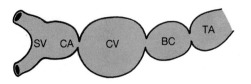

Fig. 13.1 The heart at the fourth week of pregnancy, divided by constrictions into sinus venosus (SV), common atrium (CA), common ventricle (CV), bulbus cordis (BC) and truncus arteriosus (TA).

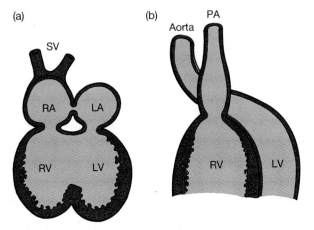

(a)   (b)

Fig. 13.2 (A) The heart at 8 weeks. The ventricles and atria are each being divided by septa into two chambers. Endocardial cushions develop from which the mitral and tricuspid valves are formed. (B) The spiral septum divides the bulbus cordis into the outflow tracts of the left and right ventricles, and the truncus arteriosus into the aorta and pulmonary arteries.

the outflow tracts of the left and right ventricles respectively, and the truncus arteriosus into aorta and pulmonary artery (Fig. 13.2B).

By the end of the eighth week, the heart has largely assumed the features which it retains until birth. The right atrium in the fetal circulation then receives blood from the superior vena cava and from the vitello-umbilical veins which later become the inferior vena cava. A proportion of the venous blood, particularly that from the superior vena cava, flows into the right ventricle, thence into the pulmonary artery and, by way of the ductus arteriosus, into the descending aorta. Only about 5% of the blood flow traverses the pulmonary circulation. Most of the highly oxygenated inferior vena caval blood is directed through the foramen ovale in the atrial septum into the left atrium and thence, by the left ventricle, into the ascending aorta. Within a few hours or, at most, days of birth the ductus arteriosus closes, and the relatively high pressure in the left atrium keeps the valve of the foramen ovale shut.

Aetiology

No aetiological factor can be found in most cases of congenital heart disease. In a minority there is evidence of either a genetic abnormality or an environmental factor affecting the mother during the early stages of pregnancy.

When congenital malformations are multiple, particularly in Down's syndrome (mongolism or Trisomy 21), Turner's syndrome and Marfan's syndrome, the heart is often involved. Congenital heart disease rarely affects more than one member of a family. If rubella occurs during the first 3 months of pregnancy, there is a considerable risk of cardiac malformation in the fetus. Other virus infections may occasionally be responsible, as may some drugs, including thalidomide, warfarin and alcohol.

THE VARIETIES OF CONGENITAL HEART DISEASE

The varieties of congenital heart disease can be divided into three types.

Communications between the left (systemic) and right (pulmonary) circulations, e.g. atrial septal defect, ventricular septal defect and persistent ductus arteriosus.

The impedance to flow is normally lower on the right side of the heart and in the pulmonary artery than it is on the left side of the heart and in the aorta. Consequently, the intracardiac pressures are relatively low on the right side. When the two sides of the heart are in communication, provided there is no other abnormality, there is a shunt of blood from left to right through the defect and an increased blood flow through the lungs. In ventricular septal defect and persistent ductus arteriosus, the volume load falls predominantly on the left ventricle, which enlarges accordingly. In atrial septal defect, the load falls on the right ventricle.

The greatly increased pulmonary blood flow frequently leads to a moderate elevation of pulmonary arterial pressure. In most cases, the resistance of the pulmonary arteries is normal but, sometimes, changes take place in the arterial walls which cause a high pulmonary vascular resistance. Severe and irreversible pulmonary hypertension may then ensue and, eventually, lead to reversal of the shunt (Eisenmenger syndrome p. 288).

Obstructive lesions, e.g. coarctation of the aorta, aortic stenosis and pulmonary stenosis.

When these lesions are isolated, they impose a burden on the related ventricle and may eventually cause cardiac failure on this account. They may be combined with abnormal communications, the most important anomaly being that of tetralogy of Fallot, in which there is pulmonary stenosis with a ventricular septal defect.

Displacement or absence of chambers, vessels or valves. These may be associated with abnormal communications or obstructions. Some displacement lesions such as dextrocardia and right-sided aorta may be unimportant. Others, such as transposition of the great arteries, are associated with a high mortality.

Abnormal communications

ATRIAL SEPTAL DEFECT (ASD)

The foramen ovale, which is unsealed in some 25% of adults, does not normally permit the flow of blood from the left atrium to the right

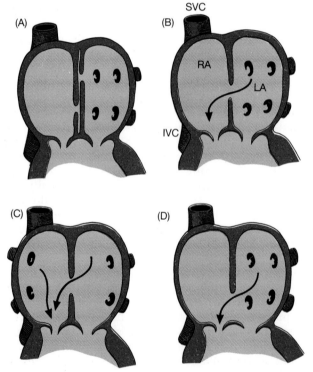

Fig. 13.3 (A) Unsealed foramen ovale. The valvar construction of the foramen ovale prevents shunting from left to right. (B) Atrial septal defect of ostium secundum type. The valve cusps are not affected. (C) Anomalous drainage of the right pulmonary veins into the right atrium, associated with an atrial septal defect of the secundum type. (D) Ostium primum defect, associated with abnormalities of the mitral or tricuspid valves.

atrium because of its valvar construction (Fig. 13.3A).

There are three types of abnormality which permit a flow of oxygenated blood into the right atrium:

- The ostium secundum defect, which may be large but does not encroach upon the atrioventricular valves. This is much the commonest variety (Fig. 13.3B).
- The ostium primum defect which is situated close to the atrioventricular valves and is often associated with abnormalities of these valves and, sometimes, with a partial or complete atrioventricular septal defect ('endocardial cushion' defect) (Fig. 13.3D). In the complete form, there is a ventricular septal defect and a common atrio-ventricular orifice.
- One or more of the pulmonary veins may be attached to the right atrium or great veins instead of the left atrium (Fig. 13.3C). There is usually an atrial septal defect as well.

The right ventricle is normally thinner and more distensible than the left and, at a given pressure level, more easily filled with blood. Therefore when both atria are in communication, blood flows preferentially into the right ventricle from both atria and the shunt through the defect is almost exclusively from left to right. The pulmonary blood flow is usually two or three times the aortic blood flow, but the distensibility of pulmonary arterioles is such that they can readily accommodate this with little or no increase in pulmonary arterial pressure. The increase of pulmonary blood flow maintained over many years, however, sometimes leads to changes in the small pulmonary vessels which increase pulmonary vascular resistance and cause severe pulmonary hypertension.

The ostium secundum type of defect seldom gives rise to disabling symptoms before the third decade of life, but breathlessness and fatigue are likely to develop before the age of 40. Symptoms are usually progressive and are exacerbated when atrial arrhythmias develop, as they commonly do. By contrast, the complete atrioventricular septal defect often presents in the first year of life with heart failure, respiratory infection, and failure to gain weight.

The arterial pulse is relatively small; the venous pressure is usually normal. The right ventricle is strikingly overactive. Splitting of the second sound is wide, and varies little with respiration. This is due to relatively late closure of the pulmonary valve as a consequence of delayed emptying of the overburdened right ventricle. A systolic murmur in the second left interspace due to high flow across the pulmonary valve is almost invariable. Larger defects cause mid-diastolic murmur at the lower left sternal edge, accentuated by inspiration, and produced by increased flow through the tricuspid valve. In the ostium primum type of defect, in which an abnormal mitral valve may permit regurgitation, there may be left ventricular

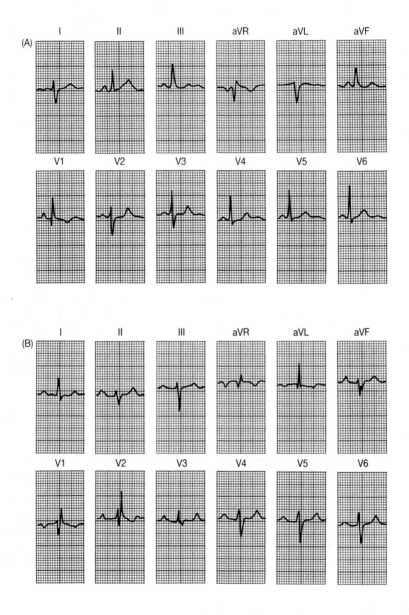

Fig. 13.4 (A) Ostium secondum atrial septal defect. The ECG typically shows an rSR' pattern, with right axis deviation. (B) Ostium primum atrial septum defect. The ECG again shows an rSR' pattern, but there is left axis deviation. In this example there is also PR prolongation.

enlargement and an apical systolic murmur.

The ECG nearly always shows the features of partial right bundle branch block ('rsr' complex). In the common ostium secundum type, there is frequently right axis deviation, whilst in the ostium primum type there is usually left axis deviation. This feature is of importance in differentiating the two types of defect (Fig. 13.4).

On the chest radiograph, the heart is usually slightly enlarged, and the pulmonary artery and its branches prominent, as are the right atrium and the right ventricle (see Fig. 5.11). The aorta is abnormally small and may not be visible. Expansile pulsation of the pulmonary arteries ('hilar dance') may be a striking feature on fluoroscopy.

Echocardiography, in ostium secundum defect, demonstrates 'paradoxical' septal motion. As a result of right ventricular overloading, the septum moves towards the right ventricle in systole instead of its usual movement towards the posterior left ventricular wall at this time.

In ostium primum, abnormalities of the mitral valve are usual.

Cross-sectional echocardiography reliably demonstrates primum and secundum defects and differentiates easily between them. Doppler ultrasound provides supporting evidence and may permit an assessment of the shunt.

These clinical features are usually sufficiently characteristic for accurate diagnosis. Confirmation by cardiac catheterization is required when the diagnosis is in doubt or surgical treatment is planned. The oxygen saturation in the right atrium is markedly higher than that in the superior vena cava, and the catheter tip may be advanced through the septal defect into the left atrium and thence to the left ventricle. In the ostium primum defect, injection of radio-opaque contrast medium into the left ventricle often reveals mitral regurgitation. When there are anomalies of the pulmonary veins (Fig. 13.3C), the anomalous veins may be entered directly from the right atrium, or, occasionally, from connections to the superior or inferior venae cavae.

Closure of an ostium secundum defect is relatively easy, carries a low mortality and is advisable in all patients with pulmonary blood flow more than twice the systemic blood flow. Correction of the ostium primum type of defect, with its associated anomalies, is more difficult and carries a higher mortality. Surgery is usually undertaken if there are symptoms or when the shunt is large. The complete atrioventricular canal may need surgical treatment in the first few months of life because of symptoms or to prevent the development of pulmonary hypertension.

VENTRICULAR SEPTAL DEFECT (VSD)

The ventricular septum consists of four components: the trabecular or muscular septum extending to the apex, the inlet or posterior septum lying between the atrioventricular valves, the outlet or infundibular septum subtending the great arteries, and the membranous septum which lies under the aortic root and abuts on to the other three components. Defects can arise in any one of these components, but the membranous septum is the most commonly affected.

Defects of the ventricular septum, which may be large in relation to the size of the heart at birth, tend to become smaller or to close in early childhood. If closure is insufficient to prevent a large shunt, the small pulmonary vessels may be damaged by being exposed to the ejectile force and pressure of left ventricular contraction. Irreversible pulmonary hypertension may be produced.

The effect of a ventricular septal defect depends upon its size and upon the impedance to blood flow imposed by the pulmonary arterial vessels. If the defect is small, the jet of blood from the high-pressure left ventricle to the low-pressure right ventricle has little haemodynamic effect. If the defect is large and the impedance of the pulmonary vessels low, a large shunt develops and the pulmonary blood flow becomes more than twice the systemic flow. If, on the other hand, there is a high pulmonary vascular resistance, the pulmonary blood flow is little or no more than the systemic and the pressure in both circuits is similar. If the pulmonary vascular resistance is very high, the shunt reverses.

In the patient with a small defect ('maladie de Roger'), there are no symptoms, but there is a loud 'tearing' pansystolic murmur accompanied by a thrill, maximal to the left side of the lower sternum.

A large left-to-right shunt at ventricular level is liable to produce cardiac failure in the second or third month after birth. The special problems associated with this type of abnormality are discussed under the section 'The diagnosis and management of the infant with heart failure and cyanosis' (p. 292). If a large shunt does not produce symptoms during infancy, there is usually little disturbance until late adolescence or early adult life. Breathlessness and fatigue may then develop and cardiac failure subsequently ensue. In the presence of a large left-to-right shunt with pulmonary blood flow greater than twice systemic, the pulse is usually small and the venous pressure normal, unless there is right heart failure. Both left and right ventricles may be hyperdynamic, and there may or may not be a systolic thrill between the apex and the left sternal edge. A pansystolic murmur is heard at this site, usually accompanied by a mid-diastolic murmur at the apex due to high flow through the mitral valve.

In patients with a high pulmonary vascular resistance, breathlessness, fatigue and cyanosis are likely to develop during the second or third decade with progression to effort syncope, recurrent haemoptysis or heart failure. The signs of the ventricular septal defect are then less obvious, although there may still be a systolic murmur between the apex and the left sternal edge. Right ventricular hypertrophy is evident; the pulmonary second sound may be accentuated and followed by the early diastolic murmur of pulmonary regurgitation.

The ECG in small defects is normal. When the left-to-right shunt is large there is usually evidence of biventricular enlargement, manifested by abnormally deep but narrow Q waves and tall R waves in the left chest leads and an rsr pattern in V1. In cases with a high pulmonary vascular resistance, the ECG pattern of isolated right ventricular hypertrophy develops.

The chest radiograph is normal with a small defect, but with a large left-to-right shunt there is some enlargement of the heart and, more specifically, prominence of the pulmonary vessels, left atrium and both ventricles.

With small defects, the cross-sectional echocardiogram is often normal. With larger defects, there is usually a 'drop-out' of septal echoes, and both left atrium and ventricle may be enlarged. Doppler ultrasound can usually provide unequivocal evidence of a ventricular septal defect and, in association with echocardiography, permit an assessment of its size and the flow through it.

Correlation of these features usually provides sufficient evidence for accurate clinical diagnosis in spite of the various forms which defects of the ventricular septum may take. Further investigation may be advisable when the diagnosis is not clear-cut and is necessary if surgical treatment is contemplated. Cardiac catheterization usually demonstrates that the oxygen saturation of right ventricular blood is higher than that in the right atrium. However, if the defect is small or if there are equal pressures in the systemic and pulmonary circulations, no shunt of oxygenated blood may be demonstrable. The injection of radio-opaque material into the left ventricle may then be necessary for the angiocardiographic visualization of the defect.

The prognosis of ventricular septal defect depends upon the age of the patient, the size of the defect, and the pulmonary vascular changes. Large ventricular septal defects are an important cause of death in the infant; in those who survive, the defect usually becomes smaller or closes. After the first year, few affected children die, but death is likely to occur in those with major defects between the ages of 20 and 40. Patients with small defects usually live a normal life span, but are exposed to the risk of infective endocarditis.

In deciding upon the appropriate therapy for a patient with ventricular septal defect, the expected prognosis must be taken into account. In all patients precautions must be taken to avoid infective endocarditis. Because the outlook in small defects is excellent, surgery is not indicated. If there is a large left-to-right shunt, the defect should be closed. When the pulmonary vascular resistance is high, surgery is usually contraindicated as it cannot correct and may, indeed, worsen the pulmonary hypertension.

PERSISTENT DUCTUS ARTERIOSUS (Fig. 13.5)

During fetal life, the ductus arteriosus permits blood to flow from the

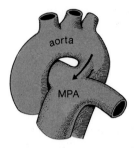

Fig. 13.5 Persistent ductus arteriosus. The shunt is from aorta to pulmonary artery because of the low resistance of the pulmonary circuit.

pulmonary artery into the aorta. Within a few hours or days or birth, it narrows and then closes.

In a few infants, the ductus arteriosus remains open and permits a large flow of blood from the high-pressure aorta to the low-pressure pulmonary artery. This may cause heart failure and death in the first few weeks of life. More commonly the ductus arteriosus undergoes partial closure and the shunt from aorta to pulmonary artery is relatively small. This gives rise to no symptoms during the first few years of life and is usually detected at a routine physical examination. A persistent ductus arteriosus of this kind may eventually become harmful for three reasons. First, it may act as a focus for infective endarteritis. Secondly, the leak of blood from the aorta to the pulmonary artery and the consequent high pulmonary blood flow may lead to cardiac failure in adolescence or adult life. Thirdly, but rarely, severe pulmonary hypertension may develop.

The patient is usually in good general health. The pulse may be of normal volume if the duct is small, but if it is large, the diastolic leak from the aorta causes a collapsing pulse. Correspondingly, the diastolic blood pressure may be low. The heart may be of normal size, or the left ventricle enlarged. The most characteristic feature of the condition is the 'continuous murmur', situated in the second left intercostal space by the sternal edge but often loudest 5–7.5 cm above or to the left of this. This murmur continues from systole into diastole and is maximum about the time of the second sound (Fig. 13.6). It seldom lasts for the whole of systole and diastole and may occupy only the latter part of systole and the earlier part of diastole. In a few instances, particularly in infants, it may occur as a crescendo in late systole only. The murmur is due to flow of blood from the aorta through the persistent ductus arteriosus into the pulmonary artery in both phases of the cardiac cycle. If the shunt is large, the increased venous return from the lungs causes a mid-diastolic murmur at the apex as it crosses the mitral valve.

The ECG is usually normal but may show the deep Q and tall R waves of left ventricular hypertrophy. The chest radiograph may show enlargement of the left ventricle, aorta and pulmonary artery, and the features of increased pulmonary blood flow. The duct can sometimes be visualized by cross-sectional echocardiography. Enlargement of the

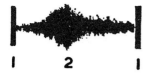

Fig. 13.6   The continuous murmur of a persistent ductus arteriosus.

left atrium and left ventricle on the M-mode echo confirms the presence of left ventricular volume overload.

The clinical diagnosis is usually easy because of the characteristic continuous murmur. Special investigation is seldom required even prior to surgical treatment. Care, however, is necessary to avoid confusion with the venous hum which is common in normal children. The hum is usually maximal to the right of the sternum below the right clavicle, diminishes or disappears when the child lies flat and can usually be abolished by compression of the jugular veins on the right side. Continuous murmurs due to other causes are rare and their maximum intensity is usually below and medial to the pulmonary area. When in doubt because of the site or quality of the murmur or the lack of correlation with the electrocardiographic and radiological features, special investigation is necessary. At cardiac catheterization there is a 'step-up' in oxygen saturation in the pulmonary artery. This can be shown to result from a persistent ductus by the passage of the catheter through it into the descending aorta, or by the angiocardiographic delineation of the ductus by the injection of contrast medium into the arch of the aorta.

Surgical treatment of a persistent ductus arteriosus by division and suture carries little risk and is the correct management in almost all patients. An alternative procedure of closure is to use a catheter occluder, which is introduced via the femoral vein. An umbrella-like device with two spring-loaded discs is positioned in the duct and left there, and the catheter removed. These procedures should be performed, if possible, before the child starts school.

In symptomatic low birth weight premature infants, the ductus frequently causes life-threatening cardiac decompensation. Although immediate surgery is probably still the most successful mode of treatment, administration of indomethacin, a prostaglandin inhibitor, can induce duct closure medically. This method is, however, not always successful.

Obstructive lesions

COARCTATION OF THE AORTA

Coarctation of the aorta is a narrowing of the lumen, usually just beyond the origin of the left subclavian artery (Fig. 13.7). It is characteristically of severe degree and is commonly associated with a bicuspid aortic valve which may be or may become stenosed or allow

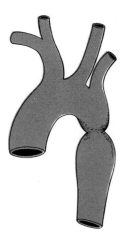

Fig. 13.7 Coarctation of the aorta. The constriction is usually in the descending aorta just below the left subclavian artery. Beyond the constriction, there is post-stenotic dilatation.

regurgitation. The ductus arteriosus may also persist, particularly if the coarctation is proximal to its attachment to the aorta.

The systolic pressure in the aorta and its branches proximal to the coarctation is raised, but this may not be obvious in early childhood; diastolic hypertension is uncommon before adult life and is seldom severe at rest. The hypertension may induce irreversible changes in the arterioles so that the blood pressure may not return to normal even after the removal of the coarctation.

Only a small volume of blood flows through the narrowed segment; much of the blood supply of the lower part of the body is by way of collateral vessels which attain great size. The blood pressure in the lower half of the body is lower than that in the upper half and the pulse wave takes longer to arrive.

The hypertension is eventually liable to cause left ventricular failure. Other risks include infection of the coarctation or of a bicuspid aortic valve, rupture or dissection of the ascending aorta, and cerebral haemorrhage. Cystic medial necrosis of the aortic wall, which is present in only a few patients with coarctation, is the deciding factor in rupture. Rupture of an intracranial aneurysm, which occurs in 5–10% of affected individuals, is the usual cause of subarachnoid haemorrhage.

Coarctation may produce no symptoms and is most often suspected during a routine medical examination when a systolic murmur is heard or hypertension detected. However, long segment narrowing in the preductal area of the aorta is associated with heart failure in infancy. In such infants, commonly, the ductus is patent, and pulmonary hypertension is present; a VSD may coexist.

The blood pressure in the upper limbs is raised; that in the legs is normal or low. The femoral arterial pulse is small and delayed in comparison with the radial pulse. In adults, collateral vessels may be

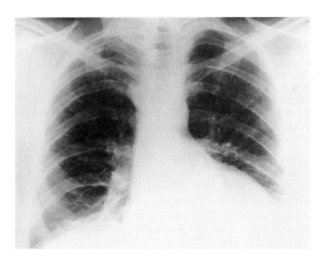

Fig. 13.8 Coarctation of the aorta. Chest X-ray in a patient with coarctation of the aorta. Prominent rib notching is apparent and the heart has a left ventricular configuration due to hypertension.

seen and felt along the borders of the scapulae and over the posterior chest wall. The left ventricle is occasionally enlarged. A systolic murmur is almost invariably heard over the area of the coarctation at about the level of the fourth intercostal space posteriorly, and tends to be louder than a systolic murmur which is often audible in the second intercostal spaces close to the sternum. A more continuous murmur may be heard over collaterals.

The ECG is usually normal; left ventricular hypertrophy is uncommon before adult years. The chest radiograph is seldom abnormal in childhood, but characteristically shows an abnormal aortic knuckle with an enlarged left subclavian artery and poststenotic dilatation of the aorta in adults. Another feature is notching of the undersides of the ribs due to the erosion by enlarged intercostal arteries (Fig. 13.8). The left ventricle may also be enlarged.

The diagnosis is usually made without difficulty on clinical grounds. It may be confirmed by intra-aortic pressure tracings above and below the coarctation and the precise anatomy can be outlined by aortography.

The correct treatment is surgical resection of the coarctation and restoration of the aorta by end-to-end anastomosis or, if necessary, by the insertion of a graft. This should be performed electively in childhood. None the less, hypertension may not be completely abolished or may recur later. Balloon angioplasty has been used with varying success in the treatment of coarctation, but is particularly effective in the 5–10% of patients who have a recurrence of the coarctation after surgery.

AORTIC STENOSIS

This condition is considered in Chapter 12.

HYPOPLASTIC LEFT HEART SYNDROME

This term is used to describe a number of disorders, such as mitral atresia and aortic atresia, in which the characteristic feature is virtual absence of left ventricular outflow. The diagnosis can usually be established by echocardiogram which reveals a small left ventricle and absent aortic valve. Life can be sustained if there is a large persistent ductus which allows blood to flow from the pulmonary artery to the aorta. Affected infants are intensely cyanosed and usually die within hours of birth. There is, as yet, no successful corrective operation; transplantation has been used successfully in some cases.

The abnormality can be detected at about the 18th week of pregnancy by fetal echocardiography; termination can then be considered.

PULMONARY STENOSIS

Pulmonary stenosis is almost invariably of congenital origin. Except when it is complicated by a ventricular septal defect (see 'tetralogy of Fallot', p. 286) the stenosis is usually confined to the valve cusps. These may be fused to form a cone-shaped structure with a narrow orifice. Beyond the obstruction the pulmonary artery is dilated; proximal to it the right ventricle is hypertrophied.

The obstruction to right ventricular emptying leads to a high right ventricular systolic pressure and a systolic pressure drop across the pulmonary valve (Fig. 13.9). In the more severe cases, right ventricular failure develops. If the foramen ovale is unsealed, or if there is an atrial septal defect, a right-to-left shunt with central cyanosis may develop as the right atrial pressure rises.

Although pulmonary stenosis may cause cardiac failure in the first few weeks of life, survival into late childhood or adult life is usual. Often the lesion is first detected on routine clinical examination in asymptomatic individuals, but some patients present with fatigue, breathlessness or syncope.

The arterial pulse may be normal or small. The jugular venous pulse is usually normal, but in severe grades it exhibits a large 'a' wave as the right atrium contracts forcibly in the face of the non-compliant hypertrophied right ventricle. On palpation, there is nearly always a systolic thrill in the second left intercostal space; the left parasternal heave of right ventricular hypertrophy can sometimes be felt. The first heart sound is normal, but it is often followed by an early systolic 'ejection' click and a loud midsystolic murmur best heard in the second left intercostal space. The second sound is normal in the mild case, but in the more severe it is split abnormally widely

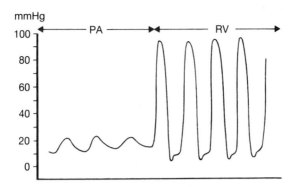

Fig. 13.9 The pressure pulse obtained as the catheter is withdrawn from pulmonary artery to right ventricle in pulmonary valve stenosis.

and the second (pulmonary) element is soft.

The electrocardiogram indicates the severity of the pulmonary valve stenosis for, in general, the greater the ECG features of right ventricular hypertrophy, the tighter the stenosis. The chest radiograph shows the post-stenotic dilatation of the pulmonary artery. In severe cases, right ventricular hypertrophy and diminution in the pulmonary vascular markings may be detected.

An accurate diagnosis can usually be made clinically. Cardiac catheterization provides confirmatory evidence; the systolic pressure difference across the pulmonary valve is a valuable index of severity, a drop of more than 50 mmHg suggesting severe stenosis (Fig. 13.9). Doppler ultrasound provides reliable evidence of the severity of the stenosis, and is particularly valuable as a means of follow-up. Unless the foramen ovale is unsealed or there is an associated atrial septal defect, no intracardiac shunting can be detected.

A minor degree of pulmonary stenosis is compatible with a normal life span. When the stenosis is more severe, death is likely to ensue sooner or later from right ventricular failure; relief of the stenosis should not be delayed too long as irreversible fibrotic changes take place in the hypertrophied right ventricle. Balloon valvoplasty is an effective and safe method of enlarging the valve orifice but the long-term results are not yet known. Surgical valvotomy is a low risk alternative.

TRICUSPID ATRESIA

In this relatively uncommon disorder, there is absence of the normal atrioventricular connection on the right side. For life to be sustained in the extra-uterine state, an atrial septal defect and a ventricular septal defect must be present. Frequently there is associated pulmonary stenosis or pulmonary atresia and, more rarely, transposition of the great arteries. The left ventricle is large and the hypoplastic right ventricle receives blood by the VSD. Cyanosis in infancy is the rule. The ECG shows left axis deviation and left ventricular hypertrophy. Cross-sectional echocardiography reveals the absent connection and can also demonstrate the VSD and ASD.

Balloon septostomy or the surgical creation of an aortopulmonary shunt is life saving in the severely affected infant. In later childhood a conduit is inserted between the right atrium and the right ventricular outflow tract or pulmonary artery (Fontan procedure).

Combined obstructive and shunt lesions

PULMONARY STENOSIS AND VENTRICULAR SEPTAL DEFECT (TETRALOGY OF FALLOT)

When pulmonary stenosis coexists with a ventricular septal defect, the stenosis may be slight and shunting exclusively from left-to-right. In most cases, however, pulmonary stenosis is severe and the ventricular septal defect large, and there is a right-to-left shunt. These abnormalities are the major features of the 'tetralogy of Fallot', of which the other components are dextroposition of the aorta (with the aortic root overriding the defect) and right ventricular hypertrophy (Fig. 13.10). The pulmonary stenosis is situated in the infundibulum of the right ventricle and, often, at the pulmonary valve as well. The infundibular stenosis tends to become more severe with advancing age and there is a progressive increase in the proportion of blood shunted from right-to-left.

In the most severe cases, symptoms start soon after birth. More frequently, cyanosis develops in the second half of the first year or not until later in childhood.

With increasing cyanosis, dyspnoea becomes more severe. The child is liable to sudden attacks of intense cyanosis, sometimes associated with syncope, for which spasm of the infundibulum of the

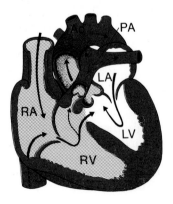

Fig. 13.10 Tetralogy of Fallot. Note infundibular pulmonary stenosis and ventricular septal defect, with right-to-left shunt at ventricular level.

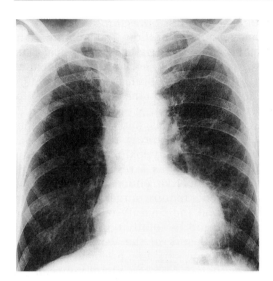

Fig. 13.11 Tetralogy of Fallot. The heart shadow is typically 'boot-shaped' with a concavity of the left heart border, instead of the normal pulmonary artery shadow. The apex is high and rounded. The lung fields are oligaemic.

right ventricle may be responsible. Children with the tetralogy of Fallot are liable to squat after exercise. It is believed that the squatting position, by compressing the abdominal aorta and the femoral arteries, increases the arterial resistance and therefore diminishes the right-to-left shunt at the ventricular level.

The child is often abnormally small and has central cyanosis with finger clubbing. The arterial pulses are small and venous pulses normal. Clinical evidence of right ventricular hypertrophy is slight. There is a loud systolic murmur accompanied by a thrill in the second or third left intercostal space unless the stenosis is so severe that virtually no blood traverses it. The second heart sound is single because the pulmonary valve component is inaudible. The electrocardiogram shows moderate right ventricular hypertrophy. The chest radiograph is characteristic in showing a 'boot-shaped' heart with a concavity on the left border in the place where the pulmonary artery is normally seen, and a prominent and elevated apex (Fig. 13.11). The pulmonary vascularity is decreased. Echocardiography shows that the aorta is large and overrides the septum, the normal continuity between the anterior aortic wall and septum being lost. Polycythaemia, secondary to the cyanosis, is usual.

The tetralogy of Fallot is the underlying lesion in 70% of children with central cyanosis over the age of 3. This frequency and the characteristic clinical, electrocardiographic and radiological features usually make the diagnosis easy in childhood. In infancy and also in later life, a confident diagnosis can less often be reached without further investigation.

On cardiac catheterization, a systolic pressure drop can be demonstrated between the body and the outflow tract of the right ventricle. Pressures in the right and left ventricles are identical. The oxygen saturation in the aorta is reduced. Injection of radio-opaque contrast medium into the right ventricle delineates the region of stenosis and demonstrates the shunt through the ventricular septal defect.

Patients with severe pulmonary stenosis and large ventricular septal defects often die in childhood and rarely reach middle age without surgery. Death may result from hypoxic episodes during childhood, from cerebrovascular accidents as a result of thrombosis promoted by polycythaemia, from infective endocarditis and from cerebral abscesses. Virtually all patients require surgery at some stage, but the type of surgery depends upon the severity of the lesion and the age. Ideally, the abnormality should be totally corrected by relief of the pulmonary stenosis and by closure of the ventricular septal defect. In severely affected infants, some surgeons prefer to perform a palliative procedure first, such as the creation of a shunt between the aorta and pulmonary circulations, either directly or by anastomosing the subclavian artery to the pulmonary artery. This increases the proportion of blood going through the lungs and thus becoming oxygenated. The child can be given several years of comparatively good health before the corrective procedure is performed.

Severe hypoxic attacks should be treated with oxygen and morphine (0.1 mg/kg). The baby should be placed in the knee–chest position. Blood pCO_2 and pH should be estimated and sodium bicarbonate given intravenously as necessary. Propranolol is possibly of value.

HIGH PULMONARY VASCULAR RESISTANCE WITH RIGHT-TO-LEFT SHUNT THROUGH A SEPTAL DEFECT OR DUCTUS ARTERIOSUS (EISENMENGER SYNDROME)

Eisenmenger originally described a patient with a ventricular septal defect with central cyanosis in the absence of pulmonary stenosis. It is now known that the reason for the right-to-left shunt in such cases is the presence of a severe pulmonary vascular disease. Because the clinical pictures of pulmonary hypertension with right-to-left shunt are so similar, irrespective of whether the shunt is at atrial, ventricular or aorto-pulmonary level, the term Eisenmenger syndrome is employed to describe all three lesions.

The cause of the pulmonary vascular disease responsible for the pulmonary hypertension is unknown. Factors which may be involved include:

- lack of regression of the fetal type of pulmonary vasculature (see p. 322);

- prolonged exposure to high pulmonary blood flow;
- prolonged exposure to high pulmonary blood pressure;
- genetic predisposition.

Although irreversible pulmonary arterial changes may develop during early childhood, they more commonly occur during adolescence. Dyspnoea and fatigue, which are usually the first symptoms, are liable to develop in late childhood, adolescence or early adult life. Other complaints include syncope, angina pectoris, oedema and haemoptysis.

On examination the patient is usually cyanosed. When the shunt is through a ductus arteriosus, the venous blood is directed into the descending aorta and only the lower limbs become cyanosed ('differential cyanosis').

The arterial pulse is usually small, due to a low stroke volume; a large 'a' wave may be present in the venous pulse, due to forceful atrial contraction in the face of right ventricular hypertrophy. On palpation, one can detect right ventricular hypertrophy and the shock of pulmonary valve closure. On auscultation, the signs are mainly those of pulmonary hypertension: a loud second heart sound, a right ventricular fourth heart sound, a pulmonary early systolic ('ejection') click and, occasionally, the early diastolic murmur of pulmonary regurgitation and the pansystolic murmur of functional tricuspid regurgitation. In atrial septal defect, the second sound remains split on expiration (because only the right ventricle is overburdened). In ventricular septal defect, there is a single second sound, because the pressure in both ventricles is identical. In persistent ductus arteriosus, there is normal splitting of the second heart sound.

The ECG shows right atrial and right ventricular hypertrophy. On the chest radiograph there are large main pulmonary arteries but small peripheral arteries, together with right ventricular and right atrial enlargement. Cross-sectional echocardiography can reliably demonstrate the ventricular or atrial septal defects in these patients.

The diagnosis is suggested by the combination of central cyanosis and pulmonary hypertension in an adolescent or young adult. The Eisenmenger syndrome differs from the tetralogy of Fallot (the commonest cardiac cause of central cyanosis in this age group) in there being no pulmonary systolic thrill or loud murmur, in the greater severity of right ventricular hypertrophy, and in the large pulmonary arteries on the chest radiograph. The diagnosis can be confirmed by demonstrating by cardiac catheterization that the pulmonary artery pressure equals the systemic pressure, and by angiocardiographic delineation of the shunt. The progress of the Eisenmenger syndrome is usually slowly downhill, death commonly occurring between the ages of 20 and 40. The main causes of death are pulmonary infarction, right heart failure and arrhythmias and, less often, infective endocarditis. Pregnancy is particularly hazardous in these patients and should be avoided or terminated early.

No surgical treatment, other than heart–lung transplantation, is of value because the major defect is the irreversible change in the small pulmonary arteries. Temporary benefit may result from the conventional treatment of cardiac failure.

Displacement lesions

TRANSPOSITION OF THE GREAT ARTERIES (Fig. 13.12)

In transposition of the great arteries, the aorta arises from the right ventricle and the pulmonary artery from the left. As a consequence, there are separate systemic and pulmonary circulations; life cannot be sustained unless there is some communication between them. Usually there is one or more of the following:

- a patent foramen ovale;
- an atrial septal defect;
- a ventricular septal defect;
- a persistent ductus arteriosus.

The infant is characteristically of normal size and well nourished. Cyanosis develops at birth or shortly thereafter. There is difficulty in completing feeds; increasing breathlessness, deep cyanosis, cardiac failure and death are usual within the first month.

On auscultation there may be a gallop rhythm and a systolic murmur.

The chest radiograph may show little abnormality at birth, but within a few days the heart becomes enlarged and the vascularity of the lung fields increased. The ECG shows little more than the right ventricular preponderance normal for this age group.

Echocardiography, especially the cross-sectional technique, is an

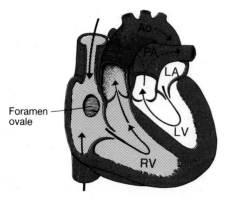

Fig. 13.12   Transposition of the great arteries. The aorta arises from the right ventricle and the pulmonary artery from the left. Life can be sustained only if communications exist between systemic and pulmonary circulations.

Foramen ovale

invaluable diagnostic tool. It permits observation of the aorta, arising from the right ventricle and lying anterior to the pulmonary artery, and also allows detection of other defects.

Transposition of the great arteries is the most common cardiac cause of cyanosis at birth and of overt heart failure in cyanotic congenital heart disease within the first few weeks of life. Accurate diagnosis at this stage is urgent; it is usually fatal to await the effects of medical treatment. Investigation should be undertaken within a matter of hours. Echocardiography is of diagnostic value in showing the abnormal connections of the great arteries. If it supports the diagnosis, it is usually then necessary to proceed to cardiac catheterization which not only enables the precise nature of the anomalies to be determined but is an essential preliminary to therapy.

In the acutely ill infant, great improvement can be achieved by producing a large defect in the atrial septum to allow mixing of the blood between systemic and pulmonary circulations (Rashkind procedure). This is done by introducing a catheter with a deflated balloon at its tip into the femoral vein and advancing it via the right atrium and foramen ovale into the left atrium. The balloon is then inflated and withdrawn abruptly so as to tear the atrial septum. This procedure is usually effective in the neonatal period and allows the child to live until the latter part of the first year of life when the venous return to the two ventricles is rerouted by the insertion of an intra-atrial baffle. This operation can be carried out with a low mortality. An alternative procedure — the 'switch' operation — is now the preferred choice for most cases in major centres. In this procedure, the surgeon detaches the aorta and pulmonary artery, and connects each to its appropriate ventricle.

EBSTEIN'S ANOMALY

In this disorder, the posteromedial part of the tricuspid valve ring is displaced towards the apex of the right ventricle. An atrial septal defect is usually present.

Dyspnoea, fatigue and arrhythmias are usual. Cyanosis may be present if there is an atrial septal defect. There are often scratchy tricuspid systolic, mid-diastolic and presystolic murmurs, arising from flow across the abnormal tricuspid valve. Tall P waves, a long PR interval and a low voltage right bundle branch block pattern are the usual ECG features. The chest radiograph shows a large right atrium and clear lung fields. Echocardiography demonstrates the abnormal position and movement of the tricuspid valve cusp.

Death usually results from arrhythmias in childhood or early adult life, but may occur later from cardiac failure or hypoxaemia.

Partial correction, with prosthetic replacement of the tricuspid valve and repair of the atrial septal defect is indicated for the disabled case but this neither restores normal function nor prevents arrhythmias.

DEXTROCARDIA

Dextrocardia refers to all situations where the heart is in the right chest. The lung and abdominal situs or arrangement may be reversed or normal. When dextrocardia exists with complete right–left reversal of the lungs and viscera then the heart is usually normal, but the ECG can be very misleading if the condition is not recognized. When the heart is in the right chest and the other organs are normally sited, or if the heart is in the left chest (laevocardia) and the other organs reversed, then the chance of complex congenital cardiac lesions is high.

RIGHT-SIDED AORTA

In this condition, the aorta turns posteriorly and runs down on the right of the trachea and the oesophagus instead of arching upwards and to the left. It may continue to descend in this direction or may cross behind the trachea and oesophagus and attain the normal left-sided course.

As an isolated anomaly it is of no clinical significance. When associated with a congenital lesion of the heart, its detection may be of diagnostic assistance for it is found in 20–25% of patients with the tetralogy of Fallot. When associated with other arterial anomalies the trachea and oesophagus may be encircled and obstructive symptoms result.

The diagnosis and management of the infant with heart failure and cyanosis

The general paediatrician and the general practitioner have the responsibility of detecting heart disease in the newborn; an expert in neonatal cardiology should be contacted without delay if there is any evidence of cyanosis or heart failure. All too frequently, the clinical evidence of heart disease is overlooked until it is too late.

Central cyanosis is a serious finding in the newborn. If it persists after exposure to oxygen therapy, and there is no evident respiratory or cerebral cause, congenital heart disease should be suspected. If the cyanosis is indeed due to congenital heart disease, the prognosis without treatment is poor. Echocardiography should be undertaken immediately. The findings of this investigation may suggest that cardiac catheterization is required: this can be combined with therapy (e.g. the Rashkind procedure, see p. 291).

The commonest causes of cardiac failure, with or without cyanosis, in the newborn, are ventricular septal defect, persistent ductus arteriosus, hypoplastic left heart, coarctation of the aorta and transposition.

The early signs of heart failure are tachypnoea, tachycardia, gallop rhythm and enlargement of the liver. Cyanosis is often present as well. The venous pressure is a poor guide to heart failure in infants. Crepitations and rhonchi are common and should not be attributed to pulmonary disease until left ventricular failure has been excluded. Oedema, which is most likely to affect the backs of the hands and feet, is a late sign, and is common in the absence of heart failure in premature infants.

Tachycardia may be difficult to assess because the pulse rate is normally fast in infants, but it seldom exceeds 140/min during sleep in the healthy baby or in those with respiratory disease. If the rate is in excess of 210/min, there is a supraventricular tachycardia requiring urgent treatment. If the heart rate is less than 50/min, heart block is almost certainly present.

Thirty per cent oxygen should be given to all infants who are cyanosed or in cardiac failure. The air should be humidified. Measurement of the blood gases and the correction of acidosis is an essential part of the proper management of heart failure in infancy. Frusemide starting with an oral dose of 2 µg/kg is first choice in severe failure. Digoxin may also be of value starting with 40–60 µg/kg by mouth or 40 µg/kg intramuscularly. Good nursing, temperature and humidity control, supportive frames or suspension in the propped-up position and tube feeding are essential in the early stages of treatment. Sedation with trimeprazine or promethazine may be required.

These medical measures are quite often successful in correcting cardiac failure due to a ventricular septal defect or persistent ductus arteriosus. The cyanotic infant is in a precarious state and may be dependent on a patent ductus; deterioration takes place as the ductus closes. This can usually be prevented by the intravenous infusion of prostaglandins.

Further reading

Anderson, R.H., Macartney, F.J., Shinebourne, E.A. & Tynan, M. (1987) *Paediatric Cardiology.* Edinburgh: Churchill Livingstone.

Perloff, J.K. (1987) *The Clinical Recognition of Congenital Heart Disease*, 3rd edn. Philadelphia: Saunders.

Hypertension and Heart Disease

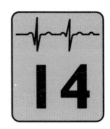

Hypertension is probably directly or indirectly responsible for 10–20% of all deaths. These deaths occur because of the deleterious effects of high blood pressure on the coronary, renal and cerebral arteries, and because of the increased work load imposed on the heart.

For reasons that will become apparent, it is impossible to define hypertension. For practical purposes, the blood pressure may be regarded as abnormally high if it persistently exceeds 140/90 mmHg in a quietly resting individual. This does not imply that individuals with raised pressure necessarily require treatment. The presence of other risk factors and evidence of adverse effects must be taken into account.

The variability of blood pressure

The level of arterial blood pressure is determined by the cardiac output and peripheral vascular resistance, two factors which vary widely from individual to individual, and within one individual at different times. Marked variations have been observed in individuals in whom the blood pressure is continuously monitored throughout the day. The mean pressure during sleep may be 30–40 mmHg lower than it is in the waking state. Factors which transiently increase pressure include anxiety and cold. Exercise leads to a brisk rise in systolic pressure but little change in the diastolic pressure. A transient doubling of systolic pressure may occur at the climax of coitus.

Certain identifiable factors are associated with persistently high blood pressure. Thus, at least in Western societies, both diastolic and systolic pressure increase with age. The blood pressure averages about 80/60 mmHg at birth and rises slowly throughout childhood. The resting blood pressure in the adolescent is often in the region of 120/70 mmHg, whilst in middle age 140/80 mmHg is more common. The systolic pressure often continues to rise into old age as the aorta becomes increasingly rigid. However, in many individuals and throughout some societies, e.g. in some Pacific islands, hypertension is virtually non-existent and there is no rise with age. In the younger age groups, males, on average, have higher pressures than females, but this tendency is reversed after the age of 45. Obese individuals tend to have pressures higher than can be accounted for by recording errors due to increased arm circumference.

The variability of arterial pressures within one individual and between individuals makes it impossible to define normality. It has been established, however, that the higher the pressure even within the 'normal' range, whether systolic or diastolic, the more likely is the occurrence of certain disease processes such as left ventricular hypertrophy and failure ('hypertensive heart disease'), coronary artery disease, cerebrovascular disease and renal disease. The blood pressure can only be regarded as pathologically high if it has caused or is likely to lead to disordered function of the cardiovascular system, brain or kidneys.

Classification by blood pressure level (Table 14.1)

Normal adult blood pressure has been defined as a systolic blood pressure equal to or below 140 mmHg together with a diastolic (fifth Korotkoff phase) equal to or below 90 mmHg.

Table 14.1   Definitions of hypertension

Diastolic pressure (mmHg)	
<85	Normal
85–89	High normal
90–104	Mild hypertension
105–114	Moderate hypertension
>115	Severe hypertension
Systolic pressure (mmHg)	
<140	Normal
140–159	Borderline isolated systolic hypertension
>160	Isolated systolic hypertension
	(disastolic <90 mmHg)

Sources: American Medical Association (1989).
   Arch Intern Med **148:** 1023, 1989.

Hypertension may be regarded as 'mild' if the diastolic pressure is between 90 and 104 mmHg, 'moderate' if between 105 and 114 mmHg, and 'severe' if above this. Hypertension is said to be in the *malignant* or accelerated phase if there is widespread arterial fibrinoid necrosis. The diastolic pressure is very high (often above 130 mmHg), with retinal haemorrhages and exudates and frequently papilloedema.

Although the unqualified term 'hypertension' generally refers to elevation of the diastolic blood pressure, it is also possible to define systolic hypertension. A systolic pressure above 160 is regarded as abnormal, even when the diastolic pressure is within normal limits.

AETIOLOGICAL FACTORS IN HYPERTENSION

In some 5% of those with high blood pressure, a cause can be identified. When the hypertension can be attributed to one of these, it is 'secondary'; when no such factor can be unearthed it is described as 'essential' or 'primary'.

Hypertension can be secondary to a large number of conditions of which the most important are the following:

- *renal disease* including glomerulonephritis, pyelonephritis, polycystic disease, renal tumours and renal artery stenosis;
- *endocrine diseases* including diseases of the adrenal gland such as primary aldosteronism, Cushing's syndrome and phaeochromocytoma;
- *coarctation of the aorta*;
- *drugs and foods* including oral contraceptives, liquorice, carbenoxolone, ACTH and corticosteroids.

The relative proportion of cases with an identifiable cause decreases with age; in the elderly, secondary hypertension is uncommon.

Essential hypertension

The cause of 'essential' hypertension remains uncertain. It is now apparent that there is no single cause and that hypertension is multifactorial. This multifactorial aetiology is supported by much epidemiological evidence which shows that there is an infinite gradation between the 'normal' and hypertensive' populations.

Genetic influences. The influence of heredity is unquestioned, hypertension being many times more common in the families of hypertensive patients than in those of normotensive individuals. Although some have suggested that hypertension is due to a single dominant gene, most of the evidence points to the influence of many genes.

Dietary influences. There is an undoubted relationship between overweight and hypertension. Weight loss in the very obese substantially lowers the blood pressure; in the less overweight it has little effect. Very low salt intake appears to protect against hypertension, but there is little evidence to incriminate excessive sodium chloride intake as a cause of high blood pressure. A high potassium intake may be protective. There is some evidence that a high intake of saturated fats may raise blood pressure. High alcohol consumption has been identified as a risk factor for hypertension, as has cigarette smoking, at least in regard to the malignant phase.

Physical activity. Physical exercise can reduce blood pressure in hypertensive subjects. This suggests that inactivity may play a role in the genesis of hypertension in some individuals.

Hormonal changes. Hormonal changes are implicated in a number of the syndromes of secondary hypertension. The possibility that hormonal changes might also be involved in the pathogenesis of essential hypertension has attracted particular interest. Attention has been concentrated on the adrenergic and renin–angiotensin systems. There is as yet no clear evidence indicating a primary role for either system in the genesis of hypertension.

Haemodynamic changes. A slight sinus tachycardia and a high cardiac output may be found in early hypertensives before there is a rise in peripheral resistance. These features may result from an excessive adrenergic influence. There is good evidence that baroreceptors are reset in hypertension, as bradycardia is not induced by the rise in pressure.

The causes of secondary hypertension

Secondary causes of hypertension are summarized in Table 14.2.

Renal disease

That renal disease can be the sole cause of hypertension has been clearly established both in animal experiments and in man. The components of the renin–angiotensin system are shown in Fig. 14.1. However, the relationship between renal disease and hypertension is complex because either may lead to the other, and it is not always easy to determine which is primary.

- *Acute glomerulonephritis.* Hypertension is almost invariable, but is transient and not often severe. The mechanism is not clear, but sodium and water retention may play a part. Cardiac failure occurs in about one-quarter of the cases, but the hypertension is seldom an important factor in this. The diagnosis can usually be made on the basis of the acute onset, the association with preceding streptococcal infection, and the presence of peripheral

Table 14.2   The causes of secondary hypertension

Renal
> Acute glomerulonephritis
> Chronic glomerulonephritis
> Chronic pyelonephritis
> Polycystic kidneys
> Renal artery stenosis
> Diabetic nephropathy

Endocrine
> Adrenal
>> Primary aldosteronism
>> Cushing's syndrome
>> Phaeochromocytoma
> Acromegaly
> Exogenous hormones
>> Oral contraceptives
>> Glucocorticoids
>> Mineralocorticoids — liquorice

Coarctation of the aorta

Pregnancy

Neurological
> Raised intracranial pressure

---

oedema and disturbed renal function.

- *Chronic glomerulonephritis.* Severe hypertension is usually a late manifestation of chronic nephritis, and develops only when there is evidence of advanced renal failure.
- *Chronic pyelonephritis.* There is evidence that chronic pyelonephritis can cause hypertension (particularly malignant hypertension) although this has been disputed. *Reflux nephropathy* is predominantly a disorder of females, and should be particularly sought for in girls with hypertension.
- *Polycystic kidneys.* Hypertension occurs in more than half of those with congenital polycystic disease of the kidneys.
- *Renal artery stenosis.* Hypertension may also be caused by *renal artery stenosis*, resulting from atheromatous narrowing, fibromuscular hyperplasia or aneurysm formation. Not infrequently, only one renal artery is involved. Renal artery angioplasty or surgery is indicated if it can be established that the renal artery disease is responsible for the high blood pressure.

Abdominal ultrasound provides a simple non-invasive means of assessing renal anatomy in patients with a suspected renal cause for

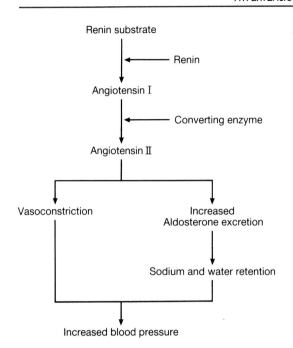

Fig. 14.1   The renin-angiotensin system.

hypertension. In patients with chronic nephritis, kidney size is reduced. In unilateral renal artery stenosis, kidney size is reduced on the side of the stenosis. In patients with pyelonephritis, there is likely to be dilatation of the calyceal system. Additional investigations in the patient with suspected renal disease may include intravenous pyelography, isotope renography, renal arteriography and renal biopsy.

Endocrine disease

Primary aldosteronism.   Aldosterone, which is secreted by the zona glomerulosa of the adrenal cortex, promotes sodium reabsorption and potassium excretion in the distal tubules of the kidney. Normally, aldosterone secretion is largely regulated by angiotensin, but in primary aldosteronism there is an overproduction of aldosterone as a result of an adrenal cortical adenoma (Conn's syndrome) or bilateral hyperplasia; angiotensin and, therefore, plasma renin levels are abnormally low. It occurs most often in young and middle-aged females. Because of the mode of action of aldosterone, the symptoms and signs are related to sodium retention, hypokalaemia and hypertension. Frequently, the patient presents with mild to moderate hypertension, but the predominant complaints are those of muscle weakness, headache, thirst and polyuria. The hypertension is seldom severe and malignant changes are rare. There is usually hypokalaemia, with a serum potassium of less than 3.0 mmol/litre, and a serum sodium that is normal or high. Characteristically, there is a metabolic alkalosis and a low serum chloride. The diagnosis should be suspected in patients with hypertension and hypokalaemia, particularly if this is associated with hypernatraemia. However, hypokalaemia is not uncommon in other hypertensive patients, particularly if they have been treated with diuretics. Furthermore, patients with malignant hypertension develop 'secondary aldosteronism' with low serum potassium. These patients usually do not have a high serum sodium.

Diagnosis. The diagnosis is suggested by:

- hypokalaemia, persisting after stopping diuretic therapy;
- excessive urinary potassium loss;
- elevated plasma aldosterone levels;
- suppressed renin levels which fail to rise on assumption of an upright posture;
- computed tomography is now the investigation of choice in establishing the presence of an adenoma and differentiating this from hyperplasia.

Management. Adenomas should be removed surgically. Patients with hyperplasia should be treated medically with spironolactone or amiloride, which antagonise the actions of aldosterone.

Phaeochromocytoma. Phaeochromocytomas arise in chromaffin tissue in the adrenal gland or elsewhere. Most are benign, but about 5% are malignant. The tumours usually secrete noradrenaline (norepinephrine), but adrenaline (epinephrine) may predominate.

Phaeochromocytomas may produce either paroxysmal or persistent hypertension. The paroxysms are associated with the sudden onset of bilateral headache, and with perspiration, palpitation and pallor (features often regarded as neurotic). The attacks usually last from a few minutes to an hour. If the hypertension is persistent, the clinical picture is that of severe hypertension, often of the malignant variety. Because of the hypermetabolic state induced by the phaeochromocytoma, the patients are rarely obese.

Diagnosis. The diagnosis should be suspected in any severe case of hypertension, particularly if the hypertension is paroxysmal. The diagnosis is confirmed by:

- excessive excretion of the catecholamine metabolite, vanilmandelic acid (VMA) in the urine is a useful screening test;
- urine and plasma catecholamine levels;
- computed tomography scan to localize the tumour.

Management. Phaeochromocytomas should be removed surgically. This is a potentially hazardous procedure and requires close control of the blood pressure and careful anaesthesia. Beta-adrenergic blocking drugs should not be used alone; they may induce an extreme alpha-adrenergic effect. This can be avoided by the initial use of an alpha-adrenergic blocking drug. The non-competitive alpha-antagonist phenoxybenzamine is frequently chosen. Once alpha-adrenergic blockade is fully established, beta-blockade can be added.

Cushing's syndrome. This results from cortisol excess and may be due to hyperplasia of the adrenal cortex, adrenal tumours, or to the excessive administration of glucocorticoids or ACTH. Adrenal hyperplasia is often the result of increased ACTH production by a pituitary microadenoma.

Hypertension, which occurs in more than 50% of cases, may be severe and proceed to the malignant phase. Other features of the syndrome are muscle weakness, osteoporosis, purple cutaneous striae, obesity of the trunk, a 'buffalo' hump, a 'moon' facies and diabetes mellitus. There may also be hirsutism, amenorrhoea, a liability to spontaneous bruising, and dependent oedema.

Diagnosis. The diagnosis should be suggested by the combination of hypertension, diabetes and truncal obesity. Outpatient screening tests include:

- excessive 24-h urinary free cortisol excretion;
- failure to suppress plasma cortisol levels following dexamethasone administration.

ACTH levels are valuable in determining the cause — being high with pituitary tumours and low if the adrenal is responsible.

Management. Treatment depends upon the aetiology of the condition. Surgical removal of one or both adrenal glands or of a pituitary tumour may be necessary. Pituitary irradiation may also be effective.

Coarctation of the aorta

See p. 281.

Oral contraception

Oral contraceptive pills give rise to an increase in blood pressure in nearly all women. This is usually slight and falls on stopping the drug. It is wise to check the blood pressure at least during the first year of administration.

HYPERTENSIVE HEART DISEASE

Pathophysiology of hypertension

The high blood pressure in essential hypertension is due to increased peripheral vascular resistance as a result of widespread constriction of the arterioles and small arteries. The cardiac output and the viscosity of the blood are normal. In the earlier stages, the hypertension is largely explicable on the basis of increased arteriolar muscle tone, but subsequently structural alterations take place in the arterioles. These changes may account for the fact that hypertension tends to beget further hypertension, and the removal of the cause of hypertension does not necessarily lead to a fall in the blood pressure to normal. The increased work of the heart imposed by the high resistance results in left ventricular hypertrophy and, eventually, left ventricular failure. As it progresses, the hypertrophy may outstrip the coronary blood supply, particularly if, as is so often the case, there is associated coronary artery disease.

Hypertension accelerates the development of atherosclerosis in the coronary, cerebral, renal and other arteries, perhaps because of long-standing mechanical stress. It often leads to the formation of microaneurysms of the cerebral arteries, especially those of the basal ganglia.

The clinical features of hypertensive heart disease

The development of hypertensive heart disease is usually a slow process; no symptoms or abnormal cardiac signs may occur for many years after high blood pressure has been detected.

The earliest symptom is dyspnoea, at first on exercise and later at rest. At a more advanced stage, the features of right heart failure may develop. Angina pectoris is common.

Abnormal cardiac signs include:

- a forcible and displaced apex beat due to left ventricular hypertrophy;
- accentuation of the aortic component of the second sound;
- added heart sounds. A fourth sound may be audible reflecting decreased ventricular compliance. As failure develops a third sound may occur.

The ECG provides useful evidence of the severity of hypertensive heart disease. In patients with mild elevation of the blood pressure, the ECG is normal. With the development of left ventricular hypertrophy, characteristic ECG changes occur:

- increase in QRS voltages with prominent R waves in left chest leads and S waves in right chest leads (see p. 25);
- ST/T changes. The T waves in the left chest leads become flattened. At a more advanced stage ST segment depression and T wave inversion develop. Coexistent coronary artery disease may complicate the appearances.

Radiographic evidence of left ventricular hypertrophy increases with the passage of time; eventually, the features of pulmonary congestion may develop.

Echocardiography is probably the most reliable technique for evaluating the severity of left ventricular hypertrophy.

Examination of the hypertensive patient

Examination should be directed to assess possible underlying causes for the hypertension and evidence of organ damage as a result of hypertension.

Blood pressure should be recorded after the patient has been lying quietly for 5 min. Clinical examination should take note of:

- features of endocrine abnormalities, particularly Cushing's syndrome;
- multiple neurofibromatoma — present in 5% of patients with phaeochromocytoma;
- inappropriate tachycardia, suggesting catecholamine excess;
- abdominal or loin bruits, suggesting renal artery stenosis;
- renal enlargement;
- radiofemoral delay, due to coarction of the aorta;
- evidence of left ventricular hypertrophy;
- evidence of left ventricular failure;
- fundal examination to detect hypertensive retinopathy.

Fundoscopy. Examination of the optic fundus is of great importance in the evaluation of patients with hypertension, for it is only in the retina that the state of the arterioles can be directly observed. The grading introduced by Keith, Wagener and Barker is widely used:

- grade 1 — increased tortuosity of the retinal arteries with increased reflectiveness, termed silver wiring;
- grade 2 — grade 1 with the addition of compression of the veins at arteriovenous crossings (AV nipping);
- grade 3 — grade 2 with the addition of flame-shaped haemorrhages and 'cotton wool' exudates;
- grade 4 — grade 3 with the addition of papilloedema — the optic disc is pink with blurred edges and the optic cup is obliterated.

Investigation of the hypertensive patient

Routine investigation of all hypertensive patients should include:

- a chest X-ray;
- an ECG;
- urinalysis. Proteinuria, hyaline and granular casts may be found when there is renal disease or malignant hypertension. There is little or no protein in the urine of patients with benign essential hypertension;
- urea and electrolytes;
- fasting blood lipids.

If there is clinical, radiological, or electrocardiographic evidence of left ventricular hypertrophy, this is best confirmed by echocardiography.

It is impractical to screen all hypertensive patients for secondary causes of hypertension. Selection of patient groups for further investigation is arbitrary, but investigation is particularly appropriate in the following groups:

- young patients under 40 years old;
- patients with malignant hypertension;
- patients resistant to antihypertensive therapy;
- patients with unusual symptoms (such as sweating attacks or weakness) which might suggest an underlying cause;
- patients with abnormal renal function, proteinuria or haematuria;
- patients with hypokalaemia off diuretic therapy.

The nature and scale of further investigations will be determined by the index of suspicion of a secondary cause for hypertension.

If concurrent ischaemic heart disease is suspected, patients should undergo exercise testing.

Prognosis

Almost all patients with untreated malignant hypertension die within 1 year. Death is usually due to uraemia, but heart failure and cerebrovascular accidents are common.

The prognosis of benign essential hypertension is relatively good in the absence of cardiac, renal or cerebral involvement. Even in such patients, the death rate from myocardial infarction and cerebrovascular accidents is much higher than that in the normotensive population. In general, the higher the blood pressure, the greater is the risk of these complications.

Other factors related to prognosis are age, sex, blood lipids, diabetes and smoking. These factors are not simply additive but multiplicative. For example, the risks of hypertension in a smoker are greater than the sum of the individual risk factors.

High blood pressure at any particular level is more sinister in the young patient than in the old, and in males than in females. Cardiac enlargement and the ECG abnormalities indicate a substantial risk of developing cardiac failure. Grade 3 retinal changes (haemorrhages and soft exudates) carry a prognosis only little better than grade 4 changes.

Proteinuria and urea retention are associated with advancing renal failure.

THE TREATMENT OF HYPERTENSION

Influence of treatment on prognosis

In the absence of treatment, cardiac failure and cerebrovascular accidents are the major causes of death, myocardial infarction and uraemia being less common, though not infrequent. Several studies have demonstrated the improvement in prognosis that results from antihypertensive therapy. This is most evident in those whose diastolic pressures exceed 105 mmHg, but some benefit is also achieved in individuals with diastolic pressures of 100 or even 95 mmHg. Such treatment has almost eliminated death from cardiac failure and has reduced the incidence of fatal and non-fatal strokes.

There is little evidence from trials that antihypertensive treatment prevents myocardial infarction. There are several possible reasons for this failure to reduce deaths from ischaemic heart disease. It is possible that treatment needs to be initiated earlier or continued longer to prevent coronary disease. It is also possible that some of the drugs used to treat hypertension may adversely influence coronary artery disease. For example thiazide diuretics cause hypokalaemia, impair glucose tolerance and have an adverse effect on blood lipids, any of which might contribute to cardiac mortality, offsetting the benefits of pressure reduction.

Which patients should be treated?

Before initiating drug therapy one must ensure that no treatable cause, such as unilateral renal disease, phaeochromocytoma or coarctation is responsible for the hypertension. If surgically correctable disorders can be excluded, one should consider the most appropriate type of treatment for the individual patient.

Most patients found on screening to have an elevated blood pressure will have mild hypertension and be free of symptoms. Treatment should not be initiated following a single elevated reading, but readings should be repeated over a period of 3–4 months.

Malignant hypertension, demonstrating retinal haemorrhages and exudates, requires urgent hospitalisation and treatment. Patients with severe hypertension (diastolic >120 mmHg) require early initiation of treatment. In most patients in whom there is evidence of secondary effects of hypertension, early drug therapy will be required.

Mild hypertension may respond to simple measures. These include:

- weight reduction;
- regular exercise;
- reduction of alcohol consumption.

All hypertensives should be strongly advised against smoking and given dietary advice to reduce cholesterol intake, to reduce overall coronary risk.

Patients found to have a diastolic pressure persistently above 100 mmHg over 3–4 months should receive pharmacological treatment. With diastolic pressures persistently in the range 95–99 mmHg, treatment may be indicated in young patients. Patients with diastolic pressures less than 95 mmHg should have their blood pressure measured annually. Recent evidence suggests a benefit in treating systolic pressures in excess of 160 mmHg in the elderly.

Drugs used in the treatment of hypertension

There are a large number of drugs in current use for the treatment of hypertension (Table 14.3); new ones are continually being added. It is only possible to mention those which, at present, seem to be of greatest value. Every physician should be familiar with the use of four or five of these drugs as patients vary from one another in their response to therapy and no one drug can be regarded as superior in all respects to others.

Although the aim should be to make the blood pressure 'normal', too great a fall in blood pressure may impair the circulation to the heart, brain or kidneys and precipitate a myocardial infarction, a stroke or renal failure.

An important consideration is the effect of treatment on the quality of life particularly in patients with mild hypertension, only an unidentifiable minority of whom will gain benefit from antihypertensive drugs.

Drugs acting on the sympathetic nervous system

Beta-adrenoceptor blocking drugs (see p. 378). These are effective antihypertensive drugs whose mode of action remains uncertain. They are more effective when combined with a diuretic or other antihypertensive drugs but are often sufficient on their own and produce no

Table 14.3 Drugs used in the treatment of hypertension

General category	Specific examples
Drugs acting on the sympathetic nervous system	
Beta-blockers	Atenolol, Metoprolol
Alpha-blockers	Prazosin, Labetalol (alpha- and beta-blocker)
Centrally acting drugs	Methyldopa, Clonidine
Diuretics	
Thiazide diuretics	Bendrofluazide, Hydrochlorothiazide
Potassium-sparing diuretics	Amiloride, Triamterene
Angiotensin converting enzyme inhibitors	Captopril, Enalapril, Lisinopril
Calcium antagonists	
Dihydropyridine group	Nifedipine, Nicardipine, Amlodipine,
Phenylalkylamine group	Verapamil
Other vasodilators	Hydralazine, Minoxidil
	Nitroprusside

marked orthostatic effects. To ensure compliance, it is best to utilize a preparation that needs to be given only once or twice a day. Provided these drugs are not prescribed for patients with obstructive airways disease or heart failure, serious complications are unusual. Minor side-effects, such as lethargy, nausea, nightmares and cold extremities are common.

Alpha-adrenoceptor blocking drugs. Prazosin is a selective antagonist of post-synaptic alpha-adrenergic receptors. It has marked arteriolar and venous vasodilating effects and the initial dose may produce profound postural hypotension. For this reason the initial dose should be taken on retiring to bed. Other alpha blockers include terazosin and doxazosin.

Labetalol. This drug blocks both alpha- and beta-adrenoreceptors and has proved useful both in essential hypertension (particularly in hypertensive emergencies) and phaeochromocytoma. It shares the same side-effects as other beta-blockers but in higher doses is more likely to cause postural hypotension.

Treatment may be started with oral labetalol in a dosage of 50–100 mg twice daily, and increased, if necessary, to a total of 800 mg a day.

Alpha-methyldopa (Aldomet, Dopamet). This drug is metabolized to alpha-methylnoradrenaline, which replaces noradrenaline in central nervous system adrenergically innervated tissues. Alpha-methylnoradrenaline is released from central adrenergic neurones and stimulates central adrenergic receptors, reducing sympathetic outflow from the central nervous system. Oral methyldopa begins to lower the blood pressure in about 4 h and its effect lasts for up to 24 h. Therapy is started with 250 mg three times a day and increased, if necessary, after a few days to 500 mg three times a day. If this dose is insufficient, a diuretic should be added. The total daily dose should not exceed 3 g. Transient sleepiness is almost invariable during the first 24 h, but a more subtle drowsiness may persist. Other complications include fluid retention, loss of libido and a Coombs' positive haemolytic anaemia.

The use of methyldopa has been largely superceded with the advent of newer antisympathetic agents with fewer side effects.

Other drugs acting on the nervous system. Drugs occasionally used include clonidine, reserpine, and the adrenergic blocking drugs, guanethidine, bethanidine and debrisoquine. The use of these agents has been largely superseded.

Diuretics

The mode of action of diuretics remains uncertain, but appears to have two components. Initially, there is a reduced plasma volume and cardiac output, but these are transient changes. With more prolonged treatment, the total peripheral resistance diminishes; this may be the result of changes in the sodium content of vessel walls.

Thiazide diuretics (see pp. 154, 386). These have been used predominantly in this context and are effective, but have the disadvantage of producing hypokalaemia and occasionally hyperglycaemia and hyperuricaemia. Another side-effect is impotence. Thiazides are best used in low doses which can maximize their antihypertensive effect, while minimizing potassium loss.

Potassium conserving diuretics (see pp. 154, 387). The potassium-conserving diuretics such as spironolactone, amiloride and triamterene have only mild antihypertensive effects but can be used together with thiazide diuretics to preserve potassium equilibrium. The loop diuretics, such as frusemide, ethacrynic acid and bumetanide, may produce a considerable reduction in blood pressure when given intravenously, but they are not ideal for long-term treatment in hypertension because their effects are relatively short-lived.

Angiotensin converting enzyme (ACE) inhibitors (see pp. 154, 384)

These drugs block the enzyme that converts angiotensin I to angiotensin II (see Fig. 14.1). They cause a fall in blood pressure by reducing systemic vascular resistance, without having any major effect on heart rate and cardiac output. This is probably mainly due to a reduction in plasma angiotensin II, but there is also a secondary fall in aldosterone.

ACE inhibitors are effective in all grades and types of hypertension, but their action is potentiated by diuretics. Profound hypotension may be induced on first commencing treatment. This should be avoided by starting with a small dose, and stopping or reducing the dosage of diuretics 1–2 days previously if these are being administered. Renal impairment may be caused, particularly in renal artery stenosis. Hyperkalaemia may occur because of the anti-aldosterone effect; the concomitant use of aldosterone antagonists or potassium supplement is generally unwise.

Cough is a particularly troublesome side-effect, occurring in some 5% of patients. Other side-effects include taste disorders, nausea, diarrhoea, rashes, cough, neutropenia, proteinuria and angioneurotic oedema.

ACE inhibitors are usually well tolerated and most patients prefer them to other antihypertensive agents.

Calcium-blocking drugs (see pp. 111, 381)

This group of drugs has become increasingly employed in the treatment of hypertension in recent years. The dihydropyridine group of calcium antagonists is most commonly used. Examples include nifedipine and nicardipine. These drugs act predominantly to relax vascular smooth muscle and hence lower peripheral vascular resistance.

Nifedipine and nicardipine are effective antihypertensive drugs, particularly when combined with other antihypertensive therapy, such as beta-adrenoreceptor blocking drugs. Verapamil also has antihypertensive actions.

Other vasodilators

Hydralazine. This is a potent arteriolar dilator and increases cardiac output and heart rate. It is best combined with a beta-adrenoceptor blocking agent. Initially 25 mg three times a day should be given; the dose may then be increased if necessary to a total daily dose of 200 mg. It has well-known side-effects of tachycardia, headache and a systemic lupus erythematosus-like reaction; these can largely be avoided by combining with other drugs so that only a small dosage is required.

Diazoxide. This is very effective in acute antihypertensive treatment (150 mg intravenously) but may cause diabetes in prolonged use. The drug is reserved for use in severe hypertension, refractory to other therapy.

Minoxidil. This is a potent vasodilator and antihypertensive. It produces a reflex tachycardia and fluid retention and should be combined with a beta-blocker and diuretic. It may cause hypertrichosis. The drug should only be used for use in severe hypertension, refractory to other therapy.

Nitroprusside. This is a very effective antihypertensive drug when given intravenously and a useful agent for hypertensive emergencies. Care must be taken in its use as a precipitous fall in blood pressure may result (see p. 376).

Choice of therapy for the individual patient

One should start therapy with a single drug which has relatively minor side-effects. Traditionally either a diuretic or a beta-blocker has been selected as the first choice agent. Typical regimes would start with either bendrofluazide 2.5 mg or atenolol 50 mg once daily. However, increasingly both ACE inhibitors and calcium antagonists are being considered as contenders for first line therapy.

Choice of an individual drug may be determined by associated disease states. In patients with angina, for example, either a beta-blocker or a calcium antagonist would be indicated to treat both angina and hypertension simultaneously. In patients with ventricular impairment, diuretics and ACE inhibitors may be preferred.

Drug side-effects may also dictate choice of therapy. Beta-blockers should be avoided in patients with asthma or severe heart failure and used with caution in patients with hyperlipidaemia. Diuretics should be avoided in diabetic patients and patients with gout. ACE inhibitors should be avoided in patients with impaired renal function.

If the response to a single drug is inadequate, a second agent should be added. Particularly useful combinations include:

- beta-blocker plus diuretic;
- beta-blocker plus dihydropyridine calcium antagonist;
- ACE inhibitor plus diuretic;
- ACE inhibitor plus dihydropyridine calcium antagonist.

Beta-blocker/Ace inhibitor and diuretic/dihydropyridine calcium antagonist combinations are less likely to be effective.

If a two-drug regimen does not give adequate blood pressure control, a third agent can be added. This is the traditional 'stepped care' approach. Increasingly, however, physicians are exploring alternative two-drug combinations before resorting to the addition of a third agent.

The patient embarking on antihypertensive treatment must be

advised that drug therapy will probably be required for the rest of his life. Regular checking of the blood pressure is essential.

Further reading

Cunningham, F.G. & Lindheimer, M.D. (1992) Hypertension in pregnancy. *New England Journal of Medicine* **326**: 927.

Frolich, E.D. *et al.* (1992) The heart in hypertension. *New England Journal of Medicine* **327**: 998.

Kaplan, N.M. (1990) *Clinical Hypertension*, 5th edn. Baltimore: Williams & Wilkins.

Sever, P., Beevers, G., Bulpitt, C. *et al.* (1993) Management guidelines in essential hypertension. *British Medical Journal* **306**: 983.

Williams, G.H. (1988) Converting enzyme inhibitors in the treatment of hypertension. *New England Journal of Medicine* **319**: 1517.

Diseases of the Aorta

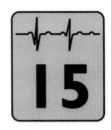

15

The aortic wall is composed of an endothelial lining or intima, a media containing smooth muscle and elastic tissue, and a fibrous adventitia. The media is largely responsible for the elasticity of the aortic wall, and the adventitia for its strength and resistance to rupture.

Dissecting aneurysm

A dissecting aneurysm (Fig. 15.1) results from the entry of blood into the media, either as a consequence of the rupture of vasa vasorum or from a tear of the aortic intima. No histological abnormality is seen in the media of most cases although cystic changes are sometimes present. Dissecting aneurysm is an important complication of the Marfan syndrome and of pregnancy, but the majority of cases occur in middle-aged or elderly men with systemic hypertension. Dissection may also occur as a result of trauma, particularly road traffic accidents. The dissection usually starts either in the ascending aorta a short distance above the aortic valve, or just beyond the origin of the left subclavian artery. The blood dissects a channel between the intima and the adventitia and usually advances distally. In so doing, it may occlude branches of the aortic arch and the descending aorta, including the renal and iliac arteries. If the dissection spreads proximally, the aortic valve may be involved, producing aortic regurgitation and, occasionally, occlusion of a coronary artery. The aneurysm usually ruptures externally into the pericardium, pleural cavity, mediastinum or retroperitoneal tissues, but sometimes it perforates the intima and the dissection 're-enters' the aortic lumen. Occasionally, the dissection becomes chronic without perforation.

 Dissecting aneurysms usually present with the sudden onset of a 'tearing' pain of extreme severity. The site of the pain depends upon the location of the dissection and moves as the dissection progresses. The pain may start in the anterior or posterior chest or in the

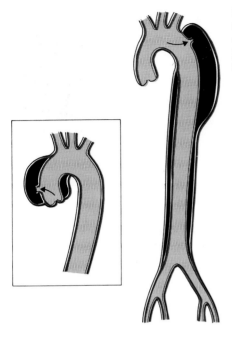

Fig. 15.1 Dissecting aneurysm of the aorta. This usually starts either a short distance above the aortic valve (left) or just below the origin of the left subclavian artery (right).

abdomen, but nearly always affects the upper back at some stage. Intervals of freedom from pain may occur; with recurrences, the pain may involve the neck, arms, chest, trunk or legs. Occasionally, the pain is slight; breathlessness or syncope may then be the presenting symptom.

Classification

Dissecting aneurysms are most simply classified into two types:

- type A — involvement of the ascending aorta with or without extension into the descending aorta;
- type B — involvement of the descending aorta without involvement of the ascending aorta.

Type A dissections account for about two-thirds of cases and type B for one-third.

Clinical features

On examination, the patient appears pale and sweaty and has a tachycardia; although he may have the appearance of shock, the blood pressure is usually within normal limits, having fallen from hypertensive levels. Other signs depend on which branches of the aorta are

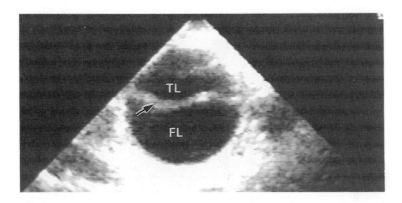

Fig. 15.2 Aortic dissection. Transoesophageal echocardiogram showing the descending aorta in cross section. A flap is demonstrated (arrowed) separating the true lumen (TL) from the false lumen (FL).

occluded. Thus, one or more of the arteries to the limbs may become impalpable. Other complications include aortic regurgitation, tamponade, hemiplegia, mental disturbances, haematuria, bloody diarrhoea and haemothorax.

Investigation

The ECG is of little diagnostic value, but pre-existing hypertension may have caused left ventricular hypertrophy. The appearances of myocardial ischaemia or myocardial infarction may be present if there has been encroachment on a coronary artery. The chest radiograph shows an increase in the width of the mediastinum. The presence of aortic dissection can be confirmed in a number of ways:

- oesophageal echocardiography — this technique is proving of particular value in the diagnosis of aortic dissection (Fig. 15.2);
- computed tomography (Fig. 15.3);
- aortic angiography.

Management

The value of the type A/type B classification (see above) lies in the differentiation of management between the two types of dissecting aneurysms. As a general rule, type A dissections are best managed by early surgery, whereas type B dissections can be managed medically.

In *type A dissections*, there is a strong likelihood of further dissection and death unless surgical repair is undertaken. Patients should first be stablized medically. Blood pressure should be lowered

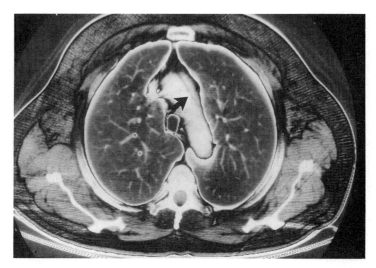

Fig. 15.3 Computed tomogram of an aortic dissection. Arrow points to detached flap in aorta.

to reduce the strain on the aorta; beta-blockers are preferred for this purpose. The choice of surgical procedure depends on the extent of dissection. If the dissection involves the aortic root, it may be necessary to insert a dacron tube graft with resuspension or replacement of the aortic valve and reimplantation of the coronary arteries.

In *type B dissections*, the risks of surgery are generally considered to exceed the risks of medical management. Antihypertensive therapy should be continued long-term to guard against the risks of recurrent dissection.

Saccular and fusiform aortic aneurysms

These are localized distensions of the wall of the aorta, being fusiform if the whole circumference of the vessel is involved and saccular if only part of it is affected.

Atherosclerotic aneurysms, which are usually situated in the descending aorta, result from atrophy of the media and adventitia with fibrous replacement. Syphilis, formerly the major cause of aortic aneurysms, has become uncommon. Syphilitic aneurysms usually affect the ascending aorta and the aortic arch, as a result of inflammatory changes in the aortic wall and subsequent fibrosis and calcification (see p. 331). Fusiform aneurysms are also seen in association with the Marfan syndrome and coarctation of the aorta. A distinctive type of aneurysm is that of the sinus of Valsalva, which will be considered separately.

Clinical features

The clinical features resulting from an aneurysm of the thoracic aorta depend upon its size and site. When the aneurysm is in the ascending aorta, there is often associated aortic regurgitation which leads to cardiac failure. As the aneurysm enlarges and encroaches upon neighbouring structures, there may be pain as a result of erosion of ribs and sternum. A pulsating mass may be seen in the front of the chest and obstruction of the superior vena cava may occur. When the aneurysm is situated in the aortic arch, wheezing, cough and hoarseness may arise from compression of the trachea, bronchus or recurrent laryngeal nerves. Aneurysms of the descending aorta are most likely to produce symptoms as a result of encroachment on the vertebrae, ribs or spinal nerves.

Investigations. Often, however, an aneurysm of the thoracic aorta is first diagnosed in an asymptomatic patient by the radiographic demonstration of a localized dilatation of the aorta. The diagnosis can be confirmed by angiography, although CT scan and transoesophageal echocardiography are also of value.

Management

Asymptomatic patients with relatively small aneurysms may survive for many years. However, the prognosis is generally poor and the patient with symptoms is unlikely to survive more than 1–2 years.

Most patients with aneurysms of the aorta have severe associated disorders such as hypertension, ischaemic heart disease or cerebrovascular disease, and death more often results from one of these than from the aneurysm. Perhaps only one-third of the patients die from aortic rupture; before surgery is undertaken, the cardiovascular and cerebral circulations must be carefully evaluated. Surgery should be considered for those aneurysms which are large or producing symptoms. Saccular aneurysms, which usually have a narrow neck, can be treated by transection of the neck with repair of the underlying aorta. If much of the aortic wall is involved, resection must be undertaken with replacement by a graft.

Aneurysm of the sinus of Valsalva

This is most commonly caused by a congenital localized absence of the aortic media, but can result from syphilitic aortitis or infective endocarditis. The aneurysm forms a thin-walled sac which in most instances protrudes into the right ventricle or right atrium (Fig. 15.4). No symptoms or signs are produced until the aneurysm ruptures. When it does so a fistula is formed between the aorta and the relevant chamber. Congenital aneurysms of the sinus of Valsalva are often

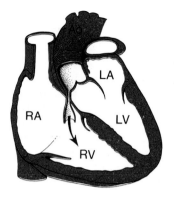

Fig. 15.4   Aneurysm of sinus of Valsalva rupturing into right atrium.

associated with other congenital lesions, particularly a ventricular septal defect.

Sudden death sometimes occurs; more often rupture causes the abrupt onset of chest pain and breathlessness. These symptoms subside over a period of days or weeks. Cardiac failure develops subsequently, but is very variable in its rate of progression.

On examination the patient may have a collapsing pulse due to the aortic diastolic leak, and there is usually a continuous systolic and diastolic murmur, resembling that of a persistent ductus arteriosus, but loudest over the sternum at the level of the third or fourth interspace.

The ECG may be normal initially, but the signs of right ventricular hypertrophy or right bundle branch block may develop later. The chest radiograph shows cardiac enlargement with pulmonary plethora. The aneurysm may be demonstrated by echocardiography, and the shunt by Doppler ultrasound. The definitive diagnosis is made by showing the leak on aortography, and by the demonstration of a left-to-right shunt on cardiac catheterization.

The ruptured sinus of Valsalva should be treated by repair of the aortic wall.

Further reading

Dalen, J.E., Pape, L.A., Cohn, L.H., Lester, J.K. (Jr) & Collins, J.J.J. (1980) Dissection of the aorta. *Progress in Cardiovascular Diseases* **23**: 237.

Liddicoat, J.E., Bekassy, S.M., Rubio, P.A., Noon, G.P. & DeBakey, M.E. (1975) Ascending aortic aneurysms. *Circulation* **52** (**Suppl. I**): 202.

Disorders of the Lungs and Pulmonary Circulation

16

PULMONARY EMBOLISM

Pulmonary thrombo-embolism can cause or aggravate heart disease, and is a common and serious complication of cardiac disorders. Pulmonary embolism, pulmonary thrombosis and pulmonary infarction are related conditions:

- *pulmonary embolism* results from the obstruction of the pulmonary arterial vessels by thrombus or by material, such as fat or air, originating in some other site;
- *pulmonary thrombosis* implies the formation of clot *in situ*;
- *pulmonary infarction* is the necrosis of a wedge of lung tissue resulting from pulmonary arterial occlusion.

Pulmonary embolism is usually a consequence of thrombophlebitis or phlebothrombosis in the leg veins but may also follow thrombosis of the pelvic veins, or clot formation in the right atrium in patients with right-sided cardiac failure, particularly if there is atrial fibrillation. Deep vein thrombosis is often asymptomatic, but the leg may be warm, tender, slightly dusky and swollen by oedema. Thrombosis is most likely to occur when there has been stasis in the veins, especially in association with childbirth, abdominal surgery, acute myocardial infarction and right-sided cardiac failure. There is a slightly increased risk in women taking oral contraceptives. Pulmonary thrombosis is uncommon except as a complication of pre-existing disease of the pulmonary arteries.

Prevention

Pulmonary embolism can be prevented by measures which prevent the development or progression of venous thrombosis. Simple measures to encourage venous flow such as the use of leg exercises and elastic stockings in those confined to bed are important and effective ways of doing so. Once thrombosis has been diagnosed treatment should be initiated with heparin, unless there are contraindications. A bolus of 5000 units may be given, followed by a continuous infusion of the drug. The dosage should be controlled by the activated partial thromboplastin time (APTT) (see p. 396). Oral warfarin should be started at the same time, as described on p. 396. The INR (BCR) should be maintained between 2.0 and 3.0, unless there is recurrent thrombo-embolism when between 3.0 and 4.5 would be appropriate. Heparin may be stopped after 5–7 days. Warfarin should be continued for 3 months for calf thrombosis and 6 months for iliofemoral thrombosis.

Clinical features

The nature of the clinical presentation with pulmonary embolism depends on the size of the embolus:

- *a small embolus* may present with non-specific features such as dyspnoea or tiredness;
- *a medium sized embolus* may cause the occlusion of a segment of the pulmonary arterial tree, causing pulmonary infarction. This may result in pleuritic pain, haemoptysis, a low-grade pyrexia and dyspnoea;
- *massive pulmonary embolism* results from the occlusion of two-thirds or more of the pulmonary arterial bed. This causes right-sided failure, a low cardiac output and a rise in venous pressure.

The physical signs of pulmonary emboli vary with the size of the embolus. Small and even medium-sized emboli may be devoid of any abnormal clinical signs. Following pulmonary infarction, signs of a pleural effusion and pleural rub may be present.

Large emboli may cause:

- hypotension and shock;
- tachycardia;
- cyanosis;
- elevation of the jugular venous pulse;
- accentuation of the pulmonary component of the second heart sound due to pulmonary hypertension;
- right ventricular third and fourth heart sounds;
- occasionally continuous, systolic and diastolic murmurs due to turbulent flow caused by the embolus.

Massive pulmonary embolism should be suspected in any patient who suddenly develops the features of shock, syncope, acute dyspnoea or chest pain, particularly if the subject has evidence of a venous thrombosis or has been confined to bed during the preceding days.

Investigations. Investigations of patients with suspected pulmonary embolism include:

- CXR;
- ECG;
- blood gases;
- ventilation–perfusion scan;
- pulmonary angiography.

The chest radiograph is seldom helpful, although it may show enlarged proximal pulmonary arteries and small peripheral ones.

The ECG in cases of mild to moderate pulmonary embolism the ECG is usually normal, except for demonstrating sinus tachycardia. In cases of severe pulmonary embolism, characteristic ECG features may be observed (Fig. 16.1):

- $S_1 Q_3 T_3$ pattern. A narrow Q wave and inverted T wave in lead III, accompanied by an S wave in lead I, all due to changes in the position of the heart caused by dilatation of the right ventricle and atrium;
- P pulmonale;
- right bundle branch block;
- 'right ventricular strain' pattern with T inversion in the leads V1 to V4;
- atrial arrhythmias.

The differential diagnosis from acute myocardial infarction may be extremely difficult. The ECG is of considerable value, but the patterns associated with massive pulmonary embolism are often misinterpreted as being those of a combination of inferior and anteroseptal infarction. The appearance of Q waves and negative T waves in lead III (but not in lead II) in association with inverted T waves from V1 to V4 strongly suggests pulmonary embolism.

Blood gases. Characteristically pulmonary embolism causes a reduced arterial pO_2 due to shunting of blood through underventilated parts of the lung. Simultaneously pCO_2 is normal or reduced due to hyperventilation.

Pulmonary scintigraphy, using radioactive technetium, is a sensitive technique for detecting perfusion abnormalities. A perfusion deficit might be due either to impaired blood flow to that segment of lung or to primary pulmonary problems, such as effusion or collapse. To improve the specificity of the method, it is generally combined with a ventilation scan using radioactive xenon gas. The demonstration of a non-perfused but ventilated zone is strongly suggestive of pulmonary embolism.

Pulmonary angiography can be undertaken in cases of diagnostic doubt or in cases of massive pulmonary embolism if surgery is

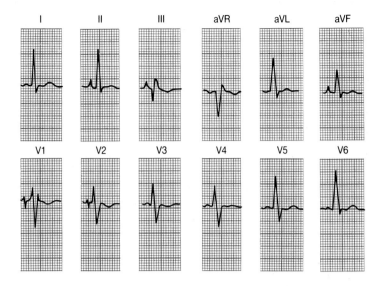

Fig. 16.1   ECG appearances in pulmonary embolism. Note tall, peaked P waves, partial right bundle branch block (rSr in V1), S in lead I, Q and negative T in III, and inverted T waves in V1 to V3.

considered. Contrast material is injected via a catheter inserted in the pulmonary artery. The procedure is potentially hazardous, but risks can be reduced by selective injections into each lung in turn or by using digital subtraction angiography to enable the volume of contrast injected to be reduced.

Management

In the majority of patients the haemodynamic consequences of pulmonary emboli are not severe. The primary objective of treatment is the prevention of further emboli. Patients are treated initially with intravenous heparin (5000 units bolus, followed by an infusion of 15 000 units/12 h, adjusted according to the patient's activated partial thromboplastin time). Warfarin therapy is commenced and heparin discontinued after 5–7 days. Wafarin should be maintained for 6 weeks to 6 months, depending on the likelihood of recurrence.

In exceptional patients who have recurrent pulmonary emboli while on warfarin, an inferior vena caval filter device can be considered. This device, inserted percutaneously via a catheter, traps clots preventing migration to the lungs.

In patients with massive pulmonary embolism, sufficient to cause severe haemodynamic compromise, two approaches are possible:

- thrombolytic therapy;
- surgical embolectomy.

Streptokinase may be administered either into a peripheral vein or directly into the pulmonary artery. A large loading dose (usually 600 000 units over 30 min) is given initially, followed by a smaller maintenance dose (100 000 units hourly), monitoring clotting parameters.

Surgical embolectomy is an alternative to thrombolytic therapy. The operation requires cardio-pulmonary bypass and experienced cardiac surgeons. Embolectomy is indicated in patients with a contraindication to thrombolysis or who continue to deteriorate despite thrombolysis.

Recurrent pulmonary emboli and thrombo-embolic pulmonary hypertension

Recurrent pulmonary embolization, which is usually associated with chronic or recurrent venous thrombosis, may appear as massive emboli, as pulmonary infarction or be silent. Eventually, the vascular obstruction may become so widespread as to cause a substantial increase in the resistance of the pulmonary arteries and lead to pulmonary arterial hypertension. Once this has become established, the prognosis is poor and most patients die within a period of 5 years. The process may sometimes be reversed or prevented from progression by permanent anticoagulant therapy.

PULMONARY HYPERTENSION

The pulmonary arterial pressure is determined by the pressure in the pulmonary capillaries, the pulmonary blood flow and the resistance of the pulmonary arteries (especially the arterioles).

The small pulmonary arteries of the fetus have a thick muscular media and the pulmonary vascular resistance of the non-aerated lung is high. This muscular layer regresses over the first 2–3 months of life. As a consequence the pulmonary vascular resistance and arterial pressure start to fall shortly after birth and within a few weeks have declined to normal adult levels.

The pulmonary arteries in the adult are relatively thin-walled, the smaller vessels having considerably less muscle in their walls than corresponding systemic arterioles. The resistance to flow is much lower and the pressure in the pulmonary artery (about 20/10 mmHg) is approximately one-seventh that in the aorta. It is believed that many of the capillaries in the lung are closed at rest, particularly those of the upper parts of the lungs. When the cardiac output increases, as on exercise, the vascular resistance falls as capillaries open and small arteries dilate. As a consequence, blood flow through the lungs can increase three-fold before any
rise in pressure occurs.

Aetiology

Pulmonary arterial hypertension (greater than 30/15 mmHg) may result from:

- an increase in pulmonary capillary pressure;
- an increase in pulmonary blood flow;
- an increase in pulmonary vascular resistance.

Elevated pulmonary capillary pressure. Passive pulmonary hypertension due to a raised pulmonary capillary pressure occurs in all conditions in which the left atrial pressure rises, such as mitral stenosis and left ventricular failure. The pulmonary artery pressure rises in proportion to the pulmonary capillary pressure.

Increased pulmonary blood flow. Pulmonary hypertension due to increased flow develops in disorders in which there are left-to-right shunts. These include septal defects and persistent ductus arteriosus. In atrial septal defect, a large pulmonary blood flow of 10–15 litres/min may be unassociated with pulmonary hypertension because there is a compensatory vasodilatation with a fall in vascular resistance. In many cases of ventricular septal defect and persistent ductus arteriosus, there is no vasodilatation, and the resistance remains normal. The pulmonary arterial pressure may therefore rise even with comparatively small shunts. With large shunts, pulmonary arterial pressure may reach systemic levels.

Increased pulmonary vascular resistance. There are a number of causes of increased pulmonary vascular resistance (Table 16.1). These diverse causes lead to increased pulmonary vascular resistance through three basic mechanisms:

- *pulmonary vasoconstriction.* Hypoxia is a potent pulmonary vasoconstrictor and is a factor in the pulmonary hypertension that occurs in respiratory disease;

Table 16.1 Causes of increased pulmonary vascular resistance

Cor pulmonale

Chronic thrombo-embolism

Eisenmenger's syndrome (p. 288)

Collagen vascular diseases

Schistosomiasis

Primary pulmonary hypertension

- *blockage* of the pulmonary arteries or arterioles by thrombosis and embolism, as in thrombo-embolism and schistosomiasis;
- *arterial medial hypertrophy*. Proliferation of the muscular medial layer of the small pulmonary arteries which are the main determinants of the pulmonary vascular resistance. The muscular proliferation may progress to fibrosis. Medial hypertrophy plays a major role in primary pulmonary hypertension and in Eisenmenger's syndrome.

Combinations of the three mechanisms are common. In mitral stenosis, for example, the initial phase of passive pulmonary hypertension is often complicated by vasoconstriction and by the obliterative changes of pulmonary embolism. In many cases of ventricular septal defect, both high blood flow and pulmonary vascular disease contribute to pulmonary hypertension. In emphysema, obliteration of the vascular bed and hypoxia are contributory factors.

Clinical features of pulmonary hypertension

Independent of causation, certain clinical features are characteristic of severe pulmonary hypertension. The symptoms include:

- dyspnoea;
- fatigue;
- syncope;
- haemoptysis;
- chest pain;
- symptoms of right-sided cardiac failure.

Abnormal features on clinical examination may include:

- elevation of the jugular venous pulse with a prominent 'a' wave;
- features of tricuspid regurgitation;
- a forceful right ventricular heave along the left sternal edge;
- a right ventricular fourth-heart sound at the lower left sternal edge;
- a loud pulmonary component to the second sound, which may be followed by an early diastolic murmur of pulmonary regurgitation (Graham Steell murmur).

Investigation. The chest X-ray may show enlargement of the proximal pulmonary arteries, right ventricle and right atrium. The peripheral lung fields appear oligaemic.

The ECG demonstrates features of right ventricular hypertrophy:

- tall peaked P waves in lead II due to right atrial enlargement;
- right axis deviation;
- a predominant R wave in lead V1;
- inverted T waves in leads V1–V3.

Management

Both management and prognosis of pulmonary arterial hypertension depend upon its aetiology and on its severity. Passive pulmonary hypertension responds well if the underlying disorder can be corrected (e.g. mitral stenosis). Pulmonary hypertension due to high pulmonary arterial flow can usually be reversed by the correction of the underlying congenital abnormality. Increased pulmonary arterial resistance due to vasoconstriction can often be diminished by relieving hypoxia or by the successful treatment of mitral valve disease. When pulmonary hypertension is due to severe pulmonary vascular disease, as in the Eisenmenger syndrome, the prognosis is poor and life is usually sustained for only a few years. In these cases, cardiac failure is progressive in spite of treatment and the only hope may lie in heart–lung transplantation.

Primary ('unexplained') pulmonary hypertension

Pulmonary hypertension is said to be primary when the aetiology cannot be determined. It is possible that small pulmonary emboli are responsible for some cases. The condition, which is rare, is most common in young women; the first symptoms are usually fatigue and exertional dyspnoea. The diagnosis is made by exclusion in patients found to have the clinical features of pulmonary hypertension. Lung biopsy can aid diagnosis, but is potentially hazardous. Characteristic 'plexiform' lesions are present in the arterioles in approximately 70% of cases.

The prognosis is poor; death is likely to occur within 5 years. Thrombosis may contribute to the progression of hypertension and anticoagulants are recommended; oral contraceptives and pregnancy must be avoided. Vasodilator therapy may prove of value in some patients, but may cause deterioration in others if there is a greater fall in systemic than pulmonary resistance. For this reason patients should be carefully monitored on first commencing therapy. Some success has recently been claimed using high doses of the calcium antagonist, diltiazem. Prostacyclin may also be of value, but is very expensive and needs to be given parenterally.

PULMONARY HEART DISEASE

The understanding of pulmonary heart disease (cor pulmonale) has been made difficult by problems of nomenclature. Here it is defined as heart disease secondary to disorders of ventilation and respiratory function. Right-sided heart failure due to pulmonary arterial disease or secondary to left-sided heart failure is not included in this definition, and is considered in the section on pulmonary hypertension (above).

The prevalence of pulmonary heart disease varies greatly between one geographical area and another. There is abundant evidence that heavy cigarette smoking and air pollution are major factors in the production of chronic bronchitis; cor pulmonale is commonest in those exposed to these influences. It is predominantly a disease of middle-aged and elderly men, and is uncommon in young men or in women of any age.

Pathogenesis of heart failure in lung disease

Lung disease causes heart disease mainly because of its effects on the pulmonary vessels. Due to a number of different mechanisms, there is an increase in pulmonary vascular resistance, leading to pulmonary hypertension, right ventricular hypertrophy and right heart failure.

These mechanisms include:

- *pulmonary arteriolar constriction* due to low alveolar oxygen tension in areas of underventilated lung;
- *anatomical reduction of the pulmonary vascular bed* from rupture of alveolar walls and from fibrotic or thrombotic obliteration of capillaries;
- *compression of pulmonary capillaries* by high intra-alveolar pressures when there is air trapping.

Pulmonary hypertension is seldom severe in pulmonary disease except when there is superadded respiratory infection.

Abnormalities in the blood gases nearly always precede the appearance of heart failure due to lung disease. Hypoxaemia is almost invariable. Even if the arterial oxygen tension is normal at rest, it is reduced on exercise. The hypoxaemia results either from disturbances in the ventilation–perfusion relationship or from interference with the diffusion of oxygen through the alveolar wall.

The carbon dioxide tension is raised when the heart failure is secondary to chronic obstructive airways disease and alveolar hypoventilation. If there is a rapid rise in carbon dioxide tension, the pH is low, but in the chronic stage of the disease the renal retention of bicarbonate maintains a normal or near normal acid–base balance.

These blood gas abnormalities are responsible for many of the characteristics of pulmonary heart disease:

- *polycythaemia* and increased blood volume due to hypoxaemia;
- *peripheral vasodilatation*, due to high carbon dioxide tension, producing a large pulse and warm extremities;
- *cerebral vasodilatation*, due to high carbon dioxide tension, which leads to a raised cerebrospinal fluid pressure, with tremor, confusion and papilloedema;

- *impaired myocardial function* due to hypoxaemia.

The more advanced symptoms of carbon dioxide retention occur mainly, if not exclusively, in patients receiving oxygen in high concentration. Such treatment is dangerous if there is carbon dioxide retention because it abolishes the hypoxaemia which is a major stimulus to respiration.

Clinical features of pulmonary heart disease

Diseases causing pulmonary heart disease cover the full spectrum of pulmonary disease including obstructive airways disease, emphysema, pulmonary fibrosis, pulmonary infiltration (e.g. sarcoidosis), pulmonary resection, skeletal abnormalities and disorders of the respiratory muscles.

The patient is commonly a cigarette-smoking middle-aged man with a long history of morning cough and sputum. There may have been recurrent attacks of winter bronchitis. These symptoms are slowly progressive until breathlessness becomes disabling. Overt cyanosis and peripheral oedema are usually late features but are sometimes the first clear manifestation of pulmonary disease. Recent worsening of cough and the production of purulent sputum is common.

The clinical features reflect pulmonary hypertension and right ventricular failure and include:

- dyspnoea;
- cyanosis;
- features of carbon dioxide retention;
- an elevated jugular venous pulse, possibly with signs of tricuspid regurgitation;
- peripheral oedema and hepatic enlargement.

Investigations

The ECG is often normal but may show P pulmonale, right axis deviation, right ventricular hypertrophy, right bundle branch block, or an rS pattern across the chest. In emphysema the QRS complexes are often small.

The radiological appearances depend upon the nature of the lung disease. When there is emphysema with an increased total lung volume, one may see a low diaphragm and a narrow heart. Enlargement of the main pulmonary artery and its major branches occurs when there is pulmonary hypertension. The radiograph is, however, often normal.

Pulmonary function tests usually demonstrate a FEV_1 below 1.5 litres and a peak expiratory flow rate less than 200 litres/min. Blood gas analysis will usually show an arterial $pO_2 < 6$ kPa (46 mmHg)).

Differential diagnosis. The pulmonary origin of cardiac failure is often overlooked, particularly when it coexists with known ischaemic, rheumatic or hypertensive heart disease. This is particularly the case with hypertension; mild hypertension is often blamed for heart failure which is secondary to chronic bronchitis and emphysema. The history of chronic cough with sputum and wheezing should suggest the possibility, as should poor chest movement and the presence of rhonchi. The diagnosis is usually best made by studies of ventilation and blood gases; carbon dioxide retention makes it almost certain that there is a pulmonary component in heart failure.

Prognosis and treatment

The prognosis is poor once cardiac failure has complicated pulmonary heart disease. Treatment may overcome individual attacks, but the subject is liable to further episodes with recurrent infection, and is unlikely to survive more than two or three such attacks over a period of a few years.

When a patient is seen in cardiac failure due to pulmonary heart disease, the major objects of treatment should be to combat respiratory infection, correct hypoxaemia and carbon dioxide retention, and relieve airways obstruction. Acute chest infections should be promptly treated with antibiotics. Beta$_2$-agonists, such as salbutamol, may have some benefit in reducing pulmonary hypertension. Corticosteroids may be of benefit in patients with reversible airways obstruction. Some patients may also benefit from the provision of long-term domiciliary oxygen. This has been shown to lower mortality in patients with chronic obstructive airways disease and persistent hypoxaemia, although improvement in pulmonary hypertension has not been convincingly demonstrated.

Diuretics are widely used for the control of right heart failure. Digoxin may also be of value.

Further reading

Flenley, D. (1981) *Respiratory Disease.* London: Baillière Tindall.

Fuster, V., Steele, P.M., Edwards, W.D., Gersh, B.J., McGoon, M.D. & Frye, R.L. (1984) Primary pulmonary hypertension. *Circulation* **70:** 580.

Harris, P. & Heath, D. (1986) *The Human Pulmonary Circulation,* 3rd edn. Edinburgh: Churchill Livingstone.

Hirsch, J., Hull, R.D. & Raskob, G.E. (1986) Clinical features and diagnosis of venous thrombosis. *Journal of American College of Cardiology* **8:** 114B.

Hirsch, J., Hull, R.D. & Raskob, G.E. (1986) Diagnosis of pulmonary embolism. *Journal of American College of Cardiology* **8:** 128B.

Systemic Disorders and the Heart

INFECTIONS AND THE HEART

Infections can affect the circulation in a variety of ways:

- direct invasion of endocardium, myocardium and pericardium;
- toxic myocarditis;
- acute circulatory failure due to toxic effects on the vasomotor centre or peripheral vessels, or to dehydration.

Infective endocarditis and pericarditis are considered in Chapter 10 and will not be discussed in detail here.

Diphtheria

Diphtheria causes an acute myocarditis in approximately 20% of subjects. The myocarditis is due to an exotoxin of the diphtheria bacillus rather than to local infection with the organism. Acute circulatory failure may occur in the first few days but the major cardiovascular effects are more common at the end of the first and during the second week. Tachycardia may be present in the absence of myocardial involvement and may be replaced by a bradycardia due to heart block. Gallop rhythm is common and there may be cardiac enlargement. The myocarditis may lead to cardiogenic shock, sometimes accompanied by cardiac failure.

ECG abnormalities often precede the clinical signs of myocarditis, the commonest change being flattening or inversion of the T waves. All grades of heart block may occur.

The presence of acute myocarditis is suggested by gallop rhythm, cardiomegaly, ECG abnormalities, heart block or cardiogenic shock.

Nearly all infants with acute diphtheritic myocarditis die; the mortality in adults is less than 25%. In those who recover from the acute attack, residual cardiac damage is almost unknown.

Diphtheria should be prevented by immunization; if it occurs the patient requires treatment with antitoxin and penicillin. Electrical pacing may be required for heart block; conduction disorders are seldom, if ever, permanent.

Tuberculosis

Tuberculosis may cause pericarditis, with or without subsequent constriction (see p. 213). It may also be responsible for heart disease secondary to pulmonary fibrosis. Tuberculous myocarditis is very rare.

Virus infections

Viruses cause both pericarditis and myocarditis. Coxsackie viruses of group B are probably the commonest organisms affecting the heart; most infections are subclinical. The clinical picture is usually one of fever, malaise and muscular pains, accompanied by evidence of pericarditis and, if there is myocarditis, tachycardia, gallop rhythm, cardiomegaly and cardiac failure. The ECG usually shows non-specific abnormalities, but there may be ST and T wave changes suggesting pericarditis or myocardial infarction. Blood levels of myocardial enzymes (such as creatine kinase) may be raised transiently. The diagnosis can be made by isolating the organism from the stool or by demonstrating a rise or fall in serum antibodies. Rest is desirable during the acute phase, and return to vigorous activity should be progressive. The patient nearly always recovers completely, but there may be residual myocardial damage and recurrences are not unusual. A myocarditis may also be associated with infectious mononucleosis, acute anterior poliomyelitis and many other virus infections.

AIDS (acquired immunodeficiency syndrome)

The heart is eventually involved in 25–50% of patients with AIDS, but only about 10% have any clinical manifestation, which usually takes the form of heart failure.

Trypanosomiasis (Chagas' disease)

Myocarditis due to infection by *Trypanosoma cruzi* is common in South America, where about 20 million people are believed to be infected. It is transmitted by the bite of infected reduviid bugs. These live in the roofs and walls of houses, and drop down on to the face of a sleeping person below. There are two major forms, acute and chronic. Acute Chagas' disease, which occurs predominantly in childhood, may be asymptomatic but can produce tachycardia, cardiomegaly and cardiac failure. Much more important is the chronic form which leads to cardiac failure of insidious onset. It particularly affects men between the ages of 20 and 40. The left ventricle is enlarged, and there may be dyspnoea, chest pain and palpitation. Eventually, right-sided heart failure develops; this is frequently complicated by thrombo-embolic events. Arrhythmias are almost invariable and complete heart block common. The ECG usually shows right bundle branch block. Death is often sudden due to ventricular fibrillation or asystole. Echocardiography shows the features of a dilated cardiomyopathy. Chagas' myocarditis should be suspected when patients who have lived in the tropical or subtropical areas of America develop arrhythmias, cardiac failure and right bundle branch block. A complement fixation test is useful in diagnosis. Treatment is essentially directed at the complications — heart failure, arrhythmias and heart block.

Toxoplasmosis

Toxoplasma gondii can give rise to a myocarditis which may complicate either the disseminated form of the disease, in which there is hepatitis, pneumonia and meningo-encephalitis, or the less acute form which resembles infectious mononucleosis with lymphadeno-pathy the most obvious abnormality. The myocarditis usually gives rise to tachycardia and may cause heart failure, pericarditis and arrhythmias. Complete recovery is unusual.

Syphilis

Cardiovascular syphilis used to be an important cause of death, but is now uncommon. It seldom affects the myocardium, although gum-mata can occur. The organism localizes in the aorta soon after the primary infection, but a latent period of 10–25 years elapses before clinical evidence of aortitis develops.

The initial lesion involves the vasa vasorum of the aorta which become obliterated. The muscle and elastic tissues of the media necrose and are replaced by scar tissue which becomes calcified. Atherosclerotic changes are frequently superimposed. The lesions are usually most severe immediately above the sinuses of Valsalva, and predominantly affect the ascending aorta. The inner aspect of the aorta appears wrinkled, with radial or parallel grooves. The process may involve the mouths of the coronary arteries producing stenosis and, occasionally, occlusion of the coronary ostia. Damage to the aortic valve ring produces dilatation with aortic regurgitation. Aortic stenosis does not occur. Aneurysms of either saccular or fusiform type may be formed.

The symptoms and signs of syphilitic disease depend mainly on whether there is coronary artery involvement, aortic valve disease or aneurysm formation. Coronary artery stenosis leads to angina pectoris and, rarely, myocardial infarction. Syphilitic aortic regurgitation may cause the clinical features of left-sided cardiac failure. Because syphilitic aortic aneurysms affect predominantly the ascending aorta and arch, the major symptoms are those of chest pain due to erosion of bone, cough and dyspnoea due to pressure on the trachea and bronchi, and hoarseness from paralysis of the left recurrent laryngeal nerve. The aneurysm may be visible in the second or third right intercostal spaces, and a systolic thrill may be palpable in this area. Occasionally, a tracheal tug pulls down the thyroid cartilage with each heart beat. There is often a loud systolic murmur over the aneurysm and the second heart sound may be accentuated.

The ECG appearances depend on the nature of the complications and are not specific. A chest radiograph shows a dilated aorta (see Fig. 5.5), often with linear calcification.

Syphilitic aortitis should be suspected if the aorta is conspicuously dilated or aneurysmal, or if there is aortic regurgitation unassociated with stenosis. The diagnosis is confirmed by serological tests specifically directed against the treponemal antigen.

The prognosis is quite good in asymptomatic syphilitic aortitis, survival for 10–20 years being probable. The patient is unlikely to live more than 2–3 years if there is angina due to coronary stenosis or left ventricular failure due to aortic regurgitation.

Syphilitic cardiovascular disease does not develop if early syphilis is adequately treated. It is uncertain whether treatment of established cardiovascular syphilis is effective in preventing progression. It is customary to give 600 mg aqueous procaine penicillin im daily for 20 days, or benzathine penicillin G 2.4 million units im weekly for 3 weeks, to control the infection. Surgery may be necessary for relief of coronary ostial stenosis, for the correction of aortic regurgitation, or for the repair of an aneurysm.

ENDOCRINE AND METABOLIC DISEASES

Hyperthyroidism

Hyperthyroidism (thyrotoxicosis) is a syndrome due to an excess of the circulating thyroid hormones T4 and/or T3. This may result from diffuse hyperplasia of the thyroid gland (Graves' disease) or single or multiple hyperactive nodules. Thyroid overactivity is associated with increased oxygen consumption, heat production, and peripheral vasodilatation. The raised cardiac output which occurs in response to these demands, and to the direct effect of thyroid hormone on the heart, is achieved mainly by tachycardia and increased myocardial contractility rather than by an enlarged stroke volume.

The heart has to support the burden of a greatly enhanced cardiac output when its own metabolic requirements are increased. The normal heart may, in these circumstances, be unable to supply an adequate circulation; a diseased heart is likely to fail.

Clear manifestations of cardiac abnormality, such as cardiomegaly or heart failure usually imply that the hyperthyroidism has aggravated underlying heart disease. This is most commonly ischaemic but it may be hypertensive or rheumatic. Occasionally, hyperthyroidism is the sole cause of heart failure.

Most of the cardiovascular features of hyperthyroidism can be accounted for by the hypermetabolic state, but it is difficult to attribute the common complication of atrial fibrillation to this cause. This arrhythmia may be due to a direct toxic effect of the thyroid hormone on the myocardium.

Symptoms

Cardiac symptoms are common in hyperthyroid patients, even in the absence of cardiac disease. Palpitation is particularly frequent, and is usually attributable to the combination of sinus tachycardia and a vigorous cardiac action. Atrial fibrillation may be responsible for irregular palpitation.

Breathlessness is also common, and can be due to hyperventilation, anxiety or left ventricular failure. Hyperthyroidism may aggravate angina pectoris in those with coronary artery disease.

Cardiovascular signs

- Sinus tachycardia is almost invariable if there is not atrial fibrillation, and persists during sleep.
- The pulse is of large volume and may have a collapsing character.
- The systolic blood pressure is frequently high, whilst the diastolic is normal or low.
- The apical impulse is vigorous, but not usually displaced.
- The heart sounds are loud.
- There is often a pulmonary midsystolic murmur, due to high flow.

Cardiac enlargement and the signs of left- or right-sided heart failure may develop if the thyroid disease is of long standing or if there is coexistent cardiac disease.

The classical features of hyperthyroidism such as weight loss, moist warm extremities, tremor, lid retraction, exophthalmos and goitre are usually present, but all these signs may be slight or absent in the older patient. There are no distinctive features on the ECG or chest radiograph.

Diagnosis

Hyperthyroidism can be recognized easily if the characteristic features are present, but the diagnosis can be difficult if the abnormalities are largely confined to the cardiovascular system. It should be suspected whenever sinus tachycardia, atrial fibrillation or cardiac failure are unexplained.

The diagnosis of hyperthyroidism is established by finding abnormally high blood levels of T4 and/or T3 (after allowance has been made for their binding proteins).

Treatment

Hyperthyroidism may be treated by antithyroid drugs (such as carbimazole, methimazole and propylthiouracil), radio-iodine or partial thyroidectomy. Radio-iodine is the most suitable therapy for most patients with thyrotoxic heart disease (except for women of child-bearing age), but surgery may be indicated if the gland is large or if there is a danger of tracheal compression.

When the rapid control of the tachycardia of hyperthyroidism is necessary, a beta-adrenoceptor blocking drug should be given.

The atrial fibrillation of thyrotoxicosis is difficult to slow adequately with digitalis alone; a beta-blocker should be added if not contraindicated. When thyroid overactivity is controlled, d.c. shock is usually effective in restoring sinus rhythm.

Heart disease in hyperthyroidism usually responds well to therapy unless it has been untreated for several years.

Hypothyroidism

Hypothyroidism is associated with reduced circulation T3 and T4, most often as a result of inflammatory destruction of the thyroid. It may, however, be secondary to reduced TSH secretion by the pituitary or hypothalamus, or to drugs such as amiodarone.

Hypothyroidism affects the cardiovascular system in several ways:

- the reduced level of body metabolism is associated with a low cardiac output, a diminished peripheral blood flow, a reduction in venous return, and sinus bradycardia;
- the deficiency of thyroid hormone seems to be responsible for

interstitial oedema and mucoid infiltration of the myocardium, and for a pericardial effusion;

- the hypercholesterolaemia characteristically present may be responsible for premature coronary atherosclerosis and ischaemic heart disease; the evidence for this is inconclusive;
- 'myxoedema coma' is associated with hypotension and bradycardia.

The patient with hypothyroidism seldom has cardiac symptoms, except for dyspnoea and angina pectoris due to coexistent coronary disease. The symptoms and signs of cardiac failure rarely, if ever, occur in the absence of some additional form of heart disease.

The pulse rate is usually between 50 and 60/min. The sluggish apex beat is difficult to feel and the heart sounds are soft.

The ECG is abnormal in showing low voltage of all components of the PQRST complexes; the T waves are flattened or inverted. The chest radiograph shows a large cardiac shadow; echocardiography often reveals that this is due to a pericardial effusion.

Hypothyroidism is usually suspected because of the general sluggishness, the cold and thickened skin, the husky voice, the coarse but scanty hair and the slow pulse, but minor forms of the disorder may easily escape detection. Blood levels of T4 and T3 are low. The most sensitive test for primary hyperthyroidism is the high serum level of thyroid-stimulating hormone (TSH) but this is not raised if hypopituitarism is responsible.

Treatment with thyroid substances is effective but may provoke angina pectoris. For this reason, in those suspected of having coronary disease, small doses (e.g. thyroxine 0.0125 mg) should be used initially and the dose should be increased very cautiously, if necessary, but not beyond 0.15 mg. The serum TSH level can be useful as a marker of the adequacy of replacement therapy. The addition of a beta-adrenoceptor blocking drug may protect the patient from angina but often fails, in which case coronary artery bypass surgery may be required.

Acromegaly

In acromegaly, hypersecretion of growth hormone from a pituitary adenoma results overgrowth in many tissues and organs, including the heart. Hypertension and accelerated atherosclerosis occur.

Diabetes

Diabetes is a metabolic disorder due to the reduced availability or effectiveness of insulin. In type 1 (insulin-dependent diabetes or

IDDM), there is a defective secretion of insulin by the pancreas, probably consequent upon infective or auto-immune damage to the islet cells. Most cases of type II diabetes (non-insulin-dependent diabetes or NIDDM) are probably genetic in origin; in this form of the disease, the tissues are relatively resistant to the actions of insulin. In both types, blood glucose is raised and there is glycosuria, but the major and most dangerous complications are predominantly cardiovascular — affecting the coronary, renal, retinal and peripheral circulations.

Diabetic patients are particularly prone to coronary heart disease, but there is also a diabetic form of cardiomyopathy. Diabetes is also commonly associated with hypertension.

Diabetes is managed with diet, insulin and hypoglycaemic agents. The actual regimen depends upon the type of diabetes, and skilled advice is required with regard to diet. The use of hypoglycaemic drugs such the sulphonylureas is controversial because of some evidence of adverse cardiac side-effects.

Carcinoid syndrome

Malignant carcinoid tumours with metastases in the liver may be associated with pulmonary stenosis and regurgitation, and with tricuspid stenosis or regurgitation, the valve cusps being fixed by fibrosis. The cardiac lesions are probably due to the actions of kinins or of 5-hydroxytryptamine (5HT, serotonin) secreted by the tumour. These substances are also responsible for the flushing attacks, telangiectasia, diarrhoea and bronchospasm characteristic of this syndrome.

The cardiac findings in the carcinoid syndrome are those of the particular valve lesion and of right-sided heart failure. The diagnosis is established either by identification of the tumour at laparotomy or by the detection in the urine of large quantities of 5-hydroxy-indole acetic acid (5-HIAA), a breakdown product of 5-HT.

Treatment is unsatisfactory, the diarrhoea may be controlled by codeine, and the flushing by ketanserin (a 5-HT blocker): cardiac failure is treated on conventional lines, valve replacement occasionally being necessary.

Haemochromatosis

In this disorder, which is mainly encountered in older males, there is excessive iron storage associated with cirrhosis of the liver, diabetes and pigmentation of the skin, and a substantial proportion of patients die from a cardiomyopathy, which may be restrictive, but is usually of the dilated congestive type. Treatment of the failure may be temporarily effective as may repeated venesection, but the prognosis is poor.

Gout

There is a statistical association between hyperuricaemia and coronary artery disease, but there is no definite evidence of an increased incidence of coronary disease in those with clinical gout. Gout may be provoked by diuretics; it may occur in severe cyanotic congenital heart disease in association with secondary polycythaemia. It occasionally causes an acute pericarditis.

Glycogen-storage disease

In this autosomal recessive disorder, excessive glycogen is deposited in skeletal and cardiac muscle. Breathlessness, feeding difficulties and muscular weakness usually develop about the third month of life and the progression of cardiac failure is relentless. The ECG and the chest radiograph demonstrate biventricular enlargement. Death occurs before the age of 3 years — usually within the first year of life.

Overweight and obesity

Overweight is associated with heart disease in a number of ways:

- overweight is a risk factor for both coronary heart disease and hypertension;
- fat arms in obese patients may cause falsely high blood pressure recordings;
- a specific Pickwickian syndrome of hypoventilation with carbon dioxide retention, hypoxia, somnolence, polycythaemia and right-sided heart failure is sometimes caused by obesity. The obesity is directly responsible for the hypoventilation because it restricts respiratory movement; improvement can be achieved by weight loss;
- overweight is assocated with sleep apnoea;
- obesity is important in patients with cardiac disease of any type because the demands on the heart are increased. Weight reduction is an essential component in the prevention and treatment of angina pectoris, hypertension, and cardiac failure.

Beri-beri

This disease is due to thiamine deficiency, which is usually the result of a diet with a high proportion of polished rice in eastern countries but is associated with alcoholism in North America and Europe. The deficiency leads to a lack of co-carboxylase which is necessary for the oxidation of pyruvic acid to acetyl coenzyme A. The citric acid cycle is inhibited and the accumulation of lactate and pyruvate may lead to peripheral vasodilatation and impaired cardiac function. The characteristic haemodynamic features are those of a low peripheral vascular resistance and a high cardiac output. Cardiac failure eventually occurs and in the later stages the cardiac output may fall.

The clinical features of beri-beri heart disease include palpitation, fatigue, breathlessness and peripheral oedema. In some cases there may be acute circulatory failure with hypotension and syncope. There is usually sinus tachycardia with a large pulse and right-sided cardiac failure. The heart is enlarged and there may be a gallop rhythm and systolic murmurs.

The neurological features are those of an ascending peripheral neuritis, commonly accompanied by mental confusion. Paraesthesiae occur in the hands and feet and there is weakness of the legs. The calf muscles are tender and areas of anaesthesia occur.

Neither the ECG, which usually shows non-specific T wave changes, nor the chest radiograph, which reveals cardiomegaly, are helpful in diagnosis. This is usually achieved by obtaining a history of nutritional deficiency or of alcoholism, and by finding evidence of both peripheral neuritis and cardiac failure. Laboratory tests show increased serum pyruvate and lactate levels and a low red blood cell transketolase level.

Most cases respond quickly to thiamine chloride, 50 mg intramuscularly per day. Subsequently, thiamine should be given orally in dose of 10–20 mg.

Alcoholic cardiomyopathy

There is increasing evidence that a large intake of alcohol, even in the absence of nutritional deficiency, can lead to cardiomyopathy. The patients are often middle-aged men who are excessively fond of both food and alcohol. The initial symptom is either breathlessness or palpitation, due to ectopic beats or atrial fibrillation. The ECG may show low, dimpled T waves. In the early stages, abstinence may reverse the picture, but otherwise there is progression with increasing cardiac failure to death.

Treatment consists of complete abstinence from alcohol and the use of conventional measures for controlling atrial fibrillation and cardiac failure.

MISCELLANEOUS DISORDERS

Rheumatoid arthritis and the connective tissue disorders

RHEUMATOID ARTHRITIS

This is accompanied by valve disease rather more often than would be expected by chance, although by no means as frequently as is rheumatic fever. Acute pericarditis and pericardial effusion are quite common; pericardial constriction is rare.

ANKYLOSING SPONDYLITIS (RHEUMATOID SPONDYLITIS)

This is associated with aortic regurgitation due to focal destruction of the elastica and media of the aorta.

REITER'S DISEASE

This is characterized by urethritis, seronegative arthritis and conjunctivitis. It is sometimes complicated by pericarditis, myocarditis and aortic regurgitation.

SYSTEMIC LUPUS ERYTHEMATOSUS

This often affects the heart, although cardiac symptoms and signs seldom dominate the clinical picture. Acute or chronic pericarditis, with or without effusion, is usually the most obvious evidence of cardiac involvement. Myocarditis sometimes develops, and may be due to disease of the small coronary vessels. Endocarditis also occurs, with large warty excrescences which may involve any of the four heart valves. These lesions seldom give rise to clinical heart disease, but may act as a focus for infective endocarditis.

POLYARTERITIS

This may result in myocardial infarction, or in cardiac failure without evidence of infarction. The heart failure may be, in part, the result of hypertension which is common in this disorder. Pericardial effusions occasionally occur.

SCLERODERMA

This may lead to cardiac failure either by producing a cardiomyopathy, usually of the constrictive type, or as a result of pulmonary heart disease secondary to diffuse pulmonary fibrosis.

PSEUDOXANTHOMA ELASTICUM

This is a familial disease affecting connective tissue associated with calcification and proliferation of the media of the coronary and peripheral arteries which may give rise to ischaemic heart disease and hypertension. The skin, particularly in certain areas such as the elbow creases and back of the neck, takes on a crêpe-like appearance with much redundant tissue. Characteristic dark 'angioid' streaks occur in the fundi.

Sarcoidosis

Sarcoid may cause heart failure, syncope due to arrhythmias and heart block, and sudden death. It can affect the heart primarily, but cardiac sarcoid more often follows lung or more general involvement.

The Marfan syndrome

This familial autosomal dominant disorder of connective tissue may result in many skeletal, cardiovascular and other abnormalities. These include great height, long limbs with spidery fingers (arachnodactyly), a high arched palate and dislocation of the lens. Defects in the synthesis, secretion and assembly of fibrillin seem to be involved; the gene for fibrillin is closely identified with the site of the Marfan gene on chromosome 15.

A weakness of the aortic media is common and leads to dilatation, aneurysm formation, and dissection. Aortic regurgitation may follow dilatation of the valve ring. Mitral valve disease may result in cusp prolapse and regurgitation.

These abnormalities can be evident in childhood but may not develop until the fifth decade.

There is no specific treatment, but contact sports and isometric exercise should be avoided. The risk of dissection can be reduced by the use of beta-blockers. Surgery may be required for the valve disorders and for progressive enlargement of the aorta, and urgently for dissection.

Cardiac tumours

Cardiac tumours are rare. The commonest is the *myxoma* which occurs most frequently in the left atrium, but occasionally in the other chambers. It varies from 1 to 8 cm in diameter, and is usually attached by a pedicle to the atrial septum. Because its position may vary with posture, transient or complete obstruction of the mitral valve may result. The tumour may prolapse into the left ventricle and cause mitral regurgitation. The haemodynamic effects of left atrial myxoma usually resemble those of mitral stenosis. The tumour may also be responsible for embolic phenomena, and can produce constitutional effects such as fever, weight loss, anaemia, finger clubbing, raised sedimentation rate and abnormal serum proteins. The obstruction of the mitral valve may lead to dyspnoea and, rarely, syncope or vertigo related to posture. Variable mitral systolic and diastolic murmurs may be heard, and there may be a loud first sound and opening snap. The diagnosis should be suspected in patients with signs of mitral stenosis, who have a history of syncope, or variable murmurs, or unexplained fever with a high ESR. The diagnosis can be most readily established by echocardiography which demonstrates a mass within the left atrium (Figs. 17.1A and B). The tumour should be removed under cardiopulmonary bypass.

Trauma

Traumatic lesions of the heart may be due to penetrating chest injuries as, for example, from gunshot wounds or stabbing, or from non-penetrating injuries produced by blows to the chest such as steering wheel accidents.

PENETRATING INJURIES

Penetrating injuries may cause lacerations of any of the heart chambers or great vessels, and death may ensue from haemorrhage or cardiac tamponade. If the victim does not die within a few hours, late complications may occur due to infective pericarditis, valve damage or intracardiac shunts. The diagnosis is usually not difficult and can be deduced from the site of the injury, the evidence of blood loss or cardiac tamponade, or ECG abnormalities.

The chest radiograph may be valuable in locating foreign bodies in or around the heart; echocardiography is useful in detecting pericardial fluid. Pericardial aspiration may relieve tamponade, but for the other serious complications, immediate surgery is usually necessary.

NON-PENETRATING INJURIES

A substantial proportion of blunt chest injuries seen in hospital have some cardiac damage. This may take the form of myocardial 'concussion' in which there is functional impairment but no structural damage, or 'contusion' in which there is myocardial necrosis. Myocardial infarction may occur from direct trauma to the muscle, or as a consequence of injury to a coronary artery. In either case, any of the complications of infarction may be seen, including arrhythmias,

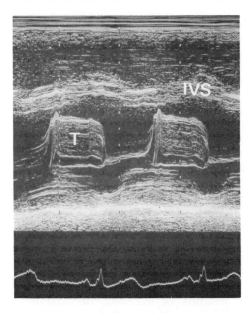

Fig. 17.1A Parasternal M-mode echocardiogram of a left atrial myxoma. Multiple echoes are seen behind the anterior mitral valve leaflet in diastole as the tumour prolapses downwards towards the left ventricle. IVS = interventricular septum. T = tumour.

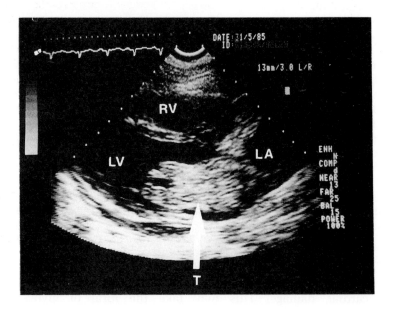

Fig. 17.1B Cross-sectional echocardiogram of myxoma. There is a large tumour (T) situated in the mitral valve orifice.

rupture, and aneurysm formation. In addition, valves and chordae tendineae may be ruptured, and haemopericardium and tamponade may occur. Aortic transection is relatively common, particularly in acceleration accidents.

Unless tamponade or murmurs develop, cardiac damage may not be suspected. Chest radiography, ECG and cross-sectional echocardiography should be undertaken in all cases of severe blunt chest trauma. Aortic damage is probably best located by computed tomography. The patient may require surgical treatment for tamponade, aortic rupture or valve regurgitation.

ANAEMIA AND THE HEART

Anaemia imposes increased demands upon the heart and, at the same time, impairs its function. It aggravates the symptoms of the patient with heart disease and has important circulatory effects even in the individual with a normal heart.

The haemodynamic effects of anaemia probably result mainly from a decrease in blood viscosity and from tissue hypoxia, which is responsible for peripheral vasodilatation. As a consequence, the peripheral arterial resistance is diminished, the diastolic pressure falls and the pulse pressure widens. Ventricular afterload is decreased. The stroke volume and cardiac output are increased when the haemoglobin falls below 7 g/100 ml blood, and both respond to exercise to a greater degree than normal. The hypoxia produces coronary vasodilatation when this is possible, but in the patient with coronary artery disease the ability to dilate is restricted. If anaemia is both severe and prolonged, fatty degeneration of the myocardium takes place.

For the reasons described, anaemia may precipitate or aggravate cardiac failure in the patient with pre-existing heart disease, and it may induce or exacerbate angina in those with coronary artery disease.

It is rare for either heart failure or angina to develop in anaemic patients with normal hearts, but signs and symptoms may occur in such patients which mimic those of heart disease. Dyspnoea, tachycardia and peripheral oedema are common in patients with chronic and severe anaemia.

Cardiovascular signs of anaemia

Anaemia may produce:

- the warm skin and bounding arterial pulse of the high output state;
- a venous hum in the neck;

- cardiac enlargement in the advanced case;
- very commonly, a systolic murmur in the second or third left intercostal space close to the sternum. This is probably due to turbulence resulting from increased flow and reduced blood viscosity;
- a loud third heart sound;
- in very severe cases, a short mitral middiastolic murmur, due to increased flow.

The ECG is usually normal, but non-specific ST and T wave changes may occur and the ST depression of myocardial ischaemia may develop.

Treatment

The clinical features of anaemia are usually readily corrected either by appropriate drug therapy, or by blood transfusion. Rapid transfusion is dangerous, particularly if there is heart failure; in this situation, it is advisable to use packed cells. If whole blood only is available, a diuretic such as frusemide 40 mg should also be given.

PREGNANCY AND THE HEART

Pregnancy imposes a substantial load on the heart and circulation. The cardiac output and blood volume increase from the sixth week onwards, until, about the 30th week, they are some 30–50% above normal levels at which they remain during the rest of pregnancy. During the last 8 weeks, the inferior vena cava may be obstructed by the uterus when the subject is supine; as a consequence, the cardiac output may fall when this position is assumed. Other factors affecting the cardiovascular system are an increased metabolic rate, a corresponding rise in oxygen consumption, the arteriovenous shunt in the uterus and an elevation in the venous pressure due to the increased blood volume.

Cardiovascular symptoms and signs of normal pregnancy

Dyspnoea, orthopnoea, and syncope are not uncommon in the normal pregnant woman. The circulatory changes of pregnancy produce characteristic signs:

- the hands are warm and the pulse is large;
- a tachycardia is present and the venous pressure slightly raised;
- the apex beat is vigorous and may be displaced outwards, partly

as a consequence of cardiomegaly and partly by the high diaphragm;

- the high flow almost always produces a soft pulmonary midsystolic murmur and a third heart sound. These are often mistaken for cardiac disease;
- the ECG often shows an axis shift and minor ST segment and T wave changes.

Heart disease in pregnancy

The circulatory burden of pregnancy frequently reveals pre-existing heart disease for the first time. Symptoms may start at about week 12 and tend to progress until they may become severe from week 24 onwards. A period of particular danger occurs after delivery, when the sudden reabsorption of blood from the uterus into the circulation may precipitate pulmonary oedema.

RHEUMATIC HEART DISEASE

Heart disease in pregnancy is frequently rheumatic; mitral stenosis is the most serious lesion encountered. Patients wih tight mitral stenosis may become breathless in early pregnancy and progress to pulmonary oedema or right-sided cardiac failure. Even those with less severe lesions may develop symptoms during the last months or shortly after delivery. Patients with mild mitral stenosis, mitral regurgitation and aortic regurgitation usually tolerate pregnancy well, but may become increasingly breathless.

The management of rheumatic heart disease in the pregnant woman depends upon a number of factors including her age, parity and religious beliefs, the stage of the pregnancy, the nature of the lesion, and the response to treatment. In the patient with severe mitral stenosis, pregnancy should be avoided or deferred until mitral valvotomy has been performed. If such a patient becomes pregnant, a decision should be made before week 16 as to whether valvotomy should be undertaken or the pregnancy terminated. As pregnancy progresses beyond this time, both termination and valvotomy become more hazardous. If the patient is seen for the first time at a later stage of pregnancy, she should be managed medically, for with adequate bed-rest, digitalis and diuretics, the maternal mortality is low.

Patients with rheumatic valve lesions other than mitral stenosis should be managed medically or have the pregnancy terminated.

Prosthetic heart valves. Prosthetic valves pose a special problem in pregnancy. Warfarin, particularly in the first trimester, may induce congenital abnormalities, but the discontinuation of anticoagulants exposes the patient to an increased risk of thrombo-embolism.

Heparin may be preferable for this early phase as well as for the last few weeks of pregnancy. The British Society for Haematology has recommended 10 000 units subcutaneously 12-hourly or 7000 units 8-hourly up to 16 weeks and from 36 weeks to delivery, with warfarin as an alternative from 16 to 36 weeks. If possible, prosthetic valves should not be inserted in women who are likely to become pregnant.

Congenital heart disease

Patients who were born with congenital heart disease are being seen with increasing frequency in pregnancy, but the cardiac abnormality is usually mild or has been corrected by surgery prior to conception. Pregnancy is tolerated well if there is an uncomplicated septal defect or persistent ductus arteriosus. Severe pulmonary hypertension of whatever aetiology is extremely hazardous, with a 25–50% risk of maternal death during the pregnancy or in the puerperium; termination in early pregnancy is to be strongly recommended.

Infective endocarditis

Normal pregnancy rarely gives rise to infective endocarditis even in those with abnormal valves. Routine antibiotic prophylaxis is probably best reserved for patients with prosthetic valves.

Toxaemia of pregnancy

Toxaemia of pregnancy is discussed in Chapter 14.

Cardiomyopathy

Cardiomyopathy ('peripartal') of unknown aetiology sometimes develops during later pregnancy or the puerperium. Although about one-third of patients recover permanently, there is a risk of progression and of recurrence during subsequent pregnancies.

Termination of pregnancy

With good medical preparation and skilled anaesthesia there is little risk in terminating a pregnancy in the presence of cardiac disease. This procedure is indicated in women with advanced heart disease and severe symptoms in early pregnancy, if they are not suitable candidates for mitral valvotomy. Termination should also be considered for those with less severe disease who would find the care of an additional child burdensome.

Sterilization

This should be considered in patients with heart disease who have completed their families or in whom further pregnancies would be harmful. It should not be undertaken lightly. The religious beliefs of the patient must be respected, the risk of psychological disturbance considered, and the possibility of surgical correction of the cardiac lesion borne in mind.

Contraception

Patients with cardiac disease may wish or need to practise contraception. Advice should be proffered to those for whom pregnancy is temporarily inadvisable.

Oral methods of contraception have the major advantage of reliability. The combined oestrogen and progestogen pill increases the risk of arterial and venous thrombosis, and exacerbates systemic hypertension and pulmonary hypertension. It should, therefore, be avoided in women known to have or be at high risk of these conditions. Women over 35 who smoke should not take the combined oral contraceptive because of the greatly increased risk of cardiovascular disease. Less information is available on the progestogen-only pill, but the risks seem to be substantially less. Intra-uterine devices are better avoided in congenital and valvar heart disease because of the risk, albeit small, of infective endocarditis.

Further reading

Acromegaly Hayward, R.P., Emanuel, R.W. & Nabarro, J.D.N. (1987) Acromegalic heart disease. *Quarterly Journal of Medicine* **237:** 41.

AIDS Acierno, L.J. (1989) Cardiac complications in acquired immunodeficiency syndrome (AIDS). *Journal of the American College of Cardiology* **13:** 1144.

Alcohol Regan T.J. (1984) Alcoholic cardiomyopathy. *Progress in Cardiovascular Diseases* **27:** 141.

Anaemia Varat, M.A., Adolph, R.J. & Fowler, N.O. (1972) Cardiovascular effects of anemia. *American Heart Journal* **83:** 415.

Carcinoid syndrome Clarke, B. & Hodgson, H.J.F. (1986) Carcinoid syndrome. *British Journal of Hospital Medicine* **35:** 746.

Coxsackie infection Reyes, M.P. & Lerner, A (1985) Coxsackievirus myocarditis. *Progress in Cardiovascular Disease* **27:** 373.

Friedreich's ataxia Child, J.S., Perloff, J.K. et al. (1986) Cardiac involvement in Friedreich's ataxia. *Journal of the American College of Cardiology* **7:** 1370.

Giant cell (cranial) arteritis Huston, K.A. & Hunder, G.G. (1980) Giant cell (cranial) arteritis. *American Heart Journal* **100:** 99.

Hypothyroidism Aber, C.P. & Thompson, G.S. (1964) The heart in hypothyroidism. *American Heart Journal* **68**: 428.

Marfan syndrome Roberts, W.C. & Honig, H.S. (1982) The spectrum of cardiovascular disease in the Marfan syndrome. *American Heart Journal* **104**: 115.

Pregnancy Metcalfe, J., McAnulty, J.H. & Ueland, K. (1986) *Heart Disease and Pregnancy*. Boston: Little Brown & Co.

Sarcoidosis Fleming, H.A. (1986) Sarcoid heart disease. *British Medical Journal* **292**: 1095.

Scleroderma Goldman, A.P. & Kotler, M.N. (1985) Heart disease in scleroderma. *American Heart Journal* **110**: 1043.

Syphilis Heggtveit, H.A. (1964) Syphilitic aortitis. *Circulation* **29**: 346.

Systemic lupus erythematosus Doherty, N.D. & Siegel, R.J. (1985) Cardiovascular manifestations of systemic lupus erythematosus. *American Heart Journal* **110**: 1257.

Thyrotoxicosis Woeber, K.A. (1992) Thyrotoxicosis and the heart. *New England Journal of Medicine* **327**: 94.

Toxoplasmosis Harvey, H.P.B., McLeod, J.C. & Twitter, J.R. (1966) Myocarditis associated with toxoplasmosis. *Australian Annals of Medicine* **15**: 169.

Trauma Taggart, D.P. & Reece, I.J. (1987) Penetrating cardiac injuries. *British Medical Journal* **294**: 1630.

Psychological Aspects of Heart Disease

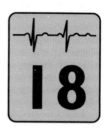

The relationship between psychological factors and heart disease is complex. Many anxious individuals believe, erroneously, that they have heart disease; anxiety and depression often complicate and aggravate organic heart disease.

PSYCHOLOGICAL FACTORS IN THE GENESIS OF HYPERTENSION AND CORONARY DISEASE

The blood pressure rises acutely on emotion; it is therefore reasonable to speculate that there is a relationship between chronic emotional stress and sustained hypertension. This would be very difficult to establish and, as yet, the evidence is equivocal. None the less, hypertensives and their normotensive children appear to have exaggerated responses to emotional stimuli, and relaxation techniques are antihypertensive in some individuals.

There has been much interest in psychological factors in coronary heart disease. Rosenman and Friedman described a 'specific overt behaviour pattern' which they designated type A, characterized by aggression, ambition, impatience and preoccupation with deadlines. They reported a high incidence of coronary disease in such individuals and have also claimed that they could be trained out of these habits after myocardial infarction, with beneficial results. Some have confirmed their observations; others have not. If what they say is true, it is surprising that coronary disease is now commonest amongst manual workers. Other psychological characteristics have been related to coronary disease — perhaps the most persuasive evidence points to suppressed anger and hostility as risk factors. There is certainly little to suggest the view that stressful occupations (traditionally doctors and lawyers) lead to coronary disease.

On the other hand, there can be no doubt of the importance of emotional stress in precipitating episodes of angina pectoris. Rarely, there is strong circumstantial evidence that emotional stress has been a contributory factor in causing myocardial infarction or fatal arrhythmias.

ANXIETY STATE AND THE HEART

Individuals with an anxiety state often have complaints suggestive of heart disease. A large number of labels have been applied to the complex of symptoms of such patients, including 'effort syndrome', 'cardiac neurosis' and 'neurocirculatory asthenia'. It was particularly common in the armed services during war-time, and has therefore been called 'soldier's heart', but it also occurs frequently in civilians.

Breathlessness, palpitation and fatigue are almost invariable, and are usually accompanied by feelings of faintness and dizziness. Chest pain is less common, but is often the reason for referral to a physician.

The breathlessness may be related to exertion, but also occurs at rest. Frequent complaints are that 'I can't take a deep breath' or 'I can't get enough air'. The palpitation is usually the awareness of a sinus tachycardia, but can be due to ectopic beats which cause the patient to think that his heart is about to stop.

The chest pain of anxiety state is usually situated in the left sub-mammary region but may be elsewhere in the left chest and may radiate to the left arm. It is sometimes provoked by effort, but tends to come on after exercise rather than during it; it can develop at rest and at night time. It often takes the form of a persistent ache lasting for hours or days; sharp momentary stabs of pain are also frequent. The patient will often say that the pain is 'in his heart'. The muscles in the area may be tender, and in some cases the pain can be abolished by infiltration with local anaesthetics.

Whilst recounting his history, the patient gives an impression of distress, and is tense or rather withdrawn in manner. Sighing respiration is common and there may be hyperventilation. Sinus tachycardia is usual, and palpation reveals a hyperdynamic heart. The hands are often sweaty but cool; there may be a coarse tremor.

The ECG confirms sinus tachycardia and may show non-specific flattening or slight inversion of T waves.

The diagnosis can usually be made from the characteristic symptoms and from observing the patient. The poor relationship of the breathlessness and pain to exertion, and the site, character and duration of the chest discomfort differentiate the syndrome from angina pectoris. The palpitation can be distinguished from that of paroxysmal tachycardia by the lack of sudden onset and by the relationship to emotion.

The prognosis with regard to the relief of symptoms is poor if it is a chronic condition or if there is a serious personality derangement. If the complaints have occurred in response to an obvious emotional stress, the outlook is relatively good. When anxiety about the heart has been induced by the thoughtless or ill-informed comments of physicians, it is particularly difficult to eradicate.

Psychiatric treatment is necessary for the more severe cases, but strong reassurance by the physician may be effective in those patients in whom cardiac symptoms predominate, particularly when an unfounded fear of organic heart disease has provoked them. The patient should be instructed to embark upon a programme of gradually increasing physical activity. Sometimes, it may be necessary to give tranquillizers such as diazepam (Valium) 2–5 mg three times a day. Propranolol in a dose of 10 or 20 mg four times a day is helpful if the palpitation of sinus tachycardia is distressing.

Psychological disturbances in patients with heart disease

Many individuals equate heart disease with total disability and death. Patients with cardiac disorders may regard themselves and be considered by others as 'invalids', even though their lesion may be of little importance or be correctable.

Fear of sudden death is common in those who experience angina and palpitation. Anxiety and depression are important causes of symptoms and disability in patients who have sustained a myocardial infarction or have undergone coronary surgery (see Chapter 7). Headache in hypertensive patients is usually due to tension and only rarely to the high blood pressure.

Excessive anxiety can be prevented by thoughtful management of the patient and his relatives. Frankness should be combined with optimism. One must be careful in one's choice of words; if such terms as angina, murmur or heart failure are to be used, they must be explained in such a way that they do not cause alarm.

Advanced heart disease can cause confusion and delirium as a result of hypoxia or hypotension or, when associated with pulmonary disease, carbon dioxide retention. Similar symptoms may arise from lignocaine overdosage, or following cardiac surgery. Depression may result from a number of cardiac drugs including methyldopa. Fatigue is common in patients on betablocking drugs. These psychological disturbances, which are secondary to medical disorders, should be treated by correcting the underlying cause.

Surgery and the Heart

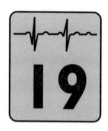

ANAESTHESIA AND GENERAL SURGERY IN PATIENTS WITH HEART DISEASE

Anaesthesia is potentially hazardous in the patient with heart disease because it may cause hypoxaemia, hypercapnia, hypotension and cardiac arrhythmias; these complications can be almost completely avoided by skilful management. The choice of anaesthetic technique is dependent on the type and severity of the cardiac lesion and the nature of the operation being undertaken.

The period of induction is particularly dangerous, as hypotension may result from the intravenous barbiturates commonly used, and endotracheal intubation may stimulate vagal reflexes with resultant bradycardia, heart block or asystole. The dose of barbiturates should be small; muscle relaxants facilitate quick intubation. Halothane may be employed for maintenance of anaesthesia but should be avoided if a fall in blood pressure is undesirable; it causes direct myocardial depression. Spinal, epidural and regional anaesthesia cause little myocardial depression, but may produce hypotension, especially in the hypovolaemic patient.

Ischaemic heart disease

Ischaemic heart disease is a major determinant of operative mortality. Hypotension may provoke serious arrhythmias or result in myocardial infarction. The risks are greatest in patients with a recent myocardial infarction. Operation within 3 months of infarction carries a 30% risk of reinfarction or cardiac death. From 3 to 6 months, this risk falls to 15%, and thereafter to 5%.

Elective surgery should therefore be avoided in the first 6 months following a myocardial infarction. If surgery is unavoidable, risks can be reduced by invasive monitoring and careful regulation of oxygenation, electrolytes and volume status.

In patients with symptoms of stable angina, surgery is in general well tolerated. Once again hypotension should be avoided. Severity of ischaemia can be assessed non-invasively pre-operatively by exercise testing. Maximum workload achieved on exercise testing is an important prognostic indicator — patients who can achieve higher workloads have fewer post-operative complications.

Patients undergoing surgery for peripheral vascular disease pose a particular problem for two reasons. Firstly, this patient population has a high incidence of serious underlying coronary disease. Secondly, patients may be incapable of performing an exercise stress test because of the development of claudication. Dipyridamole thallium imaging (p. 82) has proved of particular value in this patient group as a means of predicting post-operative complications. Patients with a positive dipyridamole thallium scan should undergo coronary angiography to determine the need for a coronary revascularization procedure prior to their peripheral vascular surgery.

Antianginal therapy should, in general, be maintained pre-operatively. For beta-blockers in particular, there is a risk of rebound phenomena if the drugs are discontinued. Oral medication should be continued up to and including the morning of operation. Post-operatively, oral medication should be resumed as soon as possible. If there is a delay in resuming oral medication, parenteral alternatives should be considered.

Hypertension

Patients with hypertension are at increased risk of major peri-operative cardiac complications. This risk is related to associated ischaemic heart disease and left ventricular impairment. Where possible, hypertension should be controlled pre-operatively. Anti-hypertensive medications should be continued up to the time of operation.

Congestive heart failure

Congestive heart failure is a major determinant of peri-operative risk. Both the symptomatic functional class, determined according to the New York Heart Association functional criteria (p. 44), and the presence of clinical signs of heart failure, such as a third sound or pulmonary crepitations, are predictive of outcome. When such features are present, treatment regimens should be optimized before undertaking elective surgery. Care should be taken to avoid excessive diuresis which may cause hypovolaemia and hypotension.

Arrhythmias

The risks associated with surgery in patients with arrhythmias are related to the risks of the underlying heart disease, rather than to the arrhythmias *per se*. There is, therefore, no evidence that simple suppression of ventricular ectopics, for example, will lower risk. The best approach for such patients is careful intra-operative and post-operative monitoring, with management of any haemodynamically compromising rhythm disturbances as they occur.

Conduction defects are a source of concern during anaesthesia, because of the possibility of progression to complete heart block. Temporary pacing is required for patients in established complete heart block or with Mobitz II second degree AV block (p. 185). Pacing is in general not required for Mobitz I second degree AV block (Wenckebach) or for patients with bifasicular block.

In patients with an implanted permanent pacemaker, special care is needed in the use of electro-cautery. There is a danger that the electrical fields caused by diathermy may cause inappropriate suppression of a demand pacemaker. Bipolar diathermy is preferable to unipolar. When unipolar diathermy is used, the indifferent electrode should be placed as far from the pacemaker generator as possible. A magnet should be available in the theatre to convert the pacemaker to fixed rate, if pacemaker inhibition should occur.

Valvular heart disease

Major surgery should, if possible, be avoided in patients with severe heart valve disease; it is better to defer general surgery until the valve lesion has been corrected. However, if prosthetic valve surgery is contemplated, it may be preferable to carry out general surgery first in order to avoid operating on a patient receiving anticoagulants.

Short-term withdrawal of anticoagulants in patients with valve prostheses is relatively safe. Oral treatment can be discontinued a few days before surgery, and patients maintained on intravenous heparin until the day of surgery. Heparin should then be resumed as early as is considered safe post-operatively, and maintained until the adequate anticoagulation on oral therapy is established once again.

In emergency operations, clotting can be restored to normal using fresh frozen plasma. Vitamin K reversal is best avoided, as this creates difficulties in re-establishing anticoagulant control post-operatively.

Estimation of risk

Attempts have been made to quantify the cardiac risk in patients undergoing general surgical procedures (Table 19.1). The most important factors in this risk table are a history of myocardial infarction in the last 6 months, and signs of heart failure. Patients can be stratified into four risk groups according to the number of points scored.

Such tables are a useful adjunct in predicting cardiac risk, but they are not a substitute for clinical judgement.

Table 19.1 Multifactorial index score to estimate cardiac risk

Criteria		Point score
History: Age >70 years		5
Myocardial infarction in last 6 months		10
Examination: S_3 or raised jugular venous pressure		11
Significant aortic stenosis		3
Electrocardiogram: Rhythm other than sinus		7
>5 ventricular ectopic beats/min		7
General: Any of the following: Respiratory failure, K^+ <3.0 mmol, HCO_3< 20 mmol, renal failure, liver dysfunction, immobilization		3
Surgery: Abdominal, thoracic, aortic		3
Emergency		4
	Total possible	53

Group	Points total	Non-fatal complications (%)	Cardiac death (%)
I	0–5	0.7	0.2
II	6–12	5	2
III	13–25	11	2
IV	>26	22	56

Source: Goldman, L., Caldera, D.L., Nussbaum, S.R. *et al.* (1977) Multifactorial index of cardiac risk in noncardiac surgical procedures. *New England Journal of Medicine* **297**: 845.

SURGERY FOR HEART DISEASE

Indications and contraindications

Most types of congenital and rheumatic heart disease are amenable to surgical treatment (for discussion of individual lesions see Chapters 12 and 13). Surgery also has a major part to play in the management of ischaemic heart disease, infective endocarditis, pericardial constriction and in diseases of the aorta. In deciding whether surgery is necessary in an individual case, one must weigh up the prognosis of the patient without surgery and the risks of morbidity and mortality imposed by surgery. For example, most patients with atrial septal defects or persistent ductus arteriosus are asymptomatic, but have a life expectancy reduced to about 40 years. Surgery in childhood is justified in these cases because the mortality is very low. At the other end of the scale, severe aortic stenosis carries a very poor prognosis and surgery should be undertaken in spite of a mortality which commonly exceeds 5%. Contraindications to surgery include poor left ventricular function, extreme pulmonary hypertension and advanced disease of other organs such as the brain, liver and lungs.

Types of cardiac surgery

Cardiac surgery may be 'closed' or 'open'. In closed-heart surgery, the circulation continues through the patient's heart throughout the operation, and the interior of the heart is not inspected. The operations are relatively simple and safe but are limited in scope to such procedures as mitral and pulmonary valvotomy, pericardectomy for pericardial constriction, division of persistent ductus arteriosus, resection of coarctation and shunt operations for tetralogy of Fallot. In experienced hands, the mortality of these operations is low, but post-operative complications include systemic embolism (after mitral valvotomy), arrhythmias, pulmonary collapse and infection, pulmonary embolism and the post-cardiotomy syndrome.

Cardio-pulmonary bypass

The vast majority of cardiac operations in the adult require cardio-pulmonary bypass. In cardio-pulmonary bypass, the heart and lungs are completely excluded from the circulation. Venous blood is drained by gravity into an oxygenator through cannulae inserted into the inferior and superior venae cavae. A pump is used to recirculate the blood through a cannula positioned in the aorta (Fig. 19.1). When operations are undertaken on the mitral valve, the aortic valve prevents regurgitation into the left ventricle of the blood pumped into the aorta by the artificial heart–lung apparatus. When operations are being carried out on the aortic valve, the aorta must be cross-clamped below the origin of the innominate artery to permit a dry surgical field. The ischaemic myocardium is protected during cross-clamping by a combination of cooling and electromechanical dissociation. Electromechanical dissociation can be achieved either by instilling a potassium-containing, crystalloid, cardioplegic solution into the aortic root (and hence into the coronary tree), or by fibrillating the heart so that contraction ceases. Cross-clamping is also necessary during the construction of coronary anastomoses in coronary artery bypass grafting.

With total cardio-pulmonary bypass, the cerebral circulation is maintained, and operations on the open heart lasting up to 5 h can be performed. The potential risks are considerable; the major hazards are cerebral air embolism, trauma to blood by the pump-oxygenator, and

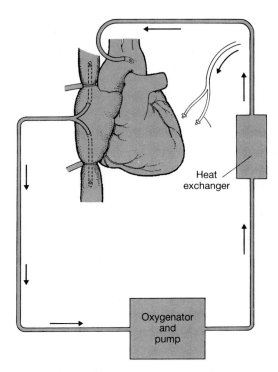

Fig. 19.1 Cardio-pulmonary bypass. Venous blood drains from cannulae in the venae cavae into an oxygenator, and is then returned to the femoral artery or aorta by a pump. The temperature of the perfusing blood can be controlled with a heat pump.

Heat exchanger

Oxygenator and pump

electrolyte and acid–base disturbances. The lungs often become abnormally stiff in the post-operative phase, and pulmonary atelectasis and infection are common. If perfusion has been inadequate, renal failure may occur. In the first few days after operation, arrhythmias are frequent.

Open-heart surgery with total bypass is suitable for all surgically treatable lesions. Because of the risks involved, it should be undertaken only by an experienced team of surgeons, anaesthetists and ancillary staff. In the best hands, the mortality of the bypass technique itself is less than 1%.

The replacement of heart valves (see also Chapter 12)

Valve replacement has proved highly successful in the management of serious valvular disease. In appropriately selected patients, valve replacement ameliorates or abolishes symptoms and causes striking haemodynamic improvement.

Replacement valves are of two types, mechanical and tissue. Mechanical prostheses take a variety of forms (Fig. 19.2):

- ball valves (e.g. Starr–Edwards);

(A)

(B)

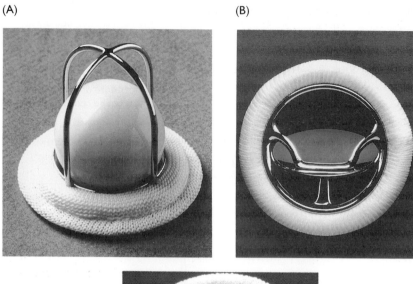

(C)

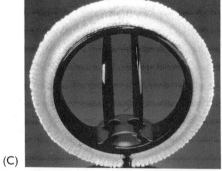

Fig. 19.2 Mechanical valve prostheses. (A) Starr–Edwards; (B) Bjork–Shiley; (C) St Jude.

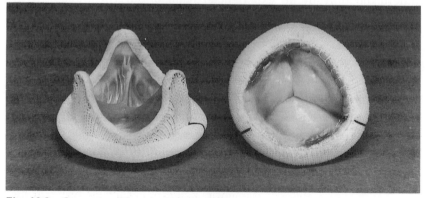

Fig. 19.3 Carpentier–Edwards tissue prosthesis.

- tilting disc valves (e.g. Bjork–Shiley);
- bi-leaflet valves (e.g. St Jude).

Most tissue valves are isolated, sterilized animal valves (heterografts). The Carpentier–Edwards prosthesis (Fig. 19.3), for example, is prepared from pig valves.

Choice of prosthesis — mechanical or tissue?

Mechanical tissue prostheses differ in their types of complications and in the need for anticoagulants. For tissue valves, the thrombo-embolic complication rate is low and there is no requirement for long-term anticoagulation. However, tissue valves are prone to failure due to a stiffening and subsequent tearing of the valve leaflets. Over a 10-year period 20–30% of patients require repeat valve replacement for this reason.

For mechanical valves the incidence of thromboembolic complications is greater. Consequently patients require long-term anticoagulation. This in itself carries a small risk of serious haemorrhagic complications. Set against this disadvantage, the incidence of valve failure is very much lower for mechanical valves than for tissue valves. Hence the likelihood of reoperation for valve failure is considerably less.

Prosthesis selection needs to be tailored to the individual patient. In a young individual with no contraindication to anticoagulation, a mechanical prosthesis is preferable. In patients in whom anticoagulants are contraindicated, tissue prostheses will be preferred. In elderly patients, in whom anticoagulants are relatively contraindicated and who are unlikely to live long enough to require a second valve replacement, tissue prostheses are once gain preferable.

Complications of prosthetic valves

Thromboembolism. The annual incidence of thromboembolic events in a patient with a metal prosthesis receiving anticoagulant therapy is approximately 1–2%. The risk of thromboembolism is generally greater following mitral and following aortic replacement. The risk of embolic problems is related to the adequacy of anticoagulant control. The INR should be maintained between 3 and 4.5.

Anticoagulant related complications. The risk of serious haemorrhagic complications related to anticoagulation is of the order of 1% per annum. For tissue valves, this is greater than the thromboembolic risk and for this reason anticoagulants are unnecessary, unless there is some additional indication for anticoagulation, such as atrial fibrillation.

Primary valve failure.   Valve failure is rare with mechanical prostheses. On the rare occasions when failure does occur, it is generally sudden and results in disastrous haemodynamic consequences, frequently resulting in the death of a patient.

In contrast, primary valve failure is common with tissue valves. The incidence of valve failure in 10 years is approximately 20–30% but an accelerated rate of failure is probable after this time. Failure is gradual and generally provides forewarning, allowing valve replacement to be undertaken before serious haemodynamic consequences ensue.

Endocarditis

Endocarditis is a particularly serious complication in prosthetic valves, because eradication of the infection with antibiotics alone is difficult. Endocarditis frequently results in the development of a paraprosthetic leak, with consequent haemodynamic deterioration. Prosthetic valve endocarditis is further discussed on page 224.

Physical findings

Prosthetic valves produce characteristic clicks. These are particularly evident in patients with mechanical prostheses. A mitral prosthesis causes a 'first sound' and 'opening snap', and an aortic prosthesis an 'ejection click' and 'aortic second sound'. Ejection murmurs are common in the case of aortic prostheses and do not indicate any abnormality of function. Regurgitant murmurs, by contrast, are always abnormal, indicating either a valvar or para-valvar leak.

Valve repair as an alternative to replacement

Despite the great success of valve replacement, the problems and complications of prosthetic valves are well recognized. In recent years there has been an increasing emphasis on conservative surgery, when feasible, as an alternative to replacement.

The mitral valve presents the greatest scope for conservation. In patients with mitral stenosis, mitral valvotomy remains the operation of choice for patients with a non-calcified valve and minimal regurgitation. The subsequent incidence of complications is much lower than would be expected for valve replacement.

Valve conservation is also possible for some regurgitant mitral lesions. Best results have been achieved in patients with mitral prolapse, although results are also encouraging in patients with ruptured chordae. Techniques include remodelling of the mitral annulus by leaflet plication, incorporation of a prosthetic ring and chordal shortening procedures.

Conservative procedures have also proved successful in the management of tricuspid disease — this generally involves the insertion of a ring prosthesis.

Intra-aortic balloon pumping (counterpulsation)

Mechanical support may be given to the circulation by a balloon introduced via a femoral artery into the descending thoracic aorta which is inflated in diastole and deflated in systole by an external pump (Fig. 19.4). This reduces afterload and increases coronary and peripheral diastolic blood flow. It greatly improves the patient with poor cardiac performance, particularly immediately after cardio-pulmonary bypass surgery. It is of value in cardiogenic shock, as after myocardial infarction, only if it allows the patient to survive until some corrective surgical procedure can be undertaken.

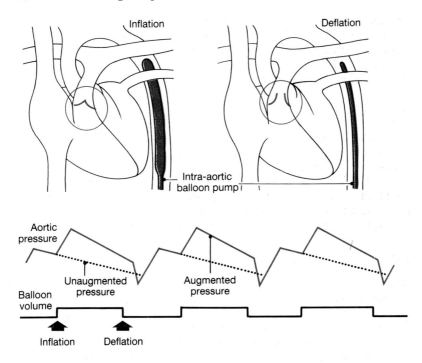

Fig. 19.4 Intra-aortic balloon pump. The balloon is inflated in diastole, following aortic valve closure. Balloon inflation augments aortic pressure without adding to cardiac workload. The balloon is deflated in late diastole. The resulting reduction in aortic pressure reduces left ventricular afterload.

Further reading

Bonchek, L.J. (1981) Current status of cardiac valve replacement. *American Heart Journal* **101:** 96.
Goodwin, J.F. (1986) Cardiac transplantation. *Circulation* **74:** 913.
Schroeder, J.S. & Hunt, S.A. (1986) Cardiac transplantation: where are we? *New England Journal of Medicine* **315:** 961.

Practical Guidelines for the Management of Cardiac Emergencies

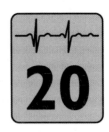

20

ACUTE MYOCARDIAL INFARCTION

The patient should be placed on a cardiac monitor and venous access established. A 12-lead ECG should then be performed. If this confirms acute myocardial infarction, the following treatment should be given.

Pain relief

Pain relief in acute myocardial infarction is of the utmost importance. Patients should be given diamorphine 5 mg i.v., accompanied by an anti-emetic such as prochlorperazine. In frail or elderly patients, or patients with a history of respiratory problems, it may be advisable to reduce the dosage of diamorphine to 2.5 mg. Conversely, in some individuals, 5 mg will not be enough to ensure pain relief and this dose may need to be repeated.

Aspirin

Aspirin is of proven benefit in reducing mortality in acute myocardial infarction. A 300-mg tablet of soluble aspirin should be given as quickly as possible. There are few absolute contraindications to aspirin. In the majority of instances, the relative contraindication of a history of peptic ulceration can be overlooked, as the benefits of treatment outweigh the risk.

Thrombolysis

A streptokinase infusion should be commenced as quickly as possible. Streptokinase (1.5 million units) is dissolved in 100 ml of saline, to be infused over 60 min. Hypotension is frequently encountered during the infusion, but in general resolves rapidly following temporary interruption of the infusion, which can then be resumed. Anaphylaxis can occur, but it is rare.

Contraindications. Recent history of stroke or intracranial bleeding is an absolute contraindication to the use of thrombolytic agents. Recent major surgery, within the last 5 days, is a further absolute contraindication. A history of peptic ulceration is in general a relative contraindication and in the majority of instances the benefits of treatment will outweigh the risks. Severe hypertension (systolic > 200 mmHg) should be reduced prior to the administration of streptokinase.

Streptokinase should not be used in a patient who has had previous streptokinase treatment more than 5 days and less than 1 year previously. In these patients tissue plasminogen activator (tPA) should be considered as an alternative.

Supportive management

If he is short of breath, oxygen therapy may be indicated. If there is evidence of failure, a diuretic should be given. Arrhythmias should be treated if these are haemodynamically compromising.

Uncertain aspects of treatment

Early beta-blockade. Before the advent of thrombolysis it was established that administration of beta-blockers intravenously in acute infarction reduced mortality by about 15%. It has yet to be demonstrated that this mortality reduction is achieved in patients receiving thrombolytic agents, but there are theoretical reasons to believe that this may indeed be the case.

Heparin. There are a number of theoretical reasons for the administration of heparin following thrombolysis. Heparin may prevent reocclusion of a reperfused artery, may reduce the incidence of left ventricular thrombus and may reduce the incidence of deep venous thrombosis during the later hospital stay. However, the evidence that heparin reduces mortality is not clearcut.

Nitrates. Nitrates have not been as extensively studied in acute infarction as other therapies. The available evidence suggests that nitrates are of benefit and that they may reduce mortality. For this reason it is common practice to give nitrates to patients with acute infarction. This can most conveniently be achieved with an intravenous infusion, which allows titration of blood pressure response. However, the benefits of nitrate therapy have yet to be proven in large-scale randomized studies.

ACE inhibitors. The role of ACE inhibitors in acute infarction is as yet uncertain.

CARDIAC ARREST

Basic life-support

Prior to commencing resuscitation, it is essential to establish that the subject is unconscious and that he has arrested. The subject should be gently shaken, while asking 'What's the problem?' or 'Are you all right?'. The rescuer should check for a pulse, palpating the carotid pulse for at least 5 s to ensure that the circulation has stopped. During the early phase of an arrest there may still be respiratory effort and the pupils may remain responsive. These features should not prevent the initiation of resuscitative measures.

Having established that the subject is pulseless, the rescuer should call for help to ring an ambulance if outside hospital, or the cardiac arrest team if in hospital. He should then commence the ABC of resuscitation:

- Airway;
- Breathing;
- Circulation;

Airway

It is necessary to open the airway by tilting the head backwards and lifting the chin. Any obvious obstruction such as dentures or vomitus should be removed.

Breathing

Mouth to mouth resuscitation can then be commenced. The chest should be seen to rise and fall with each ventilation.

When resuscitation aids are available, these should be used. An airway should be inserted and a bag valve mask unit substituted for mouth to mouth respiration.

Circulation

Chest compressions should be delivered to the sternum at a rate of 60–80/min. If only one rescuer is available, 15 chest compressions should be given followed by two ventilations. When two rescuers are available a compression : respiration ratio of 5 : 1 should be used.

For external cardiac massage, the patient must be lying on a firm surface, either on the floor or on a board placed behind his chest. The heel of one hand should be placed on the lower part of the sternum and the heel of the other hand placed immediately on top of it. The sternum is then rhythmically depressed by about 3–5 cm 60 times or more per minute.

Advanced life-support

Basic life-support is a holding measure until definitive treatment of the patient's underlying rhythm disturbance can restore cardiac

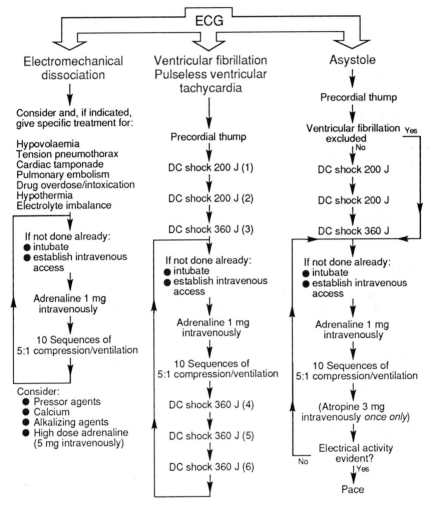

Fig. 20.1 Resuscitation guidelines.

Ventricular fibrillation:
  (1) The interval between shocks 3 and 4 should not exceed 2 minutes.
  (2) Adrenaline should be given during each loop, i.e. every 2 to 3 min.
  (3) Continue loops for as long as defibrillation is indicated.
  (4) After 3 loops consider:
    • an alkalizing agent
    • an antiarrhythmic agent.

Asystole:
  If no response after 3 cycles consider high-dose adrenaline (5 mg intravenously).

output. Out of hospital, ambulance personnel equipped with a defibrillator can provide definitive treatment. In hospital, this is the role of the cardiac arrest team.

Guidelines for the sequence of resuscitative procedures have been laid down by the European Resuscitation Council Working Party (Fig. 20.1). These recommendations provide algorithms for treating different modes of cardiac arrest. Patients are divided into three categories according to their presenting arrhythmia:

- ventricular fibrillation;
- apparent asystole;
- electro-mechanical dissociation.

With many defibrillators, application of the paddles to the chest wall allows an ECG rhythm strip to be recorded, categorizing the underlying rhythm disturbance. In other cases the rhythm can be established by attaching the patient to a cardiac monitor. If this cannot be achieved immediately, it should be assumed that the patient is in ventricular fibrillation and the patient should be shocked, as this is the most likely cause of arrest.

Management of ventricular fibrillation

The patient should receive three shocks in rapid succession of 200, 200 and 360 J. If these shocks do not restore sinus rhythm, 1 mg of adrenaline should be given intravenously, followed by 10 sequences of 5 : 1 compression/ventilation and three further 360 J shocks. The sequence of compression/ventilation and shocks is repeated until a normal rhythm is restored. Adrenaline has been given precedence over lignocaine, because animal models have suggested that it may improve cerebral perfusion.

In many in-hospital arrests, when resuscitation facilities are immediately at hand, it is appropriate to give the first three shocks prior to commencing ventilation or external cardiac massage. If the initial three shocks are unsuccessful, then a protracted arrest is likely. The patient should be intubated. External cardiac massage should be given with at least 15 cardiac compressions between each further shock.

In cases of *protracted ventricular fibrillation* further injections of adrenaline 1 mg i.v. should be given every 3 min. Different defibrillator paddle positions should be tried in the hope that a higher current density across the heart will be achieved, terminating the fibrillation. It may also be advisable to change the defibrillator. Other antiarrhythmic drugs should be considered, such as bretylium 400 mg i.v. or amiodarone 300 mg i.v. Intravenous magnesium may also be appropriate.

Apparent asystole

True asystole is uncommon early in cardiac arrest. When asystole does occur, it is generally a result of prolonged arrest and indicates a very poor prognosis. On occasions it is possible to be misled, if the gain control has been turned back on a monitor, and to interpret ventricular fibrillation as asystole. For this reason, the guidelines recommend that unless the physician is certain the underlying rhythm is true asystole, the patient should be defibrillated.

In cases of true asystole patients should first be given 1 mg of adrenaline i.v. followed by up to 3 mg of atropine i.v. Emergency pacing should be considered if facilities for this are available.

Electro-mechanical dissociation

Electro-mechanical dissociation is frequently a late event in cardiac arrest and indicates a poor prognosis. When electro-mechanical dissociation is the presenting feature, it suggests the possibility of underlying left ventricular rupture and it is unlikely that the patient will be resuscitated. However, there are also other causes of electro-mechanical dissociation which should not be overlooked, as these disorders are potentially remediable. Treatable causes of electro-mechanical dissociation include:

- hypovolaemia;
- pneumothorax;
- cardiac tamponade;
- pulmonary embolism.

Appropriate treatment depends on recognition of the specific underlying cause.

Management post-arrest

After resuscitation from a cardiac arrest the patient must be carefully monitored, preferably on a coronary care unit. If the patient remains unconscious, it will certainly be necessary to protect his airway and may be necessary to provide ventilatory support. Blood gasses should be checked frequently. Electrolytes should also be checked and hypokalaemia corrected. Following an arrest due to ventricular fibrillation, potassium should be maintained in the high/normal range.

MANAGEMENT OF TACHYARRHYTHMIAS

For all tachyarrhythmias, if the patient is severely compromised haemodynamically, cardioversion is the most appropriate treatment.

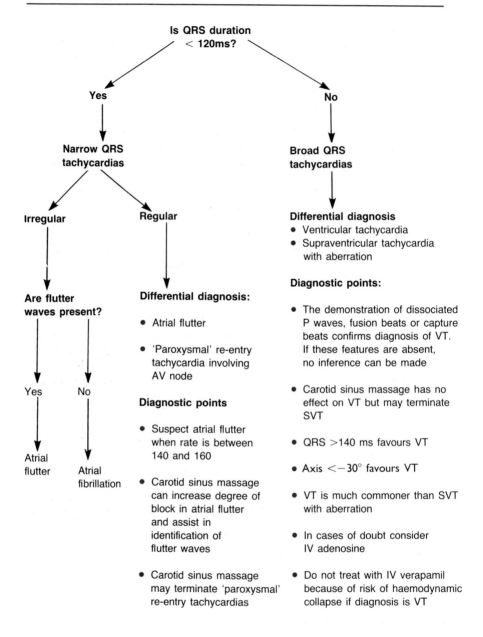

Is QRS duration < 120ms?

Yes

No

Narrow QRS tachycardias

Broad QRS tachycardias

Irregular

Regular

Are flutter waves present?

Yes   **No**

Atrial flutter   Atrial fibrillation

Differential diagnosis:

- Atrial flutter

- 'Paroxysmal' re-entry tachycardia involving AV node

Diagnostic points

- Suspect atrial flutter when rate is between 140 and 160

- Carotid sinus massage can increase degree of block in atrial flutter and assist in identification of flutter waves

- Carotid sinus massage may terminate 'paroxysmal' re-entry tachycardias

Differential diagnosis
- Ventricular tachycardia
- Supraventricular tachycardia with aberration

Diagnostic points:

- The demonstration of dissociated P waves, fusion beats or capture beats confirms diagnosis of VT. If these features are absent, no inference can be made

- Carotid sinus massage has no effect on VT but may terminate SVT

- QRS >140 ms favours VT

- Axis <−30° favours VT

- VT is much commoner than SVT with aberration

- In cases of doubt consider IV adenosine

- Do not treat with IV verapamil because of risk of haemodynamic collapse if diagnosis is VT

Fig. 20.2 Diagnostic algorithm for some common tachyarrhythmias.

In less severely compromised patients, drug management may be considered. Drug selection is determined by the nature of the arrhythmia. A simple diagnostic algorithm to aid in the diagnosis of a number of common arrhythmias is presented in Fig. 20.2.

Ventricular tachycardia

Rapid ventricular tachycardias cause cardiac arrest and management is similar to ventricular fibrillation. In less severely compromised patients, intravenous drug treatment should be considered, before resorting to cardioversion. Lignocaine is the drug of first choice. It is relatively non-toxic and is unlikely to cause haemodynamic deterioration or to exacerbate the arrhythmia. In patients failing to respond to lignocaine, cardioversion is the safest option. Alternatively, another class I antiarrhythmic agent can be administered. Flecainide (up to 2 ml/kg i.v. over 10 min) is one possibility but care needs to be taken because of the drug's negative inotropic effects and potential pro-arrhythmic action.

Undiagnosed broad complex tachycardias

The majority of broad complex tachycardias are ventricular in origin. A minority are supraventricular, with accompanying bundle branch block. The diagnostic features of ventricular tachycardia are described on p. 182. If the diagnosis remains in doubt, the patient should be given intravenous adenosine. This terminates the majority of supraventricular tachycardias and is without effect on ventricular tachycardias (Table 20.1)

Adenosine should be administered as a series of increasing intravenous boluses, successive doses being determined by response of the arrhythmia. The recommended initial bolus dose for adults is 3 mg over 2 s. If the tachycardia does not terminate within 1–2 min, a second bolus dose of 6 mg should be given. If after a further 1–2 min, this too is unsuccessful a third bolus dose of 12 mg should be given.

Table 20.1 Response to adenosine

Arrhythmia	Response
'Paroxysmal' supraventricular tachycardia	Termination
Atrial fibrillation, atrial flutter	Transient increase in AV block
Ventricular tachycardia	No effect
Atrial fibrillation in Wolff–Parkinson– White syndrome	No effect

Transient side-effects, particularly chest discomfort and dys-pnoea, are common. Occasionally there may be excessive bradycardia in heart block, but this generally lasts only a few seconds. Adenosine is best avoided in patients on therapy with dipyridamole and may be ineffective in patients receiving theophylline.

Torsades de pointes tachycardia

This arrhythmia is generally a manifestation of drug toxicity or metabolic disturbance. It is frequently multifactorial in origin. Episodes causing collapse and loss of consciousness may require d.c. shock, although the arrhythmia generally takes the form of recurrent, self-terminating episodes of tachycardia. The precipitating cause should be identified and corrected. Correction of hypokalaemia is particularly important. In many cases, bradycardias contribute to the genesis of the arrhythmia. This should be treated by pacing, at a rate of 90–100 beats/min. Atrial pacing is satisfactory but is more prone to lead displacement than ventricular pacing, which is more commonly chosen. If pacing cannot be easily instituted, then an isoprenaline infusion should be considered as an alternative.

Atrial fibrillation

If the patient is severely compromised haemodynamically, cardiover-sion may be appropriate. However, in many cases atrial fibrillation occurs because the patient is ill in other ways and in these circumstances the arrhythmia is likely to recur after cardioversion. If cardioversion is undertaken, the initial shock strength should not be less than 100 J.

In many cases drug treatment of the arrhythmia is appropriate. A number of options are possible. These options are alternatives — different antiarrhythmic drugs should not be combined:

- digoxin 1 mg i.v. in 100 ml saline over 2 h (or 0.5 mg orally repeated after 2 h). Digoxin limits the ventricular response rate but has no direct action to restore sinus rhythm;
- flecainide up to 2 mg/kg i.v. over 10 min. Flecainide is effective in restoring sinus rhythm in the majority of patients with acute onset atrial fibrillation. However the drug should be used with caution because of its negative inotropic effects and potential pro-arrhythmic action.
- amiodarone 300 mg i.v. over 30 min followed by 1200 mg in 24 h. Amiodarone is effective in restoring and maintaining sinus rhythm. The drug has the disadvantage of causing thromboph-lebitis when given via a peripheral line and should hence be administered via a central line.

It should be appreciated that many cases of atrial fibrillation terminate spontaneously without the need for any treatment. This is particularly true following myocardial infarction. Episodes of atrial fibrillation related to alcohol abuse are also, in general, self-limiting and specific antiarrhythmic treatment is unnecessary.

When intervening either pharmacologically or with cardioversion to restore sinus rhythm, the possibility of systemic embolism should be considered. There is a risk of thrombus formation in the fibrillating atria, particularly during prolonged episodes of fibrillation, with subsequent embolism on restoring sinus rhythm. If atrial fibrillation is not causing haemodynamic compromise, a safer approach may be to control the ventricular response rate and anticoagulate the patient with warfarin, prior to elective cardioversion in 1 month.

Atrial flutter

The same agents used for ventricular rate control in atrial fibrillation can also be used for rate control in atrial flutter. However, pharmacological treatment is less often successful in restoring sinus rhythm and hence cardioversion may be more appropriate. The initial shock strength should be 25 J and this succeeds in reverting the majority of patients. In some patients it is possible to terminate the arrhythmia by atrial pacing.

Paroxysmal supraventricular tachycardia

This term encompasses a number of different arrhythmias, due to reentry tachycardias involving conduction through the AV node (p. 169). If the patient is severely compromised cardioversion is appropriate, in which case a 25-J shock is generally sufficient. In most instances the patient is sufficiently well to consider drug treatment. Verapamil is usually the drug of choice — 5 mg i.v. over 30 s repeated after a further minute if necessary. Intravenous verapamil must not be given to patients who are receiving beta-blockers. Intravenous adenosine (see p. 369 for dosage) is becoming increasingly popular as an alternative (Fig. 20.3).

Atrial fibrillation in Wolff–Parkinson–White syndrome

Patients are frequently severely compromised haemodynamically. Cardioversion may well be necessary (100-J shock). In patients well enough to consider drug treatment, flecainide (up to 2 mg/kg i.v. over 10 min, maximum total dose 150 mg) is the most appropriate therapy.

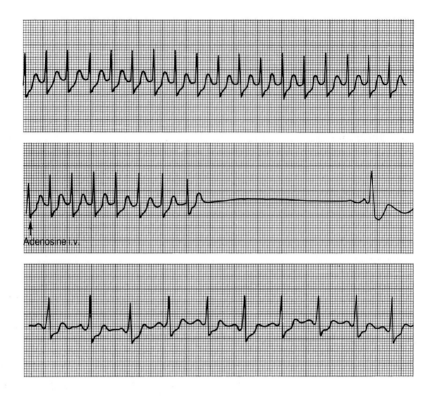

Fig. 20.3 A narrow complex supraventricular tachycardia is terminated by a bolus of intravenous adenosine. There is a three second pause on restoration of sinus rhythm. With resumption of sinus rhythm a delta wave is apparent, revealing the underlying diagnosis of Wolff–Parkinson–White syndrome. Continuous rhythm strips.

MANAGEMENT OF PULMONARY OEDEMA

A venous line should be inserted and the patient should be monitored. If there is an underlying cardiac rhythm disturbance, this should be corrected. Specific measures for the treatment of pulmonary oedema include:

Oxygen

Oxygen (40%) should be given to correct hypoxaemia. Most patients are hypocapnic and CO_2 retention is rarely a problem, but in occasional patients with obstructive airways disease and CO_2

retention, it may be necessary to use a lower inspired oxygen concentration.

Diamorphine

The standard dose of diamorphine is 5 mg given intravenously. It may be necessary to reduce this dose in elderly or frail patients. The dinmorphine should be accompanied by an anti-emetic, such as prochlorperazine.

Nitrates

Administration of a sublingual tablet of glyceryl trinitrate has an immediate effect to lower pulmonary pressures and reduce pulmonary oedema.

Frusemide

The patient should be given intravenous frusemide. The usual dose would be 40 mg, but this may be increased in patients already on diuretic therapy. The immediate benefits of frusemide are related to a direct effect to reduce pulmonary pressures — the benefits from diuresis take longer to occur.

In cases of refractory pulmonary oedema inotropic therapy should be considered. Aminophylline 250 mg i.v. over 10 min is frequently effective. Alternatively, patients may be commenced on a dobutamine infusion, commencing at 5 µg/kg/min.

MANAGEMENT OF PULMONARY EMBOLISM

General management and pain relief

Opiates such as diamorphine are appropriate, but care is needed in hypotensive patients. Hypoxaemia is likely and high concentrations of oxygen (at least 40%) should be administered. It is usual to have high right-sided filling pressures following pulmonary embolism. Any decrease in the right-sided filling pressure is likely to lead to a further decrease in cardiac output. For this reason diuretics and vasodilators should be avoided. If right-sided pressure should fall, it may become necessary to give intravenous fluids to maintain cardiac output.

Anticoagulation

The patient should be heparinized to prevent further embolism. Therapy should be initiated with a bolus of 5000–10 000 units, followed by a maintenance infusion of 1000 units/h, adjusted according to the activated partial thromboplastin time (APTT). The APTT should be maintained at approximately twice the control value.

Thrombolysis

In patients with severe haemodynamic compromise, thrombolytic therapy should be given to dissolve the embolus. A loading dose of 600 000 units of streptokinase should be given over 30 min, followed by a maintenance infusion of 100 000 units hourly, with subsequent adjustment in accordance with clotting parameters.

Embolectomy

Pulmonary embolectomy is rarely undertaken. Its use is confined to patients who continue to deteriorate despite thrombolytic therapy or patients in whom there is an absolute contraindication to the use of thrombolytic agents.

MANAGEMENT OF CARDIAC TAMPONADE

General management

The management of cardiac tamponade depends upon clinical circumstances. In many cases, haemodynamic compromise may be relatively mild and no action may be required other than simple observation. As in pulmonary embolism, patients with cardiac tamponade have high right-sided filling pressures. Diuretics and vasodilators should be avoided. Further elevation of right-sided pressures with intravenous fluids may be of value and gain a temporary improvement in cardiac output while awaiting more definitive therapy.

In other cases of more severe haemodynamic compromise, intervention may be necessary. If the patient is not critical and if there is an underlying cause of tamponade which is likely to recur, formal surgical drainage with the formation of a pericardial window to the pleural cavity is most appropriate.

In cases of severe haemodynamic compromise, where urgent action is required, pericardial aspiration is indicated. In all but the most severe emergencies, the pericardial effusion should be defined with an echocardiogram. This facilitates assessment of the best approach for drainage, which in most cases will be subcostal. In a few cases, however, there may be a greater separation of pericardium from myocardium over the apex and in these circumstances an apical approach should be considered.

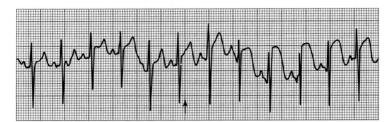

Fig. 20.4 Pericardial aspiration. An ECG has been recorded by attaching a V lead of an ECG machine to the aspiration needle. The development of marked ST elevation indicates that the tip of the needle is in direct contact with myocardium.

Pericardial aspiration — subcostal approach

The patient should be sitting at an angle of 45° with his back supported. Local anaesthetic is infiltrated just to the left of the xiphisternum. An 18- or 16-gauge aspiration needle is then inserted, directed towards the left shoulder. Prior echocardiography can demonstrate the correct angulation of the needle. A sterile, insulated wire with a crocodile clip at each end is attached to the needle and to a V lead of an appropriate ECG machine. The needle is advanced slowly applying gentle suction until either pericardial fluid is aspirated or ST elevation becomes apparent on the electrocardiogram recorded from the needle — ST elevation indicates that the needle has contacted the myocardium (Fig. 20.4). A sudden 'give' will usually be felt when the pericardial space is entered. If blood is withdrawn it should be observed for clotting to determine whether the specimen has been obtained from a cardiac chamber — fluid from a haemopericardium will not clot. Once the needle is in the pericardial space a guide wire is passed and the needle replaced by a blunt cannula or a catheter such as a pigtail catheter.

TEMPORARY CARDIAC PACING

Temporary cardiac pacing is most frequently undertaken using The Seldinger technique via a subclavian approach. The skin is anaesthetized about 1 cm below the mid-point of the clavicle, a local anaesthetic infiltrated upwards underneath the clavicle and then medially towards the sternal notch. A longer needle attached to a saline-filled syringe is then substituted and passed in the same direction, whilst aspirating. When the subclavian vein is entered a guide wire is passed through the needle and along the vein, under fluoroscopic guidance to the right atrium. The needle is then withdrawn and an introducer passed over the guide wire. The guide wire itself is then withdrawn and a bipolar temporary pacing wire passed through the sheath.

The pacing wire is passed to the right atrium. In general, it is difficult to advance the pacing wire directly across the tricuspid valve and this can only be achieved by forming a loop in the right atrium. The wire should be positioned along the floor of the ventricle with its tip in the apex. The pacing threshold is then determined by attaching the wire to an external pacemaker box. In general the threshold should be less than 1 V, at a pulse duration of 0.5 ms. Occasionally, particularly in patients with a right ventricular infarction, it may be necessary to accept higher thresholds.

Complications of temporary pacing

Pneumothorax. After any subclavian venous puncture, a chest X-ray should be requested to check for a pneumothorax. Angling the exploring needle as close as possible to the undersurface of the clavicle minimizes the risk of pneumothorax. In patients with severe respiratory disease, in whom a pneumothorax might provoke respiratory failure, alternative pacing routes should be considered (see below).

Subclavian artery puncture. Even in the most experienced hands it is possible to puncture the subclavian artery rather than the subclavian vein. If arterial puncture should occur, serious consequences are rare. The exception, however, is in thrombolysed patients, where severe bleeding may result. As the subclavian artery is inaccessible to apply pressure, bleeding may be difficult to control. For this reason, where possible, subclavian access should be avoided, when temporary pacing becomes necessary following thrombolysis in acute myocardial infarction. Venous access for pacing can also be achieved by the antecubital vein, the femoral vein or the jugular vein.

Lead displacement. This results in loss of capture or variable capture and necessitates reposition of the pacing wire.

Lead perforation. This may occur acutely during lead positioning or due to gradual erosion over a number of days. It causes a rise in the threshold and may result in loss of pacing. The threshold should be checked every day in a patient with a temporary wire to detect any change in threshold which might indicate perforation. When perforation occurs it may result in pericardial pain and may, occasionally, cause cardiac tamponade.

HYPERTENSIVE CRISIS

If the diastolic blood pressure exceeds 140 mmHg, there is considerable danger of stroke or hypertensive encephalopathy and urgent treatment is necessary to lower the blood pressure. Urgent treatment is also required in patients with bilateral fundal haemorrhages or exudates.

Although urgent control of blood pressure is desirable, excessively rapid reduction may be equally dangerous. Rapid pressure reduction may result in hypoperfusion of the brain, and cause irreversible cerebral damage.

For patients who are alert and in no immediate danger, oral therapy alone may be satisfactory. Nifedipine, 10 mg orally or sublingually, lowers the blood pressure by about 25% in 30 min. The dose may be repeated in a further 30 min if needed. In occasional patients the fall in blood pressure may be excessive and result in cerebral ischaemia.

If more urgent control of blood pressure is required, this can be achieved by parenteral drug administration. A nitroprusside infusion is frequently chosen and provides a rapid pressure reduction in all patients. The starting dose is 0.25 µg/kg/min, which can be titrated up according to response. Great care is necessary, because a slightly excessive dose may cause severe hypotension and result in cerebral ischaemia. One of the advantages of nitroprusside is that the hypotensive effect disappears in minutes once the drug is stopped. Direct intra-arterial pressure measurements are indicated to guard against excessive pressure reduction.

Labetalol is sometimes chosen as an alternative for its combined alpha- and beta-antagonism. The drug is best given as an infusion with a starting dose of 2 mg/min. The infusion should be continued until a satisfactory blood pressure response is achieved and then stopped. The effective dose is usually in the range 50–200 mg.

Further reading

Adult advanced cardiac life support: The European Resuscitation Council Guidelines 1992 (abridged) (1993) *British Medical Journal* **306**: 1589.
Guidelines for basic life support (1993) *British Medical Journal* **306**: 1587.

Appendix — Commonly Used Cardiovascular Drugs

Some commonly used cardiovascular drugs are listed. Dosage, major contraindications and common side-effects are also listed but this list is not exhaustive and referral to the British National Formulary or individual data sheets is recommended for further information.

Beta-blockers

Indications	Contraindications	Side-effects
• Hypertension (p. 306)	• Bradycardia	• Bronchospasm
• Stable angina (p. 111)	• Heart block	• Heart failure
• Unstable angina (p. 115)	• Heart failure	• Heart block
• Acute myocardial infarction (p. 363)	• Asthma	• Tiredness
• Prophylaxis post-myocardial infarction (p. 137)		• Cold extremities
• Arrhythmias (p. 204)		• Depression
		• Impotence

Agent	Dose	Comments
	Note: regimens used in the management of angina and hypertension may differ. For angina, smaller doses are in general given more frequently and the total daily dose is less than for the management of hypertension	

Non-cardioselective beta-blockers

Agent	Dose	Comments
Propranolol	Oral, 40–120 mg tds. Intravenous, 1 mg over 1 min, if necessary repeated at 2-min intervals; maximum 5 mg. (Excessive bradycardia can be countered by injection of atropine 0.6–2.4 mg)	
Sotalol	80–160 mg bd	Sotalol differs from other beta-blockers in prolonging action potention duration and having a class III antiarrhythmic action (p. 203)
Nadolol	40–240 mg once daily	
Oxprenolol	40–160 mg tds	This drug has intrinsic sympathomimetic activity, i.e. it acts as a partial agonist and, with low sympathetic drive, increases heart rate
Pindolol	2.5–5.0 mg tds	This drug has marked intrinsic sympathomimetic activity
Timolol	5–15 mg tds	

Agent	Dose	Comments
Cardioselective beta-blockers		
Atenolol	25–100 mg once daily	This drug has a low lipid solubility leading to decreased distribution across the blood–brain barrier. Hence it has fewer CNS side-effects
Metoprolol	50–100 mg bd	Metoprolol has a shorter half-life than atenolol. The short half-life is an advantage in situations where there may be concern about the safety of beta-blockade
Acebutolol	200–400 mg bd	Possesses intrinsic sympathomimetic activity
Bisoprolol	5–20 mg once daily	This agent is highly selective for $beta_1$ adrenoceptor sites and hence is more cardioselective than the other agents in this group
Other beta-blockers		
Labetalol	50–200 mg bd	This drug blocks both alpha- and beta-receptors. It has modest sympathomimetic activity
Xamoterol	200 mg once or twice daily	This drug has very marked intrinsic sympathomimetic activity and has been used in the treatment of mild heart failure

Calcium antagonists

DIHYDROPYRIDINES

Indications	Contraindications	Side-effects
• Hypertension (p. 309)	• Hypotension	• Excessive tachycardia
• Stable angina (p. 112)	• Severe failure	• Occasional exacerbation of angina
• Prinzmetal's angina (p. 93)	• Aortic stenosis	• Facial flushing and ankle oedema
	• Unstable angina in the absence of a beta-blocker	

Agent	Dose	Comments
Nifedipine	10–20 mg tds	
Nicardipine	20–40 mg tds	
Amlodipine	5–10 mg daily	This drug has a much longer half-life than other dihydropyridines and can be used as a once daily dose

BENZOTHIAZEPINES

Indications	Contraindications	Side-effects
• Stable angine (p. 112) • Unstable angina (p.115)	• Heart block • Severe failure	• Slowing of AV node conduction • Rashes • Negative inotropism

Agent	Dose	Comments
Diltiazem	60–120 mg tds	The drug's suppression of AV node conduction prevents the tachycardia which occurs with dihydropyridines like nifedipine

PHENYLALKYLAMINES

Indications	Contraindications	Side-effects
• Hypertension (p. 309) • Stable angina (p. 112) • Hypertrophic cardiomyopathy (p. 222) • Rate control in atrial fibrillation and atrial flutter (p. 176) • Termination or prophylaxis of supraventricular tachycardias (p. 171)	• Heart failure • AV node block • Beta-blockade — particularly with iv verapamil • Broad complex tachycardias • Acute myocardial infarction	• Negative inotropism • AV node block • Constipation

Agent	Dose	Comments
Verapamil	Orally 40–120 mg tds Intravenously 5–10 mg over 1 min	

Nitrates

Indications	Contraindications	Side-effects
• Stable angina (p. 110) • Prinzmetal's angina (p. 93) • Unstable angina (p. 111) • Acute myocardial infarction (p. 363) • Heart failure (p. 155)	• Hypotension • Hypertrophic obstructive cardiomyopathy • Aortic stenosis • Mitral stenosis • History of migraine	• Hypotension • Headache

Agent	Dose	Comments
Sublingual glyceryl trinitrate (GTN)	Tablet strength usually 0.3, 0.5 or 0.6 mg	Tablets can be taken both to terminate episodes of pain and prophylactically to prevent episodes
GTN spray	0.4 mg metered dose	As for sublingual GTN
Buccal GTN	1–5 mg tds	
Transdermal GTN	5–25 mg in 24 h	Patches should be removed overnight

Agent	Dose	Comments
Isosorbide dinitrate	10–20 mg tds	Latest dose should be no later than 6 o'clock in the evening to provide a nitrate-free interval overnight
Isosorbide mononitrate	10–40 mg bd	Dosage should be asymmetrical with the second dose in the early afternoon to provide a nitrate-free interval overnight
Slow release isosorbide mononitrate	40–60 mg od	

Angiotensin-converting enzyme inhibitors

Indications	Contraindications	Side-effects
• Hypertension (p. 308) • Heart failure (p. 155) • Post-infarction (pp. 363, 95)	• Renal failure (creatinine > 200 μmol/l) • Bilateral renal artery stenosis	• Hypotension, particularly in patients on high doses of diuretics • Deterioration of renal function • Hyperkalaemia • Cough

Agent	Dose	Comments
Captopril	6.25 mg test dose Maintenance 12.5–50 mg bd	
Enalapril	2.5 mg test dose Maintenance 5–20 mg daily	
Lisinopril	2.5 mg test dose Maintenance 5–20 mg daily	

Diuretics

LOOP DIURETICS

Indications	Contraindications	Side-effects
• Left ventricular failure (p. 154) • Congestive heart failure (p. 154)	• Hypovolaemia • Severe renal impairment	• Hypovolaemia • Hypokalaemia • Ototoxicity • Gout and impairment of renal function

Agent	Dose	Comments
Frusemide	Oral, 40–160 mg in single or divided doses; intravenous 40 mg by slow injection, with further doses according to response	
Bumetanide	Oral, 1.0–5.0 mg daily in single or divided doses, intravenous, 1 mg with further doses according to response	

THIAZIDE DIURETICS

Indications	Contraindications	Side-effects
• Hypertension (p. 308) • Congestive heart failure (p. 154)	• Impaired renal function • Gout • Diabetes	• Hypokalaemia • Hyponatraemia • Glucose intolerance • Hyperuricaemia

Agent	Dose	Comments
Bendrofluazide	2.5–10 mg daily	Low doses should be used for treating hypertension. The maximum hypotensive effect is usually achieved with 2.5 mg

Agent	Dose	Comments
Hydrochlorothiazide	25–100 mg daily	and higher doses only serve to cause additional lowering of potassium
		As for bendrofluazide use a low dose for treating hypertension
Metolazone	1–5 mg daily	Extreme care is necessary when used with loop diuretics, as a very vigorous diuresis ensues

POTASSIUM-SPARING DIURETICS

Indications	Contraindications	Side-effects
• Combination with loop and thiazide diuretics (pp. 154, 308)	• Renal failure	• Hyperkalaemia • Gynaecomastia in the case of spironolactone

Agent	Dose	Comments
Amiloride	2.5–20 mg daily	Generally used in combination therapy with other diuretics
Triamterene	50–200 mg daily	Generally used in combination therapy
Spironolactone	25–200 mg in divided doses	Frequently causes GI disturbance

Cardiac Glycosides

Indications	Contraindications	Drug interactions	Side-effects
• Control of ventricular rate response in atrial fibrillation (p. 176)	• Renal failure	• Increased blood levels with quinidine, verapamil, amiodarone, propafenone	• Arrhythmias
• Left ventricular failure and congestive cardiac failure (p. 151)	• Hypokalaemia • Wolff–Parkinson–White Syndrome • Hypertrophic cardiomyopathy	• Diuretic-induced hypokalaemia	• Anorexia, nausea and vomiting • Visual disturbance

Agent	Dose
Digoxin	*Loading* Oral, 0.5 mg repeated after 2 h; intravenous, 1 mg in 100 ml over 2 h *Maintenance* 0.25 mg daily

Vasodilators

Indications	Contraindications	Side-effects
• Hypertension (p.309) • Heart failure (p. 155)	• Hypotension • Aortic stenosis • Hypertrophic obstructive cardiomyopathy	• Excessive hypotension

Agent	Dose	Comments
Nitroprusside	Intravenous infusion of 0.25 µg/kg/min increasing to 10 µg/kg/min depending on the response	Degraded by light. Care must be taken to avoid excessive hypotension
Hydralazine	25–50 mg bd	High doses may cause systemic lupus erythematosus
Prazosin	Initial dose 0.5 mg daily, maintenance 0.5–10 mg bd	Postural hypotension may occur with the first dose. This should be taken on retiring to bed. Tolerance may occur

Antiarrhythmic drugs

CLASS IA

Indications	Contraindications	Side-effects
• Ventricular arrhythmias (p. 205) • Supraventricular arrhythmias (p.204)	• Excessive bradycardias • AV block • Impaired left ventricular function	• Negative inotropism • Pro-arrhythmia

Agent	Dose	Comments
Quinidine	200–400 mg tds	May cause QT prolongation and Torsades de pointes. May cause thrombocytopenia
Procainamide	Intravenous, not to exceed 100 mg/min, repeated at 5-min intervals with ECG and blood pressure monitoring; maximum 1 g Oral, 1–1.5 g tds, preferably controlled by monitoring plasma concentrations	Hypotension with intravenous infusion. Systemic lupus erythematous-like syndrome with longterm oral therapy
Disopyramide	Intravenous, 2.0 mg/kg over 5 min to a maximum of 150 mg Oral 100–250 mg tds	Contraindicated in atrial flutter — may slow the atrial rate through a Class I effect while speeding up AV conduction through anti-cholinergic effects, resulting in 1:1 AV node conduction and acceleration of the ventricular response rate

CLASS IB

Indications	Contraindications	Side-effects
• Ventricular tachycardia (p. 369) • Ventricular fibrillation (p. 366)	—	In high doses may cause CNS side-effects

Agent	Dose	Comments
Lignocaine	Intravenous, 100-mg bolus, wherever necessary repeated after 1–2 min. Maintenance infusion 4 mg/min for 30 min, 3 mg/min for a further 30 min and thereafter 1–2 mg/min	—
Mexiletine	200–250 mg tds	Resembles lignocaine in structure and actions and can be used in the chronic treatment of arrhythmias when intravenous lignocaine has succeeded acutely

CLASS IC

Indications	Contraindications	Side-effects
• Ventricular arrhythmias (p. 205) • Supraventricular arrhythmias (p. 204)	• Because of the risk of pro-arrhythmia, use of these drugs should be confined to life-threatening arrhythmias • Myocardial depression • AV block	• QRS prolongation • Depression of left ventricular function • Pro-arrhythmia

Agent	Dose	Comments
Flecainide	Intravenous, 2 mg/kg over 10 min to a maximum of 150 mg. Oral, 100 mg bd	CNS and gastrointestinal side-effects are common
Propafenone	150–300 mg tds	

CLASS II — see section on beta-blockers

CLASS III

Indications	Contraindications	Side-effects
• Ventricular arrhythmias (p. 205) • Supraventricular arrhythmias (p. 204)	QT prolongation	Arrhythmia, particularly Torsades de pointes

Agent	Dose	Comments
Amiodarone	Intravenous infusion, 300 mg over 30 min followed by 900 mg over 24 h via a central line Oral loading 200 mg tds for 1 week reducing to a maintenance of 200 mg daily	The drug has extensive side-effects, of which the most serious is pulmonary fibrosis. During chronic oral therapy pulmonary, thyroid and liver function tests should be monitored

Bretylium   400 mg i.v. over 10 min   Hypotension may occur during
                                         intravenous loading

Sotalol — see section on beta-blockade   Hypotension may occur. The drug takes
                                          up to 20 min to be maximally effective

CLASS IV

Verapamil — see section on calcium antagonists

ADENOSINE

Indications	Contraindications	Side-effects
• Supraventricular tachycardias (p. 203) • Diagnosis of broad complex tachycardias (p. 369)	• Theophylline treatment • Dipyridamole treatment	• Chest discomfort • Transient heart block

Adenosine

Dose

3 mg bolus dose. If no effect on tachycardia
increase to 6 mg bolus dose. If still no effect
then increase to 12 mg bolus dose.

393

Thrombolytic agents

Indications	Contraindications	Side-effects
• Acute myocardial infarction (p. 131)	• Recent GI bleeding • Cerebrovascular accidents • Severe hypertension	• Minor and major bleeding complications, particularly cerebral haemorrhage

Agent	Dose	Comments
Streptokinase	1.5 million units in 100 ml saline infused over 60 min	Hypotension is frequent, but generally resolves rapidly with a temporary interruption of the infusion, which can then be restarted at a later stage. Rarely, anaphylaxis may occur. Streptokinase should not be readministered within a time period of 5 days to 1 year after previous streptokinase therapy, as the presence of antibodies is likely to reduce the efficacy of further treatment.
Anistreplase (APSAC)	30 units over 5 min via bolus injection	This agent is a derivative of streptokinase. Anaphylaxis occurs rarely but the same 5 day–1 year time window exclusion, following previous streptokinase therapy, still applies
Alteplase (tissue plasminogen activator)	10 mg over 2 min followed by 50 mg over 1 hour and a further 40 mg over subsequent 2 hours. Dosage reduced in patients weighing less than 67 kg to total dose of 1.5 mg/kg	tPA carries a marginally higher risk of haemorrhagic stroke than streptokinase. It can be used when repeated administration of streptokinase or anistreplase is contra-indicated

Antiplatelet drugs

Indications	Contraindications	Side-effects
• Unstable angina (p. 115) • Acute myocardial infarction (p. 131) • Prophylaxis post-MI	• History of GI bleeding	• Dyspepsia and GI bleeding

Agent	Dose	Comment
Aspirin	150 mg daily	

Anticoagulants

Indications	Contraindications	Side-effects
• Mitral valve disease (p. 250) • Left ventricular aneurysm (p. 132) • Atrial fibrillation (p. 176) • Mechanical valve prostheses (p. 359) • DVT prophylaxis (p. 132) • DVT treatment (p. 319) • Pulmonary embolism (p. 321)	• Bleeding disorders • Hypertension • Active peptic ulceration	• Minor and major bleeding complications

Agent	Dose	Comments
Warfarin	Typically 10 mg, 10 mg and 5 mg on successive days on commencing treatment. Subsequent dosage adjusted according to prothrombin time	Warfarin should be avoided in pregnancy. Drug interactions
Heparin	DVT prophylaxis, 5000 units bd subcutaneously. Acute MI post-thrombolysis, 12 500 units bd subcutaneously. Full i.v. heparinization 5000–10 000 units loading dose followed by infusion of 1000 units/h, adjusted according to the activated partial thromboplastin time (APTT)	

Lipid lowering drugs

Indications	Contraindications	Side-effects
• Hypercholesterolaemia (p. 97)	• Specific to individual agents	Specific to individual agents

Agent	Dose	Comments
Cholestyramine	4–8 g tds	Gastrointestinal symptoms
Bezafibrate	200 mg tds	

Gemfibrozil	600 mg bd	
Simvastatin	10–40 mg daily	The drug causes a reversible myositis. Serum transaminase and creatine kinase levels should be checked periodically. If a progressive rise occurs the drug should be discontinued. Contraindicated in patients with active liver disease.
		Myositis is more common in patients on cyclosporin, gemfibrozil or nicotinic acid

References

British National Formulary.
Association of the British Pharmaceutical Industry Data Sheet Compendium, Datapharm Publications, 1991.

Index